S0-AQJ-837

2

CURRENT CLINICAL TOPICS IN INFECTIOUS DISEASES

JACK S. REMINGTON, M.D.

Professor of Medicine
Division of Infectious Diseases
Stanford University School of Medicine

Chief, Division of Allergy,
Immunology and Infectious Diseases
Palo Alto Medical Research Foundation

MORTON N. SWARTZ, M.D.

Professor of Medicine
Harvard Medical School

Chief, Infectious Disease Unit
Massachusetts General Hospital

McGraw-Hill Book Company

New York St. Louis San Francisco Auckland Bogotá Guatemala Hamburg
Johannesburg Lisbon London Madrid Mexico Montreal New Delhi Panama Paris
San Juan São Paulo Singapore Sydney Tokyo Toronto

NOTICE

Medicine is an ever-changing science. As new research and clinical experience broaden our knowledge, changes in treatment and drug therapy are required. The editors and the publisher of this work have made every effort to ensure that the drug dosage schedules herein are accurate and in accord with the standards accepted at the time of publication. Readers are advised, however, to check the product information sheet included in the package of each drug they plan to administer to be certain that changes have not been made in the recommended dose or in the contraindications for administration. This recommendation is of particular importance in regard to new or infrequently used drugs.

THE LIBRARY OF CONGRESS HAS CATALOGED THIS SERIAL PUBLICATION AS FOLLOWS:
RC111
C87
Current clinical topics in infectious diseases. 1-
    New York, McGraw-Hill Book Co., c1980-
        v.   ill.   25 cm.
    Annual.
    Key title: Current clinical topics in infectious diseases, ISSN 0195-3842.
    1. Communicative diseases—Periodicals.
    [DNLM: 1.   Communicable Diseases—periodicals.   W 1 CU786T]
RC111.C87   616.9′05   80-643590
ISBN 0-07-051851-3   MARC-S

CURRENT CLINICAL TOPICS IN INFECTIOUS DISEASES 2

Copyright © 1981 by McGraw-Hill, Inc. All rights reserved. Printed in the United States of America. No part of this publication may be reproduced, stored in a retrieval system, or transmitted, in any form or by any means, electronic, mechanical, photocopying, recording, or otherwise, without the prior written permission of the publisher.

234567890 HDHD 8987654321

This book was set in Electra by Bi-Comp, Incorporated. The editors were Richard S. Laufer and John J. Fitzpatrick; the production supervisor was Jenet C. McIver. The designer was Elliot Epstein.
Halliday Lithograph Corporation was printer and binder.

To our fellows

Contents

List of contributors

John E. Bennett, M.D.
Head, Clinical Mycology Section, Laboratory of Clinical Investigation, National Institute of Allergy and Infectious Diseases, National Institutes of Health, Bethesda, Maryland

James D. Cherry, M.D.
Professor of Pediatrics and Chief, Division of Pediatric Infectious Diseases, The Center for the Health Sciences, UCLA School of Medicine; Attending Physician, Department of Pediatrics, UCLA Hospital and Clinics, Los Angeles, California

David S. Feingold, M.D.
Professor of Medicine and Dermatology, Boston University School of Medicine; Chief, Dermatology Section, Boston Veterans Administration Medical Center, Boston, Massachusetts

Janet J. Fischer, M.D.
Professor of Medicine, Division of Infectious Diseases, Department of Medicine, University of North Carolina School of Medicine; Attending Physician, Infectious Diseases Service (Medicine), Medical Service, North Carolina Memorial Hospital, Chapel Hill, North Carolina

Joseph E. Geraci, M.D.
Professor of Medicine, Division of Infectious Diseases, Mayo Clinic and Mayo Foundation, Rochester, Minnesota

William L. Hewitt, M.D.
Professor of Medicine and Chief, Division of Infectious Diseases, Department of Medicine, The Center for the Health Sciences, UCLA School of Medicine, Los Angeles, California

Richard B. Hornick, M.D.
Professor of Medicine, University of Rochester School of Medicine and Dentistry; Chairman, Department of Medicine, Strong Memorial Hospital, Rochester, New York

O. Wayne Houser, M.D.
Associate Professor of Radiology, Mayo Medical School; Consultant, Department of Radiology, Mayo Clinic and Mayo Foundation, Rochester, Minnesota

Ernest Jawetz, M.D., Ph.D.
Professor of Microbiology and Medicine, School of Medicine, University of California, San Francisco, California

Lisa G. Kaplowitz, M.D.
Fellow, Division of Infectious Diseases, Department of Medicine, University of North Carolina School of Medicine, Chapel Hill, North Carolina

Jerome O. Klein, M.D.
Professor of Pediatrics, Boston University School of Medicine; Associate Director, Department of Pediatrics, Boston City Hospital, Boston, Massachusetts

J. T. Lie, M.D.
Professor of Pathology, Mayo Medical School; Consultant in Pathology and Anatomy and Cardiovascular Diseases, Mayo Clinic and Mayo Foundation, Rochester, Minnesota

William R. McCabe, M.D.
Professor of Medicine and Microbiology, Boston University School of Medicine; Director, Maxwell Finland Laboratory for Infectious Diseases, Boston City Hospital, Boston, Massachusetts

Richard N. Olans, M.D.
Clinical Instructor in Medicine, Boston University School of Medicine; Director of Infectious Diseases, Malden Hospital, Malden, Massachusetts

David G. Piepgras, M.D.
Assistant Professor of Neurological Surgery, Mayo Medical School, Mayo Clinic and Mayo Foundation, Rochester, Minnesota

Jack S. Remington, M.D.
Professor of Medicine, Division of Infectious Diseases, Stanford University School of Medicine; Chief, Division of Allergy, Immunology and Infectious Diseases, Palo Alto Medical Research Foundation, Palo Alto, California

Randall J. Ryser, M.D.
Assistant Resident in Medicine, Strong Memorial Hospital, Rochester, New York

John N. Sheagren, M.D.
Professor of Internal Medicine, University of Michigan Medical School; Chief, Medical Service, Veterans Administration Medical Center, Ann Arbor, Michigan

P. Frederick Sparling, M.D.
Professor of Medicine and Bacteriology and Chief, Division of Infectious Diseases, University of North Carolina School of Medicine, Chapel Hill, North Carolina

Thomas A. Stamey, M.D.
Professor of Surgery, Stanford University School of Medicine; Chairman, Division of Urology, Stanford University Hospital, Stanford, California

Morton N. Swartz, M.D.
Professor of Medicine, Harvard Medical School; Chief, Infectious Disease Unit, Massachusetts General Hospital, Boston, Massachusetts

John A. Washington II, M.D.
Professor of Microbiology and Laboratory Medicine, Mayo Medical School; Head, Section of Clinical Microbiology, Mayo Clinic and Mayo Foundation, Rochester, Minnesota

Walter R. Wilson, M.D.
Assistant Professor of Medicine and Microbiology, Mayo Medical School; Consultant in Internal Medicine and Infectious Diseases, Mayo Clinic and Mayo Foundation, Rochester, Minnesota

Preface

As literature in the field of infectious diseases has increased in complexity and volume, a need has become evident for timely, concise summaries and critical commentaries on subjects pertinent to the student and practitioner of medicine, the specialist in infectious diseases, and those in allied fields. It is our intention that this series provide the reader with a true update of information in very specific areas of infectious diseases which require reevaluation.

Each author was requested to confine his chapter to a relatively narrow subject, to deal only with contemporary questions and problems, to gather and synthesize the information on recent advances which is now spread diffusely among numerous journals, to offer a critical evaluation of this information, to place the information into perspective by defining its present status, and to point out voids in the information and thereby indicate directions for further study. All of this was to be done within the most rigid deadlines to ensure that the chapters be written and published in less than a year. We are extremely grateful to the contributing authors, each of whom is a recognized authority in his field, for consenting to undertake such an admittedly difficult task.

Because this "update" concept is relatively new to the authors and editors, we found it impossible at times to adhere to a given format. In the chapter on Rocky Mountain Spotted Fever, for example, it was necessary to broaden the scope of presentation to provide a clearer view of the *typical* and *atypical* clinical features of this disease in order to better define some of the current issues in diagnosis and management. Similarly, in the chapter on coryneform bacterial infections the focus was not only on the clinical and therapeutic aspects of disease produced by this group of organisms, but also, necessarily, on the bacteriology and ecology of these previously poorly understood and often overlooked potential pathogens.

Current Clinical Topics in Infectious Diseases 2 is the second of a series which will be published annually. Each text in the series will include updates of a variety of subjects covering the wide scope of clinical infectious disease problems including bacteriology, mycology, virology, parasitology, and epidemiology.

JACK S. REMINGTON
MORTON N. SWARTZ

Acute epiglottitis, laryngitis, and croup

JAMES D. CHERRY

Epiglottitis, laryngitis, and croup are three different clinical disease entities which are considered together because they all result from infection in the region of the larynx. All have some degree of upper airway narrowing which causes hoarseness or stridor on inspiration. Epiglottitis is truly one of the few infectious disease emergencies; although it is considered mainly an illness of children, its incidence in adults appears to be increasing.

The term *croup* is frequently used in an inclusive way for several different respiratory illnesses characterized by varying degrees of inspiratory stridor resulting from obstruction in the region of the larynx. While this discussion covers only infectious illnesses, it should be made clear at the outset that noninfectious problems can cause acute obstructive problems in the supraglottic, laryngeal, and subglottic regions. Specifically important in this regard is allergic disease (acute angioneurotic edema of the epiglottis) and a foreign body at any level within the upper airway.

The etiology and therapy of laryngitis and croup have changed remarkably over the last 50 years. Unfortunately, since the clinical approach to laryngitis and croup today frequently fails to use all the available knowledge, therapeutic programs often are not optimal. The purpose of this review is to emphasize the emergency nature of epiglottitis and to analyze the events which have caused confusion over the management of laryngitis and croup.

ACUTE EPIGLOTTITIS

Definition

Acute epiglottitis is an illness caused in most instances by infection with *Haemophilus influenzae* type B; it is characterized by inflammation and edema of the epiglottis and frequently also the aryepiglottic folds and ventricular bands at the base of the epiglottis. The disease occurs mainly in children and is a pediatric-otolaryngologic emergency. It is characterized by rapid onset and progression. Without treatment death results from respiratory obstruction.

1

Etiology

The etiologic agent which is clearly of most importance in epiglottitis is *H. influenzae* type B. What is less clear, however, is the role of other infectious agents in this illness. Confusion has arisen because of the assigned significance given to organisms recovered from various anatomic sites. In many studies organisms recovered from the throat or the surface of the epiglottis are considered causative. This interpretation must be accepted with caution, as surface bacteria may be part of the normal mucosal flora and may not have got there by extension from the infection within the epiglottis. Table 1 lists the blood, epiglottic, and throat and nasopharyngeal bacteriologic findings in 17 published studies involving 939 children and adolescents. Similar data for 42 adult cases are presented in Table 2.

Children In the majority of pediatric cases blood cultures grew *H. influenzae* type B. There is a notable difference in isolation rate between the different studies, but in 10 studies in which 75 percent or more of the patients had blood cultures performed, the isolation rate for *H. influenzae* type B was 86 percent.

Agents other than *H. influenzae* type B have only very rarely been recovered from the blood of children with epiglottitis (2, 4, 7, 12, 17). *Streptococcus pneumoniae* has been recovered from two children, and in one of these instances *H. influenzae* was concomitantly isolated. One child had a group A streptococcus recovered from the blood, and another had an *H. influenzae* strain which was not type B (4, 17). *Staphylococcus aureus* was recovered from the blood of an unusual case involving a neonate (7).

As noted in Table 1, there is a great difference between the various studies in the results of cultures from the epiglottis. Margolis et al. (13), Milko et al. (9), and Branefors-Helander and Jeppsson (11) noted *H. influenzae* type B in over 83 percent of instances of culture of the epiglottis. These findings indicate that the surface of the epiglottis is usually infected with *H. influenzae* type B; the lesser isolation rate in other studies probably is the result of poor technique, previous antibiotic therapy, and a general lack of interest in etiology on the part of the clinicians involved. Cultures of the throat or nasopharynx in epiglottitis reveal a variety of microorganisms and therefore cannot be used to incriminate a specific agent as the pathogen. The recovery of *H. influenzae* type B in pure culture or as the predominant organism is highly suggestive, however.

Adults In adults as well as children *H. influenzae* type B is the major etiologic agent (Table 2). However, as noted in Table 2, there may be a greater etiologic spectrum in adults than in children. Of the 11 positive blood cultures noted in Table 2, 7 were *H. influenzae* type B, 1 was *H. influenzae* of unspecified type, 2 were *Haemophilus parainfluenzae*, and 1 was a *Strep. pneumoniae*. Cultures from the epiglottis suggest that *Strep. pneumoniae* is also an important etiologic consideration in the disease in the adult.

Table 1 Bacteriologic findings of blood, epiglottic, and nasopharyngeal or throat cultures in 17 published studies of epiglottis in children and adolescents

Ref.	Period	Blood cultures				Epiglottic cultures		Nasopharyngeal or throat cultures	
		No. of patients	Positive for H. influenzae type B		Other bacteria isolated	H. influenzae	Other	H. influenzae	Other
			No.	%					
1	1937–1946	28	25	89		3 of 3		In all but 1 case; 23 of 27 type B	
2	1946–1954	42	16	69	1 Strep. pneumoniae	11 type B	1 Strep. pneumoniae, 1 beta strep	17	2 Staph. aureus
3	1950–1959	37	2	100		2 of 30 predominant type B; 4 type B with other organisms	9 alpha strep and Branhamella catarrhalis with 4 also having staph; most cultures mixed flora (strep, staph, Strep. pneumoniae, B. catarrhalis, and diphtheroids)		

3

Table 1 Bacteriologic findings of blood, epiglottic, and nasopharyngeal or throat cultures in 17 published studies of epiglottitis in children and adolescents (continued)

Ref.	Period	Blood cultures				Epiglottic cultures		Nasopharyngeal or throat cultures	
		No. of patients	Positive for H. influenzae type B No.	%	Other bacteria isolated	H. influenzae	Other	H. influenzae	Other
4	1957–1977	175	47	28	60	1 H. influenzae not type B	83 type B, 6 not type B	27 beta strep, 22 Staph. aureus, 16 B. catarrhalis, 5 Pseudomonas aeruginosa, 5 micrococcus, 3 Strep. pneumoniae		
5	1958–1975	72	29	10	34*				Isolated from 39% (nose, throat, or epiglottis)	
6	1964–1972	55	33	20	6†					
7	1964–1973	97	6	1	17	Staph. aureus in 1 neonate	8	35 normal flora; 11 alpha strep, 8 Neisseria, 7 beta strep, 7 Staph. aureus, 1 Strep. pneumoniae, 3 other	1	22 normal flora, 6 Staph. aureus, 1 Neisseria
8	1968–1974	61	51	36	71				11 isolated, 34 not isolated	

4

No.	Years									
9	1968–1973	41	33	33	100		Type B isolated from all with positive blood cultures	In other 8 patients *Staph. aureus*, *Strep. pneumoniae*, and strep strains recovered		
10	1968–1978	64	64	41	64			Wide variety of organisms recovered		Wide variety of organisms recovered; 3 no growth, 1 normal flora
11	1968–1970	16	14	13	93‡		Type B from 10 of 12 cultures; 1 not type B	1 normal flora	Type B, 10 of 14 cultures	
12	1969–1977	57	56	48	86	*H. influenzae* and *Strep. pneumoniae* in 1 child			88% of airway cultures	Majority of airway cultures had mixed flora
13	1970–1974	32	32	30	94		27 of 32 type B	1 *Klebsiella*		
14	1971–1977	98	79	77	96					
15	1972–1975	23	23	23	100				Throat cultures positive in all cases for type B	
16	1974	14	8	4	50				2	
17	1976–1977	27	27	24	89§		18 of 27 positive			9 normal flora

* Eight of negative had prior antibiotics.
† Seven of thirteen negative had prior antibiotics.
‡ One negative had prior antibiotics.
§ Two of negative had prior antibiotics.

Table 2 Bacteriologic findings of blood, epiglottic, and nasopharyngeal or throat cultures in 13 published studies of epiglottitis in adults

Ref.	Date of publication or year of study	No. of patients	Blood cultures	Epiglottic cultures	Nasopharyngeal or throat cultures
11	1968–1970	9	2 *H. influenzae* B; 1 *Strep. pneumoniae*; 5 no growth; 1 not cultured	3 *H. influenzae* B; 1 *Strep. pneumoniae*; 4 normal flora plus *H. influenzae*; 1 normal flora ·	2 *H. influenzae* B; 4 normal flora; 3 no growth
18	1957–1966	5	1 *H. influenzae* B	3 *H. influenzae* B; 1 *Staph. aureus*, 1 profuse *Strep. pneumoniae* with alpha strep and micrococcus	
19	1963–1973	17	No cultures obtained	2 alpha strep and *Neisseria*; 1 beta strep, alpha strep, and *Neisseria*	12 normal flora; 3 *Strep. pneumoniae*; 2 beta strep (most cultures obtained after antibiotics started)

20	1967	H. influenzae type not specified		
21	1968	H. influenzae B		
22	1968	H. influenzae B		Light growth *Staph. aureus*
23	1969	No cultures obtained	Pure culture of *Strep. pneumoniae* in 1 patient	Normal flora in 1 patient
24	1971	*H. parainfluenzae*		*H. parainfluenzae*
25	1971	No cultures obtained	Normal flora	Normal flora
26	1973	*H. parainfluenzae*		Nonhemolytic streptococci
27	1976	No growth		Normal flora
28	1978	*H. influenzae* B		*H. influenzae* B
29	1979	*H. influenzae* B		Normal flora plus group A strep

Epidemiology

The incidence of acute epiglottitis has never been carefully evaluated. An analysis of hospitalized cases in St. Louis suggests a yearly rate of approximately 6 cases per 100,000 persons under 16 years of age (30); the rate in children from 2 to 5 years of age is in the range of 20 cases per 100,000. About 1 per 1000 admissions of pediatric inpatient services is for epiglottitis (7), and 5 to 10 percent of children admitted with acute upper airway obstruction have epiglottitis (30, 31).

In any one geographic area there are marked differences in the yearly prevalence of cases of epiglottitis (4–7, 12, 31). No intercity yearly prevalence pattern or national or international cycle can be demonstrated. Seasonal prevalence apparently varies in different localities and is not marked. The greatest number of cases in three studies were observed in the winter and spring (2, 5, 6). Baxter (31) noted the greatest number of cases during the summer and in November. Cohen and Chai (4) found no seasonal trend.

The age incidence as compiled from seven studies is presented in Figure 1 (2, 4, 6–8, 12, 31). Of these cases 27 percent occurred during the third year of life and 72 percent occurred in children from 1 to 5 years of age. The disease is more common in boys than in girls. Of 611 cases in 8 studies, 58 percent were boys (2, 4–8, 12, 31).

Pathophysiology

Epiglottitis is characterized by cellulitis and marked edema due to bacterial infection which involves the epiglottis, the aryepiglottic folds, and the ventricu-

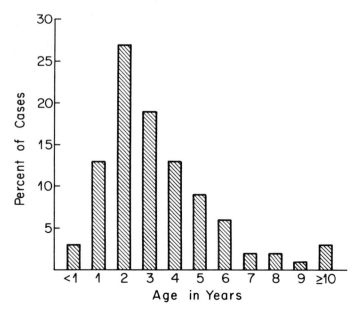

Figure 1   The age incidence of epiglottitis. Compiled from seven studies with 539 cases (2, 4, 6–8, 12, 30).

lar bands (1, 3, 11, 14, 19–21, 23, 25, 32, 33). Frequently the surface mucosa has abrasions, small ulcerations, and abscesses. The mechanism by which bacterial infection of the epiglottis occurs is unknown. Since bacteremia is virtually universal in this illness, it is tempting to suggest that supraglottic involvement is a secondary event. However, the short duration of fever, the usual absence of another respiratory focus of infection (pharyngitis, otitis media), and the rarity of epiglottitis in patients with other septicemic diseases (meningitis, arthritis, nonfacial cellulitis) suggest that bacteremia is a secondary event in epiglottitis.

Epiglottitis probably arises from the direct invasion by *H. influenzae* and other agents. What facilitates this invasion is unknown. It is possible that mild trauma relating to food intake results in a mucosal surface susceptible to invasion. It also seems quite possible that viral infection might damage the mucosal surface so that secondary bacterial infection could occur. Gardner et al. (34) noted a 21-month-old child who had a mild coryzal illness for about 1 week before the sudden, fatal occurrence of epiglottitis. At necropsy this child was found to be infected with respiratory syncytial virus as well as *H. influenzae* type B. Unfortunately, virologic investigation has not been reported in other studies of epiglottitis.

In epiglottitis major symptomatology is related to progressive obstruction of the airway due to cellulitis and edema of the epiglottis and its supporting structures. With progression, the epiglottis tends to curl posteriorly and inferiorly. Inspiration aggravates the situation by drawing the swollen epiglottis down into the laryngeal inlet. There is no difficulty on expiration.

Histologic examination reveals edema, hemorrhage, and diffuse infiltration with polymorphonuclear leukocytes. Microabscesses are noted. The epithelial mucosal surface is ulcerated to varying degrees. In several adults, epiglottic abscesses have been observed (19).

Serologic studies in patients with epiglottitis have indicated that in most instances acute phase serums are devoid of bactericidal and hemagglutinating antibody; following infection, seroconversion regularly occurs (11, 13, 35). Whisnant et al. (36) studied HLA and erythrocyte antigens in patients with *H. influenzae* epiglottitis and meningitis in an attempt to see whether there was a genetic predisposition in either disease. In the epiglottitis patient group the Ms erythrocyte gene was decreased in frequency and the Ns gene increased. Of the tissue antigens HLA-A28 was more commonly noted in patients with epiglottitis than in the control population.

Clinical diagnostic characteristics

Although careful history will occasionally reveal the occurrence of a trivial antecedent upper respiratory illness (1, 10), the classic onset of epiglottitis is abrupt and progression of disease is rapid (1–29). The total duration of illness before hospitalization is usually less than 24 h and may be as short as 2 h. Cohen and Chai (4) analyzed 142 medical records of children with epiglottitis and noted that the duration of illness before tracheotomy was 12 h or less in 73 percent and greater than 24 h in only four patients.

The usual presentation of acute epiglottitis includes the sudden onset of fever, severe sore throat, dysphagia, and drooling. There is airway obstruction which is rapidly progressive and is manifested by distress on inspiration, a choking sensation, irritability, restlessness, and anxiety. The patient usually is not hoarse, but the speech is muffled or thick-sounding. The patient with epiglottitis does not want to lie down and if forced to do so will exhibit great anxiety and become worse. The patient insists on sitting up and assumes a characteristic posture with the arms back, the trunk leaning forward, the neck hyperextended, and the chin pushed forward. This posture maximizes the diameter of the obstructed upper airway.

In contrast with laryngotracheitis, in which marked stridor on inspiration regularly occurs, the degree of stridor in epiglottitis is not great. This lack of stridor often leads the unwary physician to underestimate the severity and rapidity of progression of the patient's illness. The air exchange becomes progressively worse, and hypoxia, hypercarbia, and acidosis develop, resulting in increased irritability, restlessness, and disorientation. If therapy is not instituted, the end result is sudden cardiorespiratory arrest.

Fever occurs in almost all patients, with the majority of temperatures between 38.8 and 40.0°C. Blood leukocytosis occurs almost without exception; the mean total count in five studies was about 20,000 cells per cubic millimeter (1, 2, 4, 6, 16). The differential cell count usually reveals over 85 percent polymorphonuclear leukocytes (1, 6, 16) with bands accounting for 10 to 20 percent. In one study 85 percent of the patients had band counts greater than 500 cells per cubic millimeter.

The clinical manifestations of epiglottitis in adults are generally similar to those observed in children; however, a greater percentage of adults have a milder illness with a more prolonged prodromal period (11, 19). Branefors-Helander and Jeppsson (11) studied 25 children and adults with epiglottitis and divided them into two groups according to the severity of illness. The moderately ill group was composed of 8 adults and 3 children, whereas the severely ill group had 13 children and only 1 adult. In a study of 17 adults Hawkins et al. (19) noted that all patients had sore throat and dysphagia but only 10 had respiratory difficulty. Nine patients had cervical swelling, a finding not usually observed in children. Six patients had pharyngitis. In spite of an apparent decreased severity of illness in adults, Hawkins and associates (19) noted a mortality rate of 32 percent in 62 patients reported in the 15 years before their study.

Extraepiglottic complications are generally considered not very common in children with acute epiglottitis. However, Molteni (5) recently reviewed 72 cases of epiglottitis seen in Denver, Colorado, and noted pneumonia in 25 percent, cervical adenitis in 25 percent, tonsillitis in 8 percent, and bilateral otitis media in 5 percent. Meningitis, arthritis, and cellulitis were not observed. Four of the twenty-five patients studied by Branefors-Helander and Jeppsson (11) developed meningitis after admission to the hospital; outside this report the occurrence of epiglottitis and meningitis is a rarity.

The hallmark of successful clinical diagnosis in acute epiglottitis is awareness of the condition and an understanding of the rapidity of its progression. The clinical picture described above (sore throat, dysphagia, drooling, anxiety, inspiratory distress without significant stridor, and the sitting position) allows a presumptive diagnosis in most cases. Definitive diagnosis is made by observation of the epiglottis. The epiglottis is fiery red and greatly swollen. In most instances in children the epiglottis can be visualized by simple depression of the tongue with a tongue blade. In older children and adults indirect or direct laryngoscopy is often necessary to establish the diagnosis. Occasionally the major swelling involves the ventricular bands and the aryepiglottic folds, so that the epiglottis will appear relatively normal.

There is some controversy over the safety of using a tongue depressor in examining the patient with epiglottitis because cardiorespiratory arrest has been reported to occur. However, in most instances of cardiorespiratory arrest in this condition that I am aware of, the arrest was the result of forcing the patient into a supine position rather than of the examination itself. In my opinion most patients with epiglottitis can be examined in the sitting position with a tongue blade. Indirect laryngoscopy can also be performed in the sitting position. In the patient with advanced disease the presumptive diagnosis is usually easy, and intraoral examination should not be done. The primary concern is the establishment of an airway.

Another aspect of diagnosis which is quite popular is the lateral neck radiograph (16, 37). However, it is my opinion and that of others that this procedure is most often a useless test which only delays the necessary definitive therapy (4, 9, 30, 33). I am personally aware of several patients who died in the x-ray department before therapy had even been instituted. The use of the lateral neck radiograph should be restricted to subacute cases in which direct or indirect examination of the epiglottis has not been diagnostic.

Laboratory diagnostic studies

Necessary laboratory studies in epiglottitis are few. All patients should have a blood culture and a culture from the surface of the epiglottis obtained before, or at the time of, onset of therapy. Cultures today have a greater degree of importance because of the changing resistance patterns of *H. influenzae* to common antibiotics. All isolates should be examined for their sensitivity to ampicillin and chloramphenicol. In patients who have received antibiotics, a search for *H. influenzae* type B antigenemia and antigenuria by counterimmunoelectrophoresis or latex agglutination is a useful alternative to culture but will not, of course, yield information about organism susceptibility (38, 39). A white blood cell count and differential is often useful.

Treatment

Organized approach   The treatment of acute epiglottitis is relatively simple in that the two main aspects of therapy are the establishment of an airway and the administration of appropriate antibiotics. However, the mortality rate in this condition varies from 0 to 32 percent (4, 19), indicating apparently great differences in implementation of treatment. Most deaths in patients with epiglottitis occur within the first few hours after arrival at a hospital. A review of the literature clearly indicates the reason for the great differences in mortality in this condition (40, 41). Hospitals and pediatric services with planned protocols for the diagnostic investigation and treatment of patients with suspected acute epiglottitis generally have good morbidity and mortality statistics.

Securing an airway The hallmark of success in all programs is the establishment of an airway in all patients in whom the diagnosis of epiglottitis is made. Cantrell et al. (41) reviewed 20 studies of epiglottitis involving 749 patients and noted the following statistics: 5 deaths in 564 patients (0.9 percent) treated with either tracheostomy or endotracheal intubation and 13 deaths in 214 patients (6.1 percent) managed medically without an artificial airway.

Bass (42) reported that 42 of 83 patients with acute epiglottitis that he evaluated required tracheotomy to survive. He notes that there was no clue or any way to predict which patients would experience sudden, abrupt, and complete airway obstruction. Margolis et al. (40) found that no mortality occurred when a program of required tracheostomy was employed in epiglottitis management; previous experience at their hospital when the decision to establish an airway was individualized revealed 4 deaths in a series of 20 patients. It is my opinion from the evidence at hand that all children with acute epiglottitis regardless of the apparent severity of illness should have the elective establishment of an artificial airway. The same approach should probably also be employed in adults afflicted with this disease. However, the experience of Hawkins et al. (19), in which only 4 of 17 adults had tracheostomy and no deaths occurred, suggests that there is greater leeway in the management of adult patients.

Tracheostomy versus nasotracheal intubation The data noted in the review by Cantrell et al. (41) suggest that tracheostomy or nasotracheal intubation are equally satisfactory treatment methods. Cohen and Chai (4) noted no deaths in 147 patients who received tracheostomy, and others have also had excellent results with this mode of therapy (15, 40, 41). Several recent publications have emphasized the safety and overall good results when nasotracheal intubation is used (9, 12, 15–17, 43–46).

Antibiotics The second major aspect of therapy in acute epiglottitis is the administration of appropriate antibiotics. Since the vast majority of cases in both adults and children are due to *H. influenzae* type B, antibiotic therapy should be directed against this organism. The mainstay of therapy in recent years for *H. influenzae* has been ampicillin or chloramphenicol. At present many strains of *H. influenzae* type B are resistant to ampicillin (47–51), and occasional strains are resistant to chloramphenicol (48, 51–53); no strains which are resistant to both ampicillin and chloramphenicol have been recovered from patients ill with disease due to *H. influenzae* type B. Because of the possibility of antibiotic failure the therapy of choice in acute epiglottitis is the intravenous administration of both ampicillin (200 mg/kg daily at 4-h intervals) and chloramphenicol (100 mg/kg daily at 6-h intervals; maximum dose 4 g per day). This antibiotic regimen will also be effective in the rare case due to *H. parainfluenzae*, *Strep. pneumoniae*, and *Strep. pyogenes*.

Other measures Expert nursing care is essential so that complications of tracheostomy or nasotracheal intubation can be prevented or recognized early and treated. Modalities of treatment frequently used in epiglottitis which have no scientific validity or rationale and which should not be permitted include the administration of steroids and intermittent positive pressure breathing with or without aerosolized racemic epinephrine (54, 55).

Prognosis and prevention

Although acute epiglottitis is a rapidly progressive and frightening disease, the prognosis in the case with airway intervention and appropriate antibiotic therapy is excellent. The prognosis is of course guarded in patients who require emergency tracheostomy following cardiorespiratory arrest. At present, prevention is not possible; the further development and widespread use of *H. influenzae* capsular polysaccharide vaccine offers some promise for the prevention of all invasive diseases due to *H. influenzae*, including epiglottitis.

LARYNGITIS AND CROUP

Definitions

In this section, infectious illnesses which involve the larynx and subglottic region are considered; a classification and definitions are presented in Table 3. The specific categories noted in Table 3 represent clearly different disease entities based upon factors of age, etiologic agents, anatomical location, pathological findings, and ecological events. Unfortunately, physicians today frequently lump these five decidedly different illnesses together and treat them similarly, leading to considerable confusion over the effectiveness of various therapeutic modalities.

History

Croup resulting from *Corynebacterium diphtheriae* infection is an ancient disease with a 1500-year history (59). Even though spasmodic croup was recognized and separated from diphtheritic croup over 150 years ago, it was not until the early years of the twentieth century that laryngotracheitis and laryngotracheobronchitis of nondiphtherial origin were noted as common and important illnesses (58). In spite of present medical sophistication, there has been a general decline in physicians' knowledge of croup; therapeutic modalities are employed without adequate attention to clinical categories of illness or an understanding of expected outcomes of disease without therapy.

Three important events in the present century have had a marked relationship to croup illnesses:

1 With the advent and widespread use of diphtheria toxoid, *C. diphtheriae* is now only a rare cause of obstructive airway diseases.

Table 3 Classification and definition of infectious illnesses involving the larynx and subglottic region (32, 56–58)

Category	Other terms	Definition
Laryngitis		Inflammation of the larynx resulting in hoarseness; usually occurs in older children and adults in association with common upper respiratory viral infection
Laryngeal diphtheria	Membranous croup; true croup; diphtheritic croup	Infection involving the larynx and other areas of the upper and lower airway due to C. diphtheriae, resulting in a gradually progressive obstruction of the airway and associated inspiratory stridor
Laryngotracheitis	False croup; virus croup; nondiphtheritic croup; acute obstructive subglottic laryngitis	Inflammation of the larynx and trachea usually due to infection with parainfluenza viral types 1 and 2 and influenza A viruses; occasionally secondary bacterial infection
Laryngotracheobronchitis and laryngotracheo-pneumonitis		Inflammation of the larynx, trachea and bronchi and/or lung; usually similar in onset to laryngotracheitis but more severe illness; frequently bacterial infection has causative role
Spasmodic croup	Spasmodic laryngitis; catarrhal spasm of the larynx; subglottic allergic edema	An illness characterized by the sudden onset at night of inspiratory stridor; associated with mild upper respiratory infection without inflammation or fever but with edema in the subglottic region

2 The mortality associated with acute laryngotracheobronchitis fell dramatically during the period of the introduction and widespread use of antibiotics.

3 The development of virologic techniques in the 1950s led to the establishment of viruses as etiologic agents in the majority of cases of laryngotracheitis.

Etiology

Laryngotracheitis and spasmodic croup It is generally acknowledged today that most cases of croup are due to viral infections. Unfortunately, with few exceptions there has been no attempt to delineate differences in etiologic spectrum by severity of illness. Specifically, the prevalence of different viruses in spasmodic croup has never been studied. In Table 4, etiologic agents are presented by frequency, epidemic occurrence, and severity of illness.

Parainfluenza virus type 1 is the most common cause of epidemic acute laryngotracheitis. Epidemics of usually mild disease are also associated with parainfluenza type 2 virus. Parainfluenza virus type 3 is the cause of sporadic but occasionally severe disease. The most severe acute laryngotracheitis has been noted with influenza A viral infections (H2N2 and H3N2 subtypes). The other viruses listed in Table 4 are usually associated with mild illness (either laryngotracheitis or spasmodic croup) without epidemic occurrence.

Laryngitis In the older child and adult, laryngitis is a common manifestation of infection with many respiratory viral agents. Of most importance is the occurrence of epidemic acute respiratory disease (ARD) in military recruits due to adenoviral types 4 and 7. Laryngitis occurs in about 30 to 50 percent of those infected. Outbreaks of illness with laryngitis as a prominent finding are also due to influenza viruses and parainfluenza virus type 1. Although laryngitis has also been noted in association with group A streptococcal pharyngitis, the frequency of occurrence of laryngitis in streptococcal infections has varied from 2 to 40 percent (70–72).

Laryngotracheobronchitis Except for *H. influenzae* in epiglottitis and *C. diphtheriae* in membranous croup, bacteria are presently not usually considered as causative agents in acute crouplike illnesses (94). On the other hand, a review of many reports on laryngotracheobronchitis written before the present antibiotic era clearly indicates bacterial infection of the trachea in many cases. The most common agent found on tracheal culture was *Strep. pyogenes*; *Staph. aureus*, *Strep. pneumoniae*, and *H. influenzae* were also implicated. Recently, bacterial infection, particularly due to *Staph. aureus*, has again been implicated in croup (80, 93). It seems likely that bacterial croup is the result of bacterial superinfection in viral disease, but there is no definitive evidence to support this opinion.

Pathophysiology

Laryngotracheitis, laryngitis, and laryngotracheobronchitis Acquisition of infection is similar to other respiratory viral illnesses with initial infection within

Table 4 Etiologic agents in laryngotracheitis, spasmodic croup, laryngitis, and laryngotracheobronchitis (60–92)

Category	Etiologic agents	Frequency*	Associated with epidemics?	Severity†
Laryngotracheitis and spasmodic croup	Parainfluenza viruses:			
	Type 1	++++	Yes	+ to +++
	Type 2	++	Yes	+ to +++
	Type 3	++	No	+ to +++
	Influenza viruses:			
	Type A	+++	Yes	+ to ++++
	Type B	+	Yes	+ to ++
	Respiratory syncytial virus and adenoviruses types 1–3, 5–7 and unspecified	++	No	+ to ++
	Rhinoviruses, *Mycoplasma pneumoniae*, several enteroviruses, herpes simplex	+	No	+
Laryngitis	Adenoviruses:			
	Types 4 and 7	++++	Yes	+ to +++
	Types 2, 3, 5, 8, 11, 14, 21	+++	No	+ to +++
	Influenza viruses type A and B	++++	Yes	+ to ++++
	Parainfluenza viruses:			
	Type 1	++	Yes	+ to +++
	Type 2, 3	+	Yes	+ to ++
	Rhinoviruses and respiratory syncytial virus	++	No	+ to ++
	Enteroviruses	±	No	+
	Strep. pyogenes	+ to +++	Yes	+ to ++
Laryngotracheobronchitis	Parainfluenza viruses types 1–3	+	No	+++
	Influenza types A and B	+	No	+++
	Strep. pyogenes; *Staph. aureus*, *Strep. pneumoniae*, and *H. influenzae*	+	No	++++
	Other bacteria	±	No	++

* ++++ = most frequent; +++ = frequent; ++ = occasional; + = rare; ± = questionable.

† ++++ = most severe; +++ = severe; ++ = not severe; + = minimal distress.

the upper air passages including the nasal and pharyngeal epithelial surfaces. Following viral multiplication at the primary site of infection, which is associated with nasal stuffiness and throat irritation, there is local downward spread to involve the larynx and trachea. Direct examination reveals redness and swelling of the lateral walls of the trachea, just below the vocal cords (84, 95). Since the subglottic trachea is surrounded by a firm cartilaginous ring, inflammatory swelling can only encroach on the airway. In the young child with small air passages this leads to signs of partial airway obstruction; in the older child and adult with laryngitis, because obstruction does not reach clinical significance, only hoarseness is noted.

With progression of disease, there is destruction of the ciliated epithelial surface of the trachea, with a fibrinous covering exudate. The vocal cords are swollen, and their mobility is impaired. In laryngotracheobronchitis and laryngotracheopneumonitis there is extension of the disease to the lower respiratory tract. The slow progression and then sudden worsening in many cases in association with the finding of pathogenic bacteria on culture suggest a scenario of viral-bacterial superinfection.

In uncomplicated laryngotracheitis, recent studies have shown that besides hypoxia resulting from subglottic obstruction there is frequently failure of gas exchange within the lung (96, 97).

Spasmodic croup In spasmodic croup the subglottic area is not inflamed; only pale watery edema is noted (98). Although spasmodic croup occurs in association with infection with common respiratory viruses, it seems likely from the above observation that direct viral involvement of the tracheal epithelium does not occur. Obstruction is the result of noninflammatory edema within the submucosa of the subglottic trachea. The reason for sudden edema at this location is unknown; it is readily reversible, and the tendency for its occurrence seems to be familial.

Clinical diagnostic characteristics

The comparative clinical characteristics of laryngitis, laryngotracheitis, laryngotracheobronchitis, spasmodic croup, and diphtheritic croup are presented in Table 5.

Laryngitis Laryngitis is an acute self-limited illness which affects older children and adults. The clinical manifestation of laryngitis is hoarseness. Laryngitis as an isolated disease almost never occurs; instead hoarseness is one common manifestation of many respiratory viral infections. Other symptoms vary with the specific viral agent. In general the most severe illnesses which are associated with fever in many instances are those due to adenoviruses and influenza viruses. These illnesses are also associated with sore throat and varying degrees of systemic disability such as headache, muscle aches and pains, and prostration. Patients who develop laryngitis in association with rhinoviral, parainfluenza viral, or respiratory syncytial viral infections usually have mini-

Table 5   Clinical characteristics of laryngitis, laryngotracheitis, (56–59, 68, 69, 71, 77–88, 90, 91, 98)

Category	Laryngitis	Laryngotracheitis
Common age of occurrence	Older children and adults	3 months to 3 years
Past and family history	Not contributory	Frequently family history of croup
Exposure history	Contact with child with febrile respiratory illness or adult with upper respiratory infection	Contact with adult with a cold or influenza or child with febrile respiratory infection
Prodrome	Usually stuffy nose or coryza	Usually coryza
Progression	Variable; 12 h to 4 days	Moderate and variable; 12–48 h
Symptoms on presentation:		
Fever	Yes (100–103°F) with adenoviral and influenza viral infections; usually minimal with other viruses	Yes; quite variable (100–105°F)
Hoarseness	Yes	Yes
Barking cough	Occasionally	Yes
Dysphagia	No	No
Inspiratory stridor	No	Yes; minimal to severe
Toxic appearance	No	Usually minimal
Signs on presentation:		
Oral cavity	Normal or mild to moderate pharnygitis	Usually minimal pharyngitis
Epiglottis	Normal	Normal
Chest retraction with inspiration	No	Yes; minimal to moderate
Radiograph	Not useful	Subglottic narrowing on PA film
Laboratory:		
Leukocyte count	Usually normal	Mildly elevated with >70% polymorphonuclear cells
Bacteriology	Usually normal flora in throat; occasionally *Strep. pyogenes* in throat	Normal throat flora; culture from larynx usually does not reveal predominant pathogen
Clinical course	Hoarseness persists at a constant degree about 4 to 7 days; occasionally persists 2–3 weeks	Degree of obstruction variable and persists 4 to 7 days; usually does not require surgical intervention

laryngotracheobronchitis, spasmodic croup, and diphtheritic croup

Laryngotracheobronchitis	Spasmodic croup	Diphtheritic croup
3 months to 3 years	3 months to 3 years	All ages
May be family history of croup	Frequently family history of croup; perhaps previous attack	No or inadequate immunization
Contact with adult with a cold or influenza or child with febrile respiratory infection	Frequently mild respiratory illness in family	Perhaps exposure to patient with febrile pharyngitis
Usually coryza	Minimal coryza	Usually pharyngitis
Usually gradually progressive; 12 h to 7 days	Sudden; always at night	Slowly for 2–3 days
Yes; quite variable (100–105°F)	No	Yes; usually 100–101°F
Yes	Yes; with attacks	Yes
Yes	Yes	Yes
No	No	Usually yes
Yes; usually severe	Yes; minimal to moderate	Yes; minimal to severe
Usually moderate; may be severe	No	Usually no
Usually minimal pharyngitis	Normal	Membranous pharyngitis
Normal	Normal	Usually normal; may contain membrane
Yes; minimal to severe	Yes; minimal to moderate	Yes; minimal to moderate
Subglottic narrowing on PA film	Not useful	Not useful
Variable; usually mildly elevated with >70% polymorphonuclear cells; may be increased band count	Normal	Usually markedly elevated with increased band count
Normal throat flora; tracheal culture often yields Strep. pyogenes, Staph. aureus, Strep. pneumoniae, or H. influenzae	Normal throat flora	Smear and culture from membrane reveals C. diphtheriae
Degree of obstruction usually severe; persists 7–14 days; frequently requires surgical intervention	Symptoms of short duration with treatment; repeat attacks common	Slowly progressive obstruction of airway; frequently requires surgical intervention

mal or no fever and minimal systemic complaints, but they usually have pronounced nasal symptomatology (rhinitis and stuffiness).

Occasionally hoarseness will persist, and in some instances this may be related to secondary bacterial infection of the upper respiratory tract; persistent symptomatology may be related to sinusitis.

Laryngotracheitis The initial symptoms of nasal dryness, irritation, and coryza in laryngotracheitis suggest the onset of a cold except that fever usually occurs. After a period of a few hours to 2 days the onset of upper airway obstructive signs and symptoms occur. Distinctive "croupy" cough (sounding like a barking seal) occurs, followed by gradual but increasing difficulty with inspiratory breathing. At this time the child usually has a hoarse voice, coryza, a normal or minimally inflamed pharynx, and a respiratory rate that is only slightly increased with a prolonged inspiratory phase. Fever usually is observed, but its degree is quite variable. Since the illness is quite variable, the speed of progression and final degree of airway obstruction can rarely be predicted. In some children only hoarseness and barking cough are observed; in these cases illness lasts from 3 to 7 days with normal states returning gradually. More severe disease is characterized by progressive obstruction in which supra- and infraclavicular and sternal retractions, cyanosis of varying degrees, and apprehension are noted. Worsening disease is characterized by increase in cardiac rate and general restlessness due to hypoxia. Without intervention, death from asphyxia will occur rapidly in a small number of severely affected children. In other children a more prolonged state of hypoxia occurs, which can result in respiratory fatigue and eventual demise due to respiratory failure. The duration of illness in the moderately severe case of laryngotracheitis is usually between 5 and 7 days, and in more severe cases 10- to 14-day periods of illness frequently occur.

Laboratory study in acute laryngotracheitis reveals a white blood cell count which is frequently elevated above 10,000 cells per cubic millimeter with greater than 70 percent polymorphonuclear cells (68). A posteroanterior chest radiograph will reveal subglottic narrowing, and a lateral neck film should reveal a normal supraglottic region.

Laryngotracheobronchitis Laryngotracheobronchitis is generally quite uncommon today, but two recent publications (58, 93) and unpublished observations (99) suggest that the disease may be more common than realized. The initial symptoms and signs in laryngotracheobronchitis, as in laryngotracheopneumonitis, are identical to those of laryngotracheitis. In most instances the lower airway involvement results from extension from above. In the usual case the child will have mild to moderately severe laryngotracheitis for 2 to 7 days and then become markedly worse rather suddenly. Occasionally signs and symptoms of both upper and lower airway obstruction occur simultaneously. Findings associated with extension of disease to the bronchi, bronchioles, and lung substance include rales, air trapping, wheezing, and an increase in respiratory rate. Six of seven children reported by Jones et al. (80) had illness of such severity that either intubation or tracheostomy was necessary. The white blood cell count in this group of patients varied from 6400 to 28,700 cells per cubic millimeter, but in all an elevation in the percentage of bands was noted.

Spasmodic croup Spasmodic croup occurs in children 3 months to 3 years old, with the onset always at night. The afebrile child who was previously well or with a very mild cold awakens from sleep with sudden dyspnea, croupy cough, and inspiratory stridor. The symptoms seem to be the result of sudden subglottic edema, and relief occurs with moist air administration and general reassurance. Repeated episodes of spasmodic croup occur in some children, and the illness tends to occur in a familial pattern. Frequently a child will have successive attacks in one evening as well as on three to four successive evenings. Attacks can be prevented by humidifying the air in the bedroom and using mild sedation at the child's bedtime.

Diphtheritic croup The main features of diphtheritic croup are presented in Table 5. This illness should be suspected in any patient with upper airway obstructive disease in whom a membrane is visible on the tonsils or pharyngeal wall. However, since laryngeal diphtheria can occur without a visible membrane in the throat, this diagnosis must be considered in any croup patient without an adequate immunization history. Diagnosis can be established by direct laryngoscopy and appropriate smear and culture.

Differential diagnosis

Since the therapeutic approach to laryngitis and croup illnesses as well as to epiglottitis, to an inhaled foreign body, or to acute angioneurotic edema involving the upper airway vary markedly, correct diagnosis is essential and occasionally lifesaving. The most important differential diagnostic problem is the separation of supraglottic problems (epiglottitis and allergic edema of the epiglottis) from subglottic disease. The important differential points in epiglottitis are the lack of a croupy cough, the presence of a swollen cherry-red epiglottis, the child's sitting posture and reluctance to lie down, and a degree of apprehension and anxiety greater than that expected from the amount of stridor. In contrast, the child with laryngotracheitis will have a normal epiglottis, will always have a seal-like barking cough, will be comfortable in a supine position, and will frequently not be greatly apprehensive in spite of retractions in which the sternum depresses 2 in or more.

Laryngotracheobronchitis or laryngotracheopneumonitis can be specifically differentiated from laryngotracheitis by the presence of an expiratory phase of distress (air trapping, resulting in prolonged expiration and wheezing) and radiographic evidence of lower respiratory involvement. In many instances the initial clinical differential diagnosis between these two entities is based upon a greater severity of illness in laryngotracheobronchitis. The need to establish an artificial airway is common in laryngotracheobronchitis and rare in laryngotracheitis. Definitive bacterial culture is made at the time of intubation or tracheostomy. Occasionally bacterial tracheitis can occur without evidence of lower respiratory tract disease.

Although spasmodic croup is a clearly distinct entity that should not be confused with other subglottic illnesses, a perusal of recent literature suggests that spasmodic croup and laryngotracheitis are frequently lumped together erroneously as "laryngotracheobronchitis" or often as "croup." This is unfortunate, as prognosis and therapy for the three illnesses are different. Spasmodic croup always occurs suddenly without fever and wakens the child from sleep. It is relieved by simple therapy. Although a rarity today, laryngeal diphtheria should be considered and ruled out in all children and adults with upper airway obstructive disease.

Specific diagnosis of viral etiology in laryngitis, laryngotracheitis, laryngotracheobronchitis, and spasmodic croup can be made by the isolation of virus from the nasopharynx. The presence of a viral agent in the nasopharynx does not of course rule out concomitant bacterial tracheitis in laryngotracheitis and laryngotracheobronchitis. Culture for bacteria from the trachea is necessary to confirm this latter diagnostic possibility.

Treatment

Laryngitis Since laryngitis is usually not an isolated disease but part of a more general upper respiratory illness, treatment is aimed at the overall event. Aspirin is useful in reducing overall discomfort, and increased fluid intake will help to liquefy secretions. The voice should be rested until hoarseness clears. The use of a vaporizer will help to liquefy secretions and provide symptomatic relief. Patients in whom throat culture is positive for *Strep. pyogenes* should be treated with penicillin or a suitable alternative. In patients with prolonged hoarseness, sinusitis should be ruled out and a search for a predominant abnormal bacterial throat flora should be made. If either is positive, therapy with appropriate antibiotics is indicated. With persistent laryngitis the patient should have laryngoscopic examination to exclude tumor, foreign body, and other chronic disease.

Spasmodic croup Spasmodic croup invariably responds to the administration of moist air. In the home this therapy can be performed by taking the child to the bathroom and turning the shower on full. Another mode of therapy is the administration of a subemetic dose of syrup of ipecac. While this method apparently works, in my experience most children have vomited spontaneously, and clearing occurs after this event. The child who has an attack of spasmodic croup is likely to have another attack the same evening or during the next few nights. These attacks can be prevented by the use of mild sedation at the child's bedtime.

All too frequently children with spasmodic croup are overtreated; many physicians are unfamiliar with the benign nature of this illness and administer steroids, intermittent positive pressure breathing (IPPB), and other unnecessary therapies.

Diphtheritic croup In diphtheritic croup primary therapy is aimed at the systemic effects of the infection. Antitoxin administration in a dosage ranging from 40,000 to 120,000 units is of most importance. Penicillin (or erythromycin) in people allergic to penicillin) should be administered; tracheotomy should be performed in patients with severely compromised airways.

Laryngotracheitis Differences of opinion relating to modalities of therapy in croup have been common for the last 50 years. Few of these controversies have been solved scientifically, but the passage of time has lessened the importance of some of the discrepant issues. Of most importance in the evaluation of therapeutic modalities in laryngotracheitis is accurate differential diagnosis, but a careful look at recent studies relating to controversial therapeutic issues suggests that in most instances children with croup were not accurately classified according to type of illness (i.e., spasmodic croup, laryngotracheitis, or laryngotracheobronchitis).

In laryngotracheitis each case must be individualized; one child will only need simple therapy (i.e., mist treatment) while another will benefit from several modalities of treatment.

MOIST AIR The mainstay of treatment in acute laryngotracheitis is the immediate institution of mist therapy. In addition every effort should be made to lessen the anxiety and apprehension of the patient and the parents. It is usually best not to separate the child from the parents. Examination should be rapid, by one physician, and all but absolutely necessary procedures should be deferred.

Mist administration will prevent desiccation of the inflamed epithelium and will help to liquefy secretions and exudate (100). This decreased viscosity makes removal of exudate by coughing easier (101). The administration of water vapor may also stimulate nasal and laryngeal receptors; this slows the respiratory rate, which can be of benefit (102).

It is common to note on pediatric wards the vigorous effort to cool nebulized air by adding ice. This is frequently barbaric, almost always not indicated, and when the air is excessively cold may even have such adverse effects as shivering and bronchospasm. The moist air should be at a comfortable temperature. Using cool mist has a historical basis. Before the advent of modern humidification devices, steam was the usual method of providing moist air. In an enclosed mist tent, steam would generate excessive temperatures and this often led to distress for the patient.

OXYGEN Oxygen should be administered to children who are hypoxemic. The studies of Neuth et al. (97) and Taussig et al. (96) indicate that hypoxemia occurs without being clinically apparent. Thus, the use of oxygen in cases of moderate severity should not be discouraged. On the other hand, the use of oxygen should not be routine since its drying effect is counterproductive in removal of exudate.

SEDATIVES Sedatives should not be employed routinely or continuously, but their judicious use early in an illness may help relieve apprehension and anxiety.

STEROIDS   From 1952 to 1969 there were at least 29 communications in the English literature on the use of corticosteroids in croup. During the 1970s racemic epinephrine therapy in croup replaced corticosteroids as the controversial literature topic. In 1979 another steroid-croup-therapy paper appeared (103), and again testimonial debate on this topic was stimulated (58, 104). The majority of the steroid-croup-therapy reports have been testimonials, but there have been at least eight prospective controlled trials (103, 105–111). In three of these trials no benefit was noted (105, 106, 109); in two slight benefit was reported but the authors' discounted their own findings (107, 108); and in three trials definite benefit was ascribed to steroid treatment. Unfortunately none of the steroid-croup-therapy studies done to date have accurately classified illness by type of disease (spasmodic croup versus laryngotracheitis versus laryngotracheobronchitis) or specific etiology. When the total experience of steroids on croup is examined objectively, it appears that neither great benefit nor harm has occurred. The most important question of whether steroids will help the severely ill child with laryngotracheitis or laryngotracheobronchitis remains unanswered. It seems unlikely that steroids could benefit the child with severe laryngotracheitis due to influenza A virus infection (67, 69) or the child with bacterial laryngotracheitis or laryngotracheobronchitis (80, 93). In both instances they could be harmful. I have seen one child with severe laryngotracheobronchitis and an adenoviral infection in whom illness seemed to be aggravated by steroid therapy (Figure 2).

RACEMIC EPINEPHRINE BY AEROSOL   The most recent innovation in croup therapy was the use of IPPB and racemic epinephrine, popularized by Adair et al. in 1971 (112). This therapy as well as the use of nebulized racemic epinephrine without IPPB was adopted at many centers, and testimonials suggested a reduction in the need to perform tracheostomies (112–117). In 1973 Gardner et al. (113) in a double blind study could find no significant benefit from nebulized racemic epinephrine compared with nebulized saline. A shortcoming of this study was the failure to categorize study patients carefully so that patients with spasmodic croup were not excluded. Using racemic epinephrine by IPPB, Taussig et al. (96) noted (1) improvement in all cases, (2) recurrence of symptoms in 2 h, (3) no change in P_{O_2} with clinical improvement, and (4) clinical similarity of treated and untreated patients 24 to 36 h after therapy. In the most important study, because a parainfluenza viral etiology was documented in over 65 percent of the children with laryngotracheitis, Westley et al. (118) noted that racemic epinephrine resulted in definite short-term improvement compared with saline.

A few guidelines regarding racemic epinephrine therapy in laryngotracheitis follow:

1   Since significant rebound frequently follows racemic epinephrine therapy, repeated therapy is often necessary and should not be used as an outpatient modality.

2   Most children will respond to moist air alone, making the use of racemic epinephrine and IPPB unnecessary.

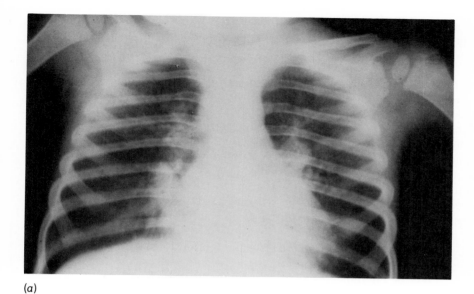

(a)

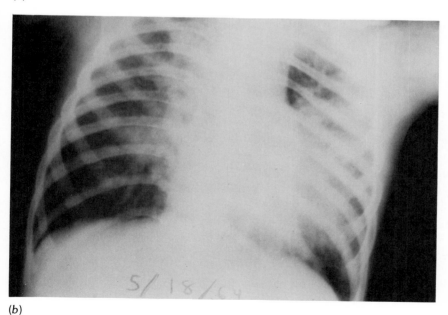

(b)

Figure 2 Progressive pneumonia in a child with laryngotracheobronchitis associated with adenoviral infection and steroid therapy. (a) Radiograph taken prior to steroid therapy. (b) Radiograph taken on the fifth day of steroid administration.

3 This therapy should be used in the hospitalized patient with severe disease as it may tide the patient over a critical period and make tracheotomy unnecessary.

ANTIBIOTICS Since in almost all instances acute laryngotracheitis is due to viral infections, the use of antibiotics does not appear to be indicated. Nevertheless, our group in St. Louis reviewed over 200 hospitalized children with croup and noted that in 85 percent of the cases antibiotics had been given (99). A review of the records indicated that in many instances the physician had a very good reason for using antibiotics, e.g., the observation of a slightly reddened or questionably enlarged epiglottis, pneumonia on radiograph, concomitant otitis media, or a markedly elevated white blood cell count.

It must also be remembered that the most dramatic reduction in croup mortality occurred during the time when clinical antibiotic use was becoming widespread. Many croup deaths in the preantibiotic era were due to secondary bacterial infections. It is my opinion that most cases of laryngotracheitis do not need antibiotic therapy, but when bacterial infection cannot be ruled out, antibiotics should be employed. In particular, patients with persistent fever (more than 4 days) or changing signs should be evaluated for secondary bacterial infection and following appropriate culture should be treated with antibiotics. The most likely pathogens are: *Staph. aureus, Strep. pyogenes, Strep. pneumoniae,* and *H. influenzae.*

TRACHEOSTOMY Tracheostomy is seldom necessary in laryngotracheitis today, but the possibility should always be considered by the physician. A planned tracheostomy will usually have a better outcome than one performed in an emergency. Although intubation is preferred by some physicians, the duration of the pathological changes within the trachea in the usual severe laryngotracheitis suggests that tracheostomy is preferable.

Laryngotracheobronchitis In general, the same treatment considerations mentioned above for laryngotracheitis apply for laryngotracheobronchitis except that since a significant number of cases have bacterial diseases, in my opinion antibiotics should be administered in all cases following appropriate cultures. Since recent reports (80, 93) indicate *Staph. aureus* as a major pathogen, therapy should be directed against this agent (oxacillin, nafcillin, etc.) as well as against *Strep. pyogenes, Strep. pneumoniae,* and *H. influenzae* (ampicillin and chloramphenicol).

Prognosis and prevention

The prognosis in croup is excellent. Only an occasional child will require tracheostomy. The following complications should be watched for: hypoxia and cardiorespiratory failure, pulmonary edema, pneumothorax, pneumomediastinum, mechanical problems relating to tracheostomy, and secondary bacterial infection.

At present croup is not preventable. The possibility of live attenuated viral vaccines against parainfluenza and influenza viruses offers promise, but research of this type at present is minimal because of ill-guided ethical restraints and a general emphasis recently on risks rather than on benefit/risk ratios.

REFERENCES

1 **Rabe EF:** Infectious croup: III. *Hemophilus influenzae* type B croup. *Pediatrics* 2:559, 1948.

2 **Berenberg W, Kevy S:** Acute epiglottitis in childhood. A serious emergency, readily recognized at the bedside. *N Engl J Med* 258:870, 1958.

3 **Vetto RR:** Epiglottitis. Report of thirty-seven cases. *JAMA* 173:88, 1960.

4 **Cohen SR, Chai J:** Epiglottitis: Twenty-year study with tracheotomy. *Ann Otol Rhinol Laryngol* 87:461, 1978.

5 **Molteni RA:** Epiglottitis: Incidence of extraepiglottic infection: Report of 72 cases and review of the literature. *Pediatrics* 58:526, 1976.

6 **Johnson GK et al:** Acute epiglottitis: Review of 55 cases and suggested protocol. *Arch Otolaryngol* 100:333, 1974.

7 **Bass JW et al:** Acute epiglottitis: A surgical emergency. *JAMA* 229:671, 1974.

8 **Benjamin B, O'Reilly B:** Acute epiglottitis in infants and children. *Ann Otol Rhinol Laryngol* 85:565, 1976.

9 **Milko DA et al:** Nasotracheal intubation in the treatment of acute epiglottitis. *Pediatrics* 53:674, 1974.

10 **Wetmore RF, Handler SD:** Epiglottitis: Evolution in management during the last decade. *Ann Otol Rhinol Laryngol* 88:822, 1979.

11 **Branefors-Helander P, Jeppsson P-H:** Acute epiglottis. A clinical, bacteriological and serological study. *Scand J Infect Dis* 7:103, 1975.

12 **Faden HS:** Treatment of *Haemophilus influenzae* type B epiglottitis. *Pediatrics* 63:402, 1979.

13 **Margolis CZ et al:** *Hemophilus influenzae* type B: The etiologic agent in epiglottitis. *J Pediatr* 87:322, 1975.

14 **Dajani AS et al:** Systemic *Haemophilus influenzae* disease: An overview. *J. Pediatr* 94:355, 1979.

15 **Oh TH, Motoyama EK:** Comparison of nasotracheal intubation and tracheostomy in management of acute epiglottitis. *Anesthesiology* 46:214, 1977.

16 **Weber ML:** Acute epiglottitis in children—treatment with nasotracheal intubation: Report of 14 consecutive cases. *Pediatrics* 57:152, 1976.

17 **Lewis JK et al:** A protocol for management of acute epiglottitis. Successful experiences with 27 consecutive instances treated by nasotracheal intubation. *Clin Pediatr* 17:494, 1978.

18 **Johnstone JM, Lawy HS:** Acute epiglottitis in adults due to infection with *Haemophilus influenzae* type B. *Lancet* 2:134, 1967.

19 **Hawkins DB et al:** Acute epiglottitis in adults. *Laryngoscope* 83:1211, 1973.

20 **Castleman B, McNeely BU:** Case 17-1967, presentation of a case. *N Engl J Med* 276:920, 1967.

21 **Johnson LW Jr.:** Death in a flyer due to acute epiglottitis and septicemia caused by *Haemophilus influenzae* type B. *Aviation Space Environ Med* February 1976, pp 187.

22 **Kringas N et al:** A case of acute epiglottitis in an adult due to *Haemophilus influenzae*, type B. *Med J Aust* 2:20, 1968.

23 **Gorfinkel HJ et al:** Acute infectious epiglottitis in adults. *Ann Intern Med* 70:289, 1969.

24 **Chow AW et al:** *Haemophilus parainfluenzae* epiglottitis with meningitis and bacteremia in an adult. *Am J Med Sci* 267:365, 1974.

25 **Robbins JP, Fitz-Hugh GS:** Epiglottitis in the adult. *Laryngoscope* 81:700, 1971.

26 **Robineau M et al:** *Haemophilus parainfluenzae* epiglottitis with positive blood cultures in an adult. *Scand J Infect Dis* 5:229, 1973.

27 **Darnell JC:** Acute epiglottitis in adults—Report of a case and review of the literature. *J Indiana State Med Assoc* 69:21, 1976.

28 **Williams NFR et al:** Acute epiglottitis and systemic infection with *Hemophilus influenzae*. *Can Med Assoc J* 118:63, 1978.

29 **Hirschmann JV, Everett ED:** *Haemophilus influenzae* infections in adults: Report of nine cases and a review of the literature. *Medicine* 58:80, 1979.

30 **Cherry JD:** Unpublished data.

31 **Baxter JD:** Acute epiglottitis in children. *Laryngoscope* 77:1358, 1967.

32 **Fearon B:** Acute obstructive laryngitis in infants and children. If the inflammatory swelling is above the glottis, severe respiratory obstruction may develop within two hours of the onset of symptoms. *Hosp Med* 4:51, 1968.

33 **Jones HM:** Acute epiglottitis: A personal study over twenty years. *Proc R Soc Med* 63:706, 1970.

34 **Gardner, PS et al:** Deaths associated with respiratory tract infection in childhood. *Br Med J* 4:316, 1967.

35 **Norden CW, Michaels R:** Immunologic response in patients with epiglottitis caused

by *Haemophilus influenzae* type B. *J Infect Dis* 128:777, 1973.

36 **Whisnant JK et al:** Host factors and antibody response in *Haemophilus influenzae* type B meningitis and epiglottitis. *J Infect Dis* 133:448, 1976.

37 **Rapkin RH:** The diagnosis of epiglottitis: Simplicity and reliability of radiographs of the neck in the differential diagnosis of the croup syndrome. *J Pediatr* 80:96, 1972.

38 **Kaldor J et al:** *Haemophilus influenzae* type B antigenuria in children. *J Clin Pathol* 32:538, 1979.

39 **Smith EWP, Ingram DL:** Counterimmunoelectrophoresis in *Hemophilus influenzae* type B epiglottitis and pericarditis. *J Pediatr* 86:571, 1975.

40 **Margolis CZ et al:** Routine tracheotomy in *Hemophilus influenzae* type B epiglottitis. *J Pediatr* 81:1150, 1972.

41 **Cantrell RW et al:** Acute epiglottitis: Intubation versus tracheostomy. *Laryngoscope* 88:994, 1978.

42 **Bass JW:** Routine tracheotomy for epiglottitis: What are the odds? *J Pediatr* 83:510, 1973.

43 **Blanc VF et al:** Acute epiglottitis in children: Management of 27 consecutive cases with nasotracheal intubation, with special emphasis on anaesthetic considerations. *Can Anaesth Soc J* 24:1, 1977.

44 **Tos M:** Nasotracheal intubation in acute epiglottitis. *Arch Otolaryngol* 97:373, 1973.

45 **Rapkin RH:** Nasotracheal intubation in epiglottitis. *Pediatrics* 56: 110, 1975.

46 **Battaglia JD, Lockhart CH:** Management of acute epiglottitis by nasotracheal intubation. *Am J Dis Child* 129:334, 1975.

47 **Syriopoulou V et al:** Increasing incidence of ampicillin resistance in *Hemophilus influenzae*. *J Pediatr* 92:889, 1978.

48 **Ward JI et al:** Prevalence of ampicillin- and chloramphenicol-resistant strains of *Haemophilus influenzae* causing meningitis and bacteremia: National survey of hospital laboratories. *J Infect Dis* 138:421, 1978.

49 **Scheifele DW:** Ampicillin-resistant *Hemophilus influenzae* in Canada: Nationwide survey of hospital laboratories. *Can Med Assoc J* 121:198, 1979.

50 **Lerman SJ et al:** Nasopharyngeal carriage of antibiotic-resistant *Haemophilus influenzae* in healthy children. *Pediatrics* 64:287, 1979.

51 **Long SS, Phillips SE:** Chloramphenicol-resistant *Hemophilus influenzae*. *J Pediatr* 90:1030, 1977.

52 **Richardson CJL et al:** Chloramphenicol-resistant *Haemophilus influenzae*. *Med J Aust* 2:429, 1979.

53 **Peel MM et al:** Chloramphenicol-resistant *Haemophilus influenzae*. *Med J Aust* 2:130, 1979.

54 **Szold PD, Glicklich M:** Children with epiglottitis can be bagged. *Clin Pediatr* 15:792, 1976.

55 **Strome M, Jaffe B:** Epiglottitis—Individualized management with steroids. *Laryngoscope* 84:921, 1974.

56 **Neffson AH:** *Acute Laryngotracheobronchitis*. New York, Grune & Stratton, 1949, pp 1–197.

57 **Davison FW:** Inflammatory diseases of the larynx of infants and small children. *Ann Otol Rhinol Laryngol* 76:753, 1967.

58 **Cherry JD:** The treatment of croup: Continued controversy due to failure of recognition of historic, ecologic, etiologic and clinical perspectives. *J Pediatr* 94:352, 1979.

59 **Top FH Sr:** Diphtheria, in Top FH Sr, Wehrle PF (eds): *Communicable and Infectious Diseases*. St. Louis, Mosby, 1972, pp 190–207.

60 **Parrott RH:** Viral respiratory tract illnesses in Children. *Bull NY Acad Med* 39:62, 1963.

61 **Horn MEC et al:** Respiratory viral infection in childhood. A survey in general practice, Roehampton, 1967–1972. *J Hyg (Camb)* 74:157, 1975.

62 **Chanock RM, Parrott RH:** Acute respiratory disease in infancy and childhood: Present understanding and prospects for prevention. *Pediatrics* 36:21, 1965.

63 **Paisley JW et al:** Type A2 influenza viral infections in children. *Am J Dis Child* 132:34, 1978.

64 **Vargosko AJ et al:** Association of type 2 hemadsorption (parainfluenza 1) virus and Asian influenza A virus with infectious croup. *N Engl J Med* 261:1, 1959.

65 **Poland JD et al:** Influenza virus B as cause of acute croup syndrome. *Am J Dis Child* 107:54, 1964.

66 **Parrott RH et al:** Serious respiratory tract illness as a result of Asian influenza and influenza B infections in children. *J Pediatr* 61:205, 1962.

67 **Forbes JA:** Severe effects of influenza virus infection. *Med J Aust* July 1958, p 75.

68 **Cherry JD:** Newer respiratory viruses: Their role in respiratory illnesses of children. *Adv Pediatr* 20:225, 1973.

69 **Howard JB et al:** Influenza A2 virus as a cause of croup requiring tracheotomy. *J Pediatr* 81:1148, 1972.

70 **Tyrrell DAJ:** *Common Colds and Related Diseases*. Baltimore, Williams & Wilkins, 1965, pp 1–197.

71 **Breese BB:** Diagnosis of streptococcal pharyngitis, in Breese BB, Hall CB (eds): *Beta Hemolytic Streptococcal Diseases*. Boston, Houghton Mifflin, 1978, pp 79–96.

72 **Mogabgab WJ:** Beta-hemolytic streptococcal and concurrent infections in adults and children with respiratory dis-

ease, 1958 to 1969. *Am Rev Respir Dis* 102:23, 1970.

73 **Banatvala JE et al:** Asian influenza in 1963 in two general practices in Cambridge, England. *Can Med Assoc J* 93:593, 1965.

74 **Person DA, Herrmann EC Jr:** Experiences in laboratory diagnosis of rhinovirus infections in routine medical practice. *Mayo Clin Proc* 45:517, 1970.

75 **Herrmann EC Jr, Habel KA:** Experiences in laboratory diagnosis of para-influenza viruses in routine medical practice. *Mayo Clin Proc* 45:177, 1970.

76 **Hope-Simpson RE, Higgins PG:** A respiratory virus study in Great Britain: Review and evaluation. *Prog Med Virol* 11:354, 1969.

77 **Dascomb HE, Hilleman MR:** Clinical and laboratory studies in patients with respiratory disease caused by adenoviruses (RI-APC-ARD agents). *Am J Med* 21:161, 1956.

78 **Stuart-Harris CH:** The adenoviruses and respiratory disease in man. *Lectures Sci Basis Med* 8:148, 1958–1959.

79 **Reilly CM et al:** Clinical and laboratory findings in cases of respiratory illness caused by coryzaviruses. *Ann Intern Med* 57:515, 1962.

80 **Jones R et al:** Bacterial tracheitis. *JAMA* 242:721, 1979.

81 **Baum HL:** Acute laryngotracheobronchitis. *JAMA* 91:1097, 1928.

82 **Brennemann J et al:** Acute laryngotracheobronchitis. *Am J Dis Child* 55:667, 1938.

83 **Brighton GR:** Laryngotracheobronchitis. *Ann Otol Rhinol Laryngol* 49:1070, 1940.

84 **Davison FW:** Acute laryngotracheobronchitis. *Arch Otol* 47:455–464, 1948.

85 **Everett AR:** Acute laryngotracheobronchitis. An analysis of 1,175 cases with 98 tracheotomies. *Laryngoscope* 61:113, 1951.

86 **Gittins TR:** Laryngitis and tracheobronchitis in children: Special reference to nondiphtheritic infections. *Ann Otol Rhinol Laryngol* 41:422, 1932.

87 **Hyde CI, Ruchman J:** Acute infectious edematous laryngitis in which recovery followed tracheotomy. *Arch Pediatr* 48:124, 1931.

88 **Johnson MC:** Acute laryngotracheobronchitis in infants. Report of three cases. *Arch Otol* 17:230, 1933.

89 **Macnab JCG:** Acute streptococcal infection of the trachea in an infant, aged fifteen months. *J Laryngol* 30:336, 1915.

90 **Orton HB et al:** Acute laryngotracheobronchitis. Analysis of sixty-two cases with report of autopsies in eight cases. *Arch Otol* 33:926, 1941.

91 **Richards L:** Fulminating laryngotracheo-bronchitis. *Ann Otol Rhinol Laryngol* 42:1014, 1933.

92 **Richards L:** A further study of the pathology of acute laryngo-tracheo-bronchitis in children. *Ann Otol Rhinol Laryngol* 47:326, 1938.

93 **Han BK et al:** Membranous laryngotracheobronchitis (membranous croup). *Am J Roentgenol Radium Ther Nucl Med* 133:53, 1979.

94 **Stern RC:** Laryngeal and tracheal infections, in Nelson WE, Vaughan VC III, McKay RJ Jr, Behrman RE (eds): *Textbook of Pediatrics.* Philadelphia, Saunders, 1979, pp 1193–1197.

95 **Szpunar J et al:** Fibrinous laryngotracheobronchitis in children. *Arch Otol* 93:173, 1971.

96 **Taussig LM et al:** Treatment of laryngotracheobronchitis (croup). Use of intermittent positive-pressure breathing and racemic epinephrine. *Am J Dis Child* 129:790, 1975.

97 **Newth CJL et al:** The respiratory status of children with croup. *J Pediatr* 81:1068, 1972.

98 **Davison FW:** Acute laryngeal obstruction in children. *JAMA* 171: 1301, 1959.

99 **Gardner HG, Cherry JD:** Unpublished data. 1973.

100 **Parks CR:** Mist therapy: Rationale and practice. *J Pediatr* 76:305, 1970.

101 **Dulfano MJ et al:** Physical properties of sputum: IV. Effects of 100 per cent humidity and water mist. *Am Rev Respir Dis* 107:130, 1972.

102 **Sasaki CT, Suzuki M:** The respiratory mechanism of aerosol inhalation in the treatment of partial airway obstruction. *Pediatrics* 59:689, 1977.

103 **Leipzig B et al:** A prospective randomized study to determine the efficacy of steroids in treatment of croup. *J Pediatr* 94:194, 1979.

104 **Bass JW et al:** Corticosteroids and racemic epinephrine with IPPB in the treatment of croup. *J Pediatr* 96:173, 1980.

105 **Eden AN et al:** Corticosteroids and croup. Controlled double-blind study. *JAMA* 200:403, 1967.

106 **Eden AN, Larkin VDP:** Corticosteroid treatment of croup. *Pediatrics* 33:768, 1964.

107 **James JA:** Dexamethasone in croup. A controlled study. *Am J Dis Child* 117:511, 1969.

108 **Skowron PN et al:** The use of corticosteroid (dexamethasone) in the treatment of acute laryngotracheitis. *Can Med Assoc J* 94:528, 1966.

109 **Sussman S et al:** Dexamethasone (16 alpha-methyl, 9 alpha-fluoroprednisolone) in obstructive respiratory tract infections in children. A controlled study. *Pediatrics* 34:851, 1964.

110 Massicotte P, Tetreault L: Evaluation de la methylprednisolone dans le traitment des laryngites aiguës de l'enfant. *Union Med Can* 102:2064, 1973.

111 Martensson B et al: The effect of corticosteroids in the treatment of pseudo-croup. *Acta Otolaryngol (Stockh)* Suppl 158:62, 1960.

112 Adair JC et al: Ten-year experience with IPPB in the treatment of acute laryngotracheobronchitis. *Anesth Analg* 50:649, 1971.

113 Gardner HG et al: The evaluation of racemic epinephrine in the treatment of infectious croup. *Pediatrics* 52:68, 1973.

114 Singer OP, Wilson WJ: Laryngotracheobronchitis: 2 years' experience with racemic epinephrine. *Can Med Assoc J* 115:132, 1976.

115 Kepes ER et al: Racemic epinephrine in postintubation laryngeal edema. *NY State J Med* 72:583, 1972.

116 Melnick A et al: Spasmodic croup in children. Personal experiences with intermittent positive pressure breathing in therapy. *Clin Pediatr* 11:615, 1972.

117 Lockhart CH, Battaglia JD: Croup (laryngotracheal bronchitis) and epiglottitis. *Pediatr Ann* 6:262, 1977.

118 Westley CR et al: Nebulized racemic epinephrine by IPPB for the treatment of croup. A double-blind study. *Am J Dis Child* 132:484, 1978.

ADDITIONAL READINGS

Burns JE, Hendley JO: Epiglottitis, in Mandell GL et al. (eds): *Principles and Practice of Infectious Diseases*. New York, Wiley, 1979, pp 463–466.

Cherry JD: Croup, in Feigin R, Cherry JD (eds): *Textbook of Pediatric Infectious Diseases*. Philadelphia, Saunders, in press.

Daum RS et al: Epiglottitis (supraglottitis), in Feigin R, Cherry JD (eds): *Textbook of Pediatric Infectious Diseases*. Philadelphia, Saunders, in press.

Gwaltney JM Jr.: Acute laryngitis, in Mandell GL et al (eds): *Principles and Practice of Infectious Diseases*. New York, Wiley, 1979, pp 441–442.

Hall CB: Acute laryngotracheobronchitis, croup, in Mandell GL et al (eds): *Principles and Practice of Infectious Diseases*. New York, Wiley, 1979, pp 442–449.

Urinary tract infections in the female: a perspective

THOMAS A. STAMEY

INTRODUCTION

As we approach the fourth decade of substantial clinical investigation into the etiology and control of urinary tract infections (UTI), one observation seems particularly relevant: *nonazotemic patients with a UTI can be cured of their infection*. At first glance this may seem like an overconfident statement, especially when one considers that about half of all bacteriuric patients can be shown to have bacterial involvement of their kidneys (1). However, virtually all patients can be cured of their UTI because these bacteria do not persist in renal tissue in the presence of adequate, sterilizing antimicrobial therapy. To be sure, there are causes of bacterial persistence within the urinary tract—at least 14 such causes in our experience at Stanford—which must be surgically eliminated in order to cure those patients who have a specific site of bacterial persistence.

First, however, let me present a brief etiologic classification of UTI that has important treatment implications for the practicing physician. Therapeutically, UTI can be divided into four categories: first infections, unresolved bacteriuria, bacterial persistence, and reinfection.

First infections

Little can be said about first infections except that most will respond to a short course of any antimicrobial agent and that less than one-third will recur in the following 18 months.

Unresolved bacteriuria: the importance of sterilizing the urine

The importance of achieving a sterile urine during antimicrobial therapy cannot be overemphasized. Until the urine has been sterilized, the type of recurrence of bacterial infection, due either to bacterial persistence or reinfection, cannot be determined. During therapy or shortly after, there must not be any—not even one—detectable organism of the original infecting strain in the urine if the clinician is to be certain that sterilization of the urine has been accomplished. The presence of even as few as 10 colonies per milliliter of the original strain raises the possibility that the infection was simply suppressed rather than sterilized. The causes of unresolved bacteriuria, i.e., the failure to sterilize the urine with antimicrobial therapy, are obviously important; the major causes, in decreasing order of importance, are the following.

Bacterial resistance to the drug selected for treatment   The clinical setting is almost invariably one in which the patient has recently received antimicrobial therapy, treatment which selected resistant bacteria among the fecal flora; the latter then went on to reinfect the urinary tract. Antimicrobial susceptibility testing is usually required in this clinical situation in order to guide antimicrobial therapy for achieving a sterile urine.

Development of resistance from initially sensitive bacteria   A less common cause of unresolved bacteriuria, the development of resistance in a previously susceptible population of organisms infecting the urinary tract, occurs in about 8 percent of patients treated with 1 g/day of tetracycline and about 7 percent of patients treated with 4 g/day of nalidixic acid (2). This form of resistance is easy to recognize clinically. Within 48 to 72 h of starting therapy, a previously susceptible population of 10^5 or more bacteria per milliliter of urine is replaced (through selection of a resistant clone undetected in the original susceptibility testing) by a comparable population of completely resistant bacteria of the same species.

Mixed bacteriuria caused by several bacterial species with different antimicrobial susceptibilities   In these mixed infections, one of the organisms acquires dominance over the other and often appears on culture plates as a pure culture of the dominant species; treatment of the dominant pathogen unmasks the presence of the second organism when the latter is resistant to the antimicrobial agent selected for therapy.

Rapid reinfection with a new, resistant species during initial therapy for the original susceptible organism   Most reinfections, even in highly susceptible females, do not occur within the first 5 to 10 days of therapy, but we have documented several instances of reinfection between the fifth and tenth day of routine therapy in highly susceptible females.

Azotemia   In patients with substantial azotemia (serum creatinine above 4 mg/dl), sterilization of the urine can be very difficult because the antimicrobial agent cannot be excreted into the urine produced by the diseased kidneys. Bioassay of antimicrobial concentrations in the urine usually demonstrates the level of the drug to be below the minimal inhibitory concentration (MIC) of the infecting strain.

Papillary necrosis from analgesic abuse   We have seen several patients with analgesic-induced nephropathy whose serum creatinine concentrations were less than 2 mg/dl but who had such severe defects in medullary concentrating capacity that bacteriuria continued despite the use of antimicrobial agents to which the infecting organism was susceptible. The bacteriuria can often be resolved by changing the antimicrobial agent to one producing even higher urinary concentrations and by encouraging the patient not to force fluids.

Giant staghorn calculi in which the "critical mass" of susceptible bacteria is too great for antimicrobial inhibition   Unresolved bacteriuria occurs in patients who have large staghorn calculi, usually associated with infection due to *Proteus mirabilis*; the number of bacteria near the surface of the stone is so great that even bactericidal drugs in nonazotemic patients are incapable of sterilizing the urine.

Once the urine has been sterilized by a few days of antimicrobial therapy, all recurrences can be divided into two groups: those in which the bacteria have persisted within the urinary tract despite a sterile urine and those due to reinfections with new organisms introduced into the urinary tract. Bacterial persistence usually requires surgical correction, and reinfections require medical prophylactic therapy.

Bacterial persistence in the presence of a sterile urine: the surgical causes of recurrent bacteriuria

Even after the urine has been sterilized, the infecting organism can still persist in a site that communicates with the urinary tract and ultimately reinfect the urine; these sites of bacterial persistence are almost invariably sites of urologic abnormalities separated from contact with normal urine and are important to recognize because surgical excision can eliminate recurrent bacteriuria. The time elapsing between cessation of antimicrobial therapy and reappearance in the urine of the same organism is usually a few days; but it may be weeks and sometimes several months, especially when the prostate is the site of bacterial persistence. Space does not allow a detailed consideration here of the causes of bacterial persistence. The 14 causes we have identified at Stanford are listed in Table 1; each of these causes has been documented, and their bacteriologic characteristics and surgical treatment have been detailed elsewhere (2). Table 1 should serve as a checklist for the clinician who seeks the cause of bacterial persistence in patients with recurrent UTI.

Reinfections: medical causes of recurrent bacteriuria

Once the causes of bacterial persistence are excluded, all other bacterial recurrences represent reinfections of the urinary tract, regardless of the time interval between sterilization of the urine and recurrence and whether the O serogroup of the *Escherichia coli* is the same or different. Since bacterial persistence within the urinary tract is relatively rare, most instances of recurrent bacteriuria

Table 1 Correctable urologic abnormalities causing bacterial persistence and recurrent UTI

1 Stones associated with infection

2 Chronic bacterial prostatitis

3 Unilateral infected atrophic kidneys

4 Vesicovaginal and vesicointestinal fistulas

5 Ureteral duplication and ectopic ureters

6 Foreign bodies

7 Urethral diverticula and infected paraurethral glands

8 Unilateral medullary sponge kidneys

9 Nonrefluxing, normal-appearing infected ureteral stumps following nephrectomy

10 Infected urachal cysts

11 Infected communicating cysts of the renal calyces

12 Papillary necrosis in a single calyx

13 Paravesical abscess with fistula to bladder

14 Labial persistence in Bartholin's ducts (?)

SOURCE: Reproduced with permission of publisher, from ref. 2.

are reinfections of the urinary tract. The basic cause of susceptibility to reinfections is a biologic one, closely related to introital colonization of the vagina with Enterobacteriaceae from the rectum. The control of reinfections is dependent on prophylactic, low-dosage antimicrobial therapy. Both introital colonization as a cause of reinfections and prophylaxis in prevention of reinfections are treated in greater detail later in this chapter.

Some additional definitions and comments

The term *chronic* should be assiduously avoided in reference to UTI. It has no meaning etiologically or therapeutically. Recurrent bacteriuria can appear to be as chronic from a series of unremitting reinfections of the urinary tract as it can appear to be from a persistent focus within an infected renal stone.

Prophylaxis is the prevention of recurrent bacteriuria by continuous antimicrobial therapy after the preceding bacteriuria has been *cured*.

The term *suppression* must not be confused with prophylaxis and probably should be limited to those examples of bacteriuria in which oral antimicrobial therapy cannot sterilize the urine but still is used to suppress multiplication of the infecting strain with the aim of decreasing symptoms. Infection stones, especially those associated with pseudomonas, are prime examples of types of bacteriuria in which there is no orally effective antimicrobial agent to achieve sterilization of the urine.

The term *relapse* should also be avoided; it is imprecise and misleading. In Europe the term is used to indicate two consecutive infections with the same organism regardless of the time between the infections and with no implication about the originating site of the infecting strain; in such a context, it is a useful term. Americans use the term to mean two consecutive infections with the identical organism within a limited time—14 days by some authors, 7 days by others. The time limitation introduces imprecision and artifact into the definition; with the 7-day limitation, a recurrent infection detected on the sixth day would be a relapse while if it were detected 48 h later it would be a reinfection. More importantly, in the United States at least, relapse is used to imply that kidney tissue is the site of bacterial persistence, an inference that is unwarranted and most surely incorrect.

The urethral syndrome is defined as a symptom complex suggesting a urinary infection (usually dysuria, frequency, urethral or suprapubic pain, occurring singly or in any combination) in a patient who does not have demonstrable bacteriuria. Two consequences are of immediate importance in this definition. First, since 20 percent of symptomatic patients with UTI will present with substantially fewer than 100,000 bacteria per milliliter of urine (3), many patients will require a suprapubic needle aspiration of the urine to prove the absence of bacteriuria. Second, since most urines are cultured aerobically only, the urethral syndrome can include patients with tuberculosis, urethral infection due to *Chlamydia trachomatis*, *Ureaplasma urealyticum* infections of the bladder, and infections of the bladder due to anaerobic or capnophilic bacteria. Once suprapubic needle aspiration of the bladder has excluded low-count bacteriuric infections of the urinary tract, tuberculosis, *Ureaplasma urealyticum*, and fastidious organisms, the most common cause of urinary frequency with urethral or suprapubic pain in our patients at Stanford is an early form of interstitial cystitis, which is usually missed on outpatient cystoscopy (4).

LOCALIZATION OF URINARY TRACT INFECTION TO THE KIDNEY OR BLADDER: DOES IT MAKE ANY DIFFERENCE?

There are three accepted techniques for distinguishing between bladder and renal bacteriuria: ureteral catheterization, bladder washout, and antibody coating of bacteria. The technique of ureteral catheterization, which we developed here at Stanford in the early 1960s (1, 5), is the most accurate and remains the standard by which Fairley's bladder-washout method (6) and Thomas's fluorescent antibody coating of bacteria (FAB test) (7) are judged. Neither of the latter two techniques will distinguish between unilateral and bilateral renal involvement, despite the fact that half of all upper tract localizations show that only one kidney is infected (1). For reasons probably related to local production of antibody by the bladder in children, the FAB test has not proved useful in young girls. Despite these limitations, the Fairley test is useful because cystoscopy is not required, and the FAB test is appealing because it is completely noninvasive. Does it make any difference whether the kidneys are involved in an infection when there are no clinical indications of renal involvement? This is an important question. In terms of clinical investigation and the natural history of UTI, it is undoubtedly useful to distinguish bladder from renal bacteriuria and to note the progression of bladder to renal involvement. From the viewpoint of the patient and the practicing clinician, however, I doubt that it makes much difference, for two reasons. First, between 1960 and 1967 we localized the site of infection in every bacteriuric patient before treatment for 10 days with appropriate antimicrobial therapy, and we proved that the urine was sterile by suprapubic aspiration of the bladder while the patient was on therapy. In the absence of the urologic abnormalities (Table 1) which cause bacteria to persist in the urinary tract, we were unable to show that upper tract infections were any more difficult to cure than infections limited to the bladdder. Because of this experience, we stopped localizing UTI except in cases of bacterial persistence where surgical excision of the infection site was planned. Second, the available data do not support the thesis that a renal infection is any more likely to recur with the same organism than it is to recur with a completely different organism. Thus, there is little or no reason to treat a renal infection any differently from a bladder infection. Guttmann, for example, analyzed the pattern of bacterial recurrence in relation to radiologic findings and found that patients who had pyelonephritic scarring showed a smaller proportion of recurrences with the same organism than those with normal intravenous urograms (8). In children, where pyelonephritic scarring and reflux are seen most often, it has long been recognized that reinfection with different bacteria is equally common in patients with ureteral reflux as in those without (9).

If bacterial persistence in the kidney were a problem following antimicrobial therapy, the frequency of bacterial recurrences should be greater in patients with radiologic abnormalities. Kunin, in a study of children (10), and Guttmann, in a study of adults (8), were both unable to show any relationship between the frequency of bacteriuric recurrences after therapy and the presence of radiologic abnormalities. Moreover, if one analyzes patients with five or more recurrent UTI in a specific follow-up period, the number of reinfections should decline and the number of recurrences with the same organism should increase as the number of consecutive recurrences increases in the population. Mabeck, however, could show no relationship between treatment failure, recurrence with the same organism, or reinfection with increasing numbers of recurrent UTI in the same population (11).

Using the FAB test in diabetic adults to distinguish renal from bladder infection, Forland et al. showed that ten of fifteen patients who were initially fluorescent-antibody-positive (FA+) recurred with a different species or O serogroup, eight of which were fluorescent-antibody-negative (FA−). Of three who recurred with the same organism, two were FA− and only one FA+ at recurrence (12).

In asymptomatic bacteriuria of pregnancy, urinary infection recurred in 10 of 35 patients who were FA+ at their original infection and in 8 of 35 patients who were FA− (13). Interestingly, all 10 recurrences from the originally FA+ patients were FA− recurrences and were actual reinfections with different bacteria. Of the 8 patients who originally had lower tract infection, half of the recurrences were FA+.

Our technique of ureteral catheterization was used to localize the site of bacteriuria in 42 patients, who were then followed for 6 months after therapy (14). The response to standard, short-term therapy of 2 weeks' duration was analyzed with culturing of all patients on the third, fourth, and fifth days of therapy as well as on multiple occasions after completion of treatment. Of the 26 patients who were rendered abacteriuric 16 had recurrences of infection with the same organism; in these 16 patients, 8 infections were of the upper tract and 8 were limited to the bladder. Cattell et al. concluded that localization studies were of no predictive value in planning the management of patients with recurrent bacteriuria.

In a recent study where C-reactive protein levels in the blood and other parameters were used to separate acute pyelonephritis from lower tract infection in children (15), 10 days of therapy in both groups was followed by an equal number of reinfections, 25 and 32 percent, respectively, and the same number of recurrences with the same organism, 6 and 4 percent, respectively. These data appear to indicate that the pattern of bacterial recurrence has little or no relation to whether the kidneys are involved in the infection. Thus bacteriologic localization data do not really alter the therapeutic approach and appear, at least at this time, to have little practical value.

SERUM VERSUS URINARY LEVELS OF ANTIMICROBIAL AGENTS

In the 1960s at Stanford, when we were localizing UTI before treatment, we compared the results of in vitro tube dilution antimicrobial susceptibilities of infecting bacteria with the outcome of therapy. When proved renal infections due to *E. coli* were treated with oral penicillin G or nitrofurantoin at the dosages shown in Table 2, and when *Pseudomonas aeruginosa* UTI were treated

Table 2 Antimicrobial concentrations in the serum and urine of adults with normal renal function

Drug	Dosage, mg PO q 6 h	Average concentration, µg/ml	
		Serum	Urine*
Penicillin G	500	<1.0	300
Nitrofurantoin	100	<2.0	150
Tetracycline	250	1.0–2.0	500
Ampicillin	250	1–2	350
Nalidixic acid	1000	20–50†	75
Gentamicin	1.0 mg/kg IM q 8 h	2–3	125
Cephalexin	250	4–6	800
Trimethoprim	100 mg PO q 8 h	0.5	90

* These values for the average antibiotic concentration in the urine are derived from the best available excretion data and are based on a 24-h urine output of 1200 ml.

† 85% bound to serum albumin.

SOURCE: Reproduced with permission of publisher from ref. 2.

with oral tetracycline (250 mg four times a day), the urines were sterilized and the infections cured despite the fact that the MICs of the infecting strains to these antimicrobial agents exceeded the serum levels attained by severalfold. We concluded, I think correctly, that the cure of UTI depended on the urinary levels of the antimicrobial agent and not the serum concentrations (1). In a later study, we prospectively treated 33 patients with 250 mg of oxytetracycline (four times day) without regard to in vitro susceptibilities (16). The serum levels of oxytetracycline drawn 1 h after a dose of the drug between the fifth and tenth day of therapy were found to be noninhibitory to the infecting strains in the 20 treatment cures and 13 treatment failures. The urine, however, was inhibitory in 18 of the 20 patients cured of their infection. These data appeared all the more convincing since it is known that tetracyclines actually interfere with the bactericidal effect of serum in vivo (17). I believe there is now general acceptance of this thesis among practicing members of the medical profession. It is regrettable that some bacteriologists, without presenting new data of their own, still cling to the older concept of the importance of tissue concentrations of antimicrobials in the treatment of urinary infections (18).

The question of serum versus urinary level unfortunately remains a practical one because of the general policy of testing susceptibility of bacteria to antibacterial agents at concentrations approximating those attainable in the serum. This prevents the physician from using drugs which are effective only at concentrations achievable in the urine (e.g., oral penicillin G for E. coli and P. mirabilis infections or tetracycline for pseudomonas infections). No one would argue about the superiority of drugs like gentamicin or trimethoprim since both their serum and urinary concentrations exceed the MIC of the infecting strain; but oral penicillin G, nitrofurantoin, and tetracycline also clearly have a useful role in the cure of urinary tract infections. Fortunately, the increasing availability of prepackaged tube dilution susceptibilities at both serum and urinary levels of antimicrobial agents should soon obviate the discrepancy cited above.

Duration of initial therapy

We have traditionally treated infections of the urinary tract for 10 days, and this provides the opportunity of obtaining a culture during therapy 1 week after first seeing the patient. There are ample data indicating that 6 weeks of therapy is no better than 2 weeks (19) and that 2 weeks is no better than 1 week (20); in children the outcome after 10 days of sulfonamide therapy was no different from that after 60 days of treatment (21). Thus, antimicrobial therapy for periods longer than 5 to 10 days to cure a specific infection seem unjustified.

Single-dose therapy   If the patient presents with acute lower tract symptoms, it appears that single-dose therapy is highly effective in curing that episode of urinary infection. In 1967, Grüneberg and Brumfitt successfully treated 22 of 25 symptomatic patients with a single dose of a "long-acting" sulfonamide (22), although Williams and Smith successfully treated only 55 of 95 pregnant patients with a single 2-g dose of a long-acting sulfonamide (23). Both these early efforts were based on the prolonged duration (serum half-life of 150 h) of the sulfonamides in the serum and urine of the patient.

The recent era of single-dose, short-acting antimicrobial therapy for urinary infections was ushered in by Ronald and his associates at Winnipeg, Canada, when they treated 100 bacteriuric women with a single 500-mg dose of kanamycin intramuscularly (24). Ronald's cases were not limited to women with acute lower tract symptoms; the Fairley bladder-washout localization of their bacteriuria showed 39 lower tract infections and 65 upper tract localizations; 92 percent of the former were cured with the single dose of kanamycin, but only 28 percent of the upper tract infections were cured with the same dosage. High rates of bacteriologic cure have been reported with what might be called single megadosage therapy; Fang et al. used 3-g doses of amoxicillin (25), as did Bailey and Abbott, who also used single-dose therapy consisting of 480 mg of trimethoprim and 2400 mg of sulfamethoxazole (26, 27). Ludwig et al. have recently reported a prospective randomized comparison of four regimens using 1- or 2-g doses of sulfisoxazole, or trimethoprim-sulfamethoxazole in doses of 160 and 800 mg or 320 and 1600 mg, respectively (28). They concluded that single-dose therapy with a number of regimens was effective in adult women with cystitis regardless of the antibody-coated bacterial status of their infection.

The therapeutic implications of the single-dose studies are obvious, and we all should treat for shorter periods of time. But what do these data mean in terms of the pathogenesis of urinary tract infections? It must be remembered that these studies are in females with acute urinary tract infections, for the most part limited to the lower urinary tract. We should not forget Mabeck's studies, which showed that 80 percent of such women achieve sterile urine with placebo therapy within 5 months and that 71 percent have a sterile urine within 1 month (11); it is not known how many were sterile within 1 week, but it must have been a substantial percentage. In this setting, then, it is not surprising that the administration of a single dose of antimicrobial therapy cures some 80 percent of symptomatic patients with lower tract infections. The clinician should not underestimate the considerable duration of antimicrobial inhibitory levels in the urine which follows single-dosage therapy, especially when that dosage is in grams rather than in milligrams or when the drug has a long half-life in the serum (e.g., trimethoprim-sulfamethoxazole). Without question, the urine of many of these patients on single-dose therapy will still contain antibacterial activity on the third day after dosing.

These surprising results indicating therapeutic efficacy in both upper and lower tract infections with single-dosage therapy should just about bury the idea that serum levels rather than urinary concentrations are of primary importance in the cure of urinary tract infections. It should no longer be surprising that 10 days of oral therapy with penicillin G or nitrofurantoin cured most upper tract infections in our 1965 study (1).

Antimicrobial agents differ markedly in their pharmacologic and microbiologic activities, even when chosen on the basis of susceptibility testing. If one selects an antimicrobial agent that is less rapid in its rate of antibacterial action (e.g., sulfonamides) or in its tissue penetration (e.g., ampicillin), then patients with bacteriuria originating in the upper tract will not be cured at the same rate as those whose bacteriuria is confined to the bladder. For one thing, the transit time of the antimicrobial agent is many times shorter in the upper tract than in the bladder. If one wishes to separate upper from lower tract infections on the basis of therapeutic efforts, methenamine should be the ideal drug because it can act only in the bladder urine and not in the renal urine. Thus, there will be all gradations of effectiveness when therapy—either single or conventional dose—is prescribed with knowledge of the localization (upper or lower tract) of the site of infection when therapy is started. The clinician should not lose sight of the need to persist with a different antimicrobial agent if bacteriuria recurs from the upper urinary tract following 5 to 10 days of therapy. I have presented elsewhere examples of where simply changing the antimicrobial agent—not the duration of therapy—was all that was required to achieve permanent sterilization of a long-standing upper tract bacteriuria (29).

PROPHYLACTIC PREVENTION OF RECURRENT BACTERIURIA

In the 1960s and early 1970s, many physicians attempted to cure recurrent UTI by treating each recurrence with increasingly potent antimicrobial agents, often even by the intravenous route. These efforts failed to recognize that the real problem was one of reinfection and that a short course of the simplest oral antimicrobial agent on an outpatient basis was just as effective as 2 weeks of hospitalization and treatment with an intravenous antibiotic. Moreover, since the basic cause of recurrent UTI is a biological problem related to colonization of the introital mucosa, it is not surprising that surgical approaches to the urinary tract such as urethral dilatations, antireflux operations on the ureters, and operations designed to open the internal vesical neck of the bladder have had little or no bacteriologic evidence to support their efficacy (2).

Since colonization of the introital mucosa of the vagina with enterobacteria from the fecal flora precedes bacteriuria (2), effective prophylaxis should be directed at either preventing introital colonization with enterobacteria or keeping the bladder urine bactericidal to the colonizing introital organism. Since the fecal Enterobacteriaeae represent the ultimate reservoir for colonization of the vaginal introitus, prophylaxis must not select for resistance of the fecal Enterobacteriaceae (30). Winberg and colleagues were the first to emphasize the relationship between resistant strains in the fecal flora, selected by oral antimicrobial therapy, and the occurrence of resistant urinary tract infections (31). Sulfonamides, tetracyclines, and ampicillin all have an adverse effect on the normally antibiotic-susceptible fecal bacteria. This adverse effect is unimportant for short-term therapy of a few days duration because most reinfections of the urinary tract do not recur that quickly; about 5 or 6 weeks is required for the resistant fecal flora (produced by administration of an oral antimicrobial agent) to revert to a normally sensitive flora. However, where months of continuous, low-dosage therapy is required for prophylaxis, the consequent adverse effects on the fecal flora simply lead to recurrent UTI resistant to antimicrobial agents.

Trimethoprim (TMP)—with or without sulfamethoxazole (SMX)—nitrofurantoin, and the methenamine salts are the only three well-studied antimicrobial agents employed for prophylaxis of UTI. The methenamine salts require large doses with ammonium chloride; they are not active in renal urine and require about 2 h of hydrolysis in the bladder to produce bactericidal levels of formaldehyde; they are much less effective in preventing reinfections than TMP or nitrofurantoin. TMP acts primarily by clearing the vaginal introitus of Enterobacteriaceae through its diffusion and ion trapping in vaginal fluid at concentrations which exceed those in the plasma (32). It also has a favorable effect through clearing the fecal flora of all Enterobacteriaceae in about 75 percent of rectal cultures obtained during prophylaxis. TMP has a long serum half-life (10 h). Prophylaxis at a dosage of one-half tablet of TMP (50 mg) or one-half tablet of TMP-SMX (40 and 200 mg) nightly is almost completely effective in preventing recurrent UTI (33). Nitrofurantoin, on the other hand, does not influence either the fecal flora or the introital carriage of Enterobacteriaceae from the rectum; its effectiveness depends exclusively on rendering the urine bactericidal and on maintaining a sensitive fecal flora. Doses of 50 or 100 mg nightly seem almost as effective as TMP-SMX (33), but missed doses are frequently associated with breakthrough infections. There is a single report on the prophylactic effectiveness of 500 mg daily of cephalexin, but little is known about the effect of this program on the intestinal or vaginal flora.

The natural history of recurrent bacteriuria in symptomatic adults shows the most effective time to begin prophylaxis is after the second recurrence in a 6-month period (3). Our routine is to stop prophylaxis every 6 months to see whether a long-term natural remission from recurrent UTI will continue without prophylaxis. It is important to leave the patient with adequate drug on hand to treat herself for a few days at full dosage and to start prophylaxis again in case a severe infection recurs when she has no recourse to immediate medical attention. Under these circumstances, I find the patient is willing to test repeatedly her natural resistance to recurrent UTI provided she is protected in this way.

INFECTIONS IN INFANCY AND CHILDHOOD

The risk of a boy's becoming ill with a symptomatic UTI in the first 11 years of life is about 1 percent; the risk for a girl is 3 percent (31). These data on symptomatic infections appear confirmed from a general practice study in which 1.5 percent of boys and 3.1 percent of girls 14 years or under presented with a UTI over a 4-year period (34). Only about 18 percent of boys with infections presenting before 1 year of age will have a recurrence on long-term follow-up, whereas two-thirds of girls will have a recurrent UTI (31). About one-third of the recurrences in girls will be asymptomatic, and there is no detectable relationship between age or site of infection in terms of the risk of recurrence; 50 percent of girls below 1 year of age and 30 percent of boys who present with their first symptomatic infection will show vesicoureteral reflux (VUR). Over 1 year of age, the corresponding figures are 30 and 18 percent. Since renal scarring is the important consequence of VUR and UTI, the intravenous urogram (IVU) is the most important examination; 13 percent of 156 boys and 4.5 percent of 440 girls had renal scarring at their first examination; the scarring was progressive in 58 percent (one-fourth of the boys and three-fourths of the girls) despite early diagnosis, successful treatment, and thorough follow-up with treatment of each recurrence (31). In our Stanford series (all girls), 17 of 40 kidneys (43 percent) with clubbing and scarring developed or increased their scarring while the patients were being treated medically for each recurrence (prophylaxis was not used); similarly, 16 of 24 kidneys (67 percent) previously clubbed and scarred showed progression following successful correction of VUR (35). These data strongly suggest that progressive scarring followed acute episodes of pyelonephritis and that about 2 years was required for a scar to develop radiologically following such a clinical episode. Of equal importance, the Stanford series also showed that successful prevention of VUR by ureteral reimplantations did not prevent recurrent bacteriuria.

What are the data on UTI detected by screening surveys, which we refer to as *screening bacteriuria* (ScBu)? In addition to the early classic studies of Calvin Kunin, two large-scale British investigations, one from Newcastle (36) and the other from Cardiff and Oxford (37), have added significant information. The Newcastle study, in which thousands of children were screened between the ages of 4 and 18, detected bacteriuria in 1 to 2 percent; VUR was present in 21 percent, and renal scars in 15 percent of those with bacteriuria. An important observation was that the incidence of renal scarring did not increase with age, confirming the Christchurch series, which suggested that most renal scarring in children occurs before the age of 4 (38) and is usually already present by the time the child is detected by the survey. It is amply clear that screening surveys in school-aged children will not prevent renal scarring because most of it has already occurred by the time of detection, a conclusion supported by both the Newcastle and the Cardiff-Oxford studies.

It is interesting that in the Newcastle study there was a 46 percent incidence of reflux in bacteriuric children with renal scarring and a 15 percent incidence in those without renal scars. Of the 39 children with renal scarring detected in the survey, 21 showed no reflux, suggesting that the original reflux had disappeared in half of those with scarred kidneys. In the 7- to 15-year follow-up of children with reflux and UTI who were treated medically with prophylactic antimicrobial therapy, VUR ceased in 71 percent; even the severest degrees of reflux (grade 4) ceased in 41 percent (39).

The Cardiff-Oxford study on ScBu children adds to our knowledge because the patients were randomly assigned to treatment or no treatment groups and the IVU was repeated 4 years later. New and/or deepening scars were found in 12 of the 44 girls (27 percent) who initially showed scarred kidneys 4 years earlier; however, 6 were in the treated and 6 in the nontreated group. All children without scars at the start of the study failed to develop scars during the 4 years of follow-up regardless of whether they were in the treated or untreated group. The risk factors for renal scarring from the Cardiff-Oxford study appeared to be (1) the presence of preexisting scars, (2) persistent UTI, and (3) vesicoureteral reflux.

It seems fair to conclude from these excellent studies on large numbers of children presenting to their physician with symptomatic UTI (31, 38) as well as large numbers detected by screening surveys (36, 37) that most renal scarring is secondary to reflux and urinary tract infection, that the renal damage is usually present by the time the infection is detected and almost always before the age of 4 years, and that most of the reflux spontaneously disappears with the passage of time. The Christchurch studies are convincing in their demonstration that renal scarring is associated only with the severest degrees of reflux. Since renal scarring occurs in about 1 in 300 schoolgirls and serious renal scarring occurs in 1 in 2000 to 5000 schoolgirls (36), it does not seem feasible to detect these very small numbers of infants with gross reflux, UTI, and susceptibility to gross scarring by screening surveys. A heightened awareness of unexplained fevers in infants by nursery personnel and the pediatrician will probably remain the best means of detecting these rare children at substantial risk of severe renal scarring.

PATIENTS AT RISK OF SERIOUS MORBIDITY AND/OR RENAL SCARRING

Excluding patients with valvular cardiac disease or prosthetic implants or who are immunosuppressed, the major categories of females with recurrent bacteriuria at increased risk of serious morbidity or diminution of renal function are presented in Table 3.

Infants and children with severe reflux and UTI

The 15 to 20 percent risk of renal scarring in bacteriuric children detected by screening surveys is discussed above.

Patients with infections due to urea-splitting bacteria which cause struvite renal stones

As long as recurrent infections in the adult woman are caused by *E. coli*, the consequences other than the usual symptoms of urinary tract infection are generally not serious. *Proteus mirabilis* and other urea-splitting bacteria, however, cause intense alkalinization of the urine, with subsequent precipitation of calcium, magnesium, ammonium, and phosphate salts and formation of branched, struvite renal calculi. The bacteriologic consequences are substantial because the bacteria persist inside the soft stones, even though the urine is readily sterilized. All the residual particles of struvite stones must be removed at the time of surgery if recurrent bacteriuria from bacterial persistence in the calculus and recurrence of the staghorn formation are to be prevented. Thus, the physician should be wary of the patient with recurrent bacteriuria due to *P. mirabilis*. To be sure, *P. mirabilis* is not an uncommon cause of bacteriuria, and most *P. mirabilis* infections of a short duration are not associated with formation of struvite stones. Almost all patients, however, with infection with *P. mirabilis* for 6 months or longer will be found to have renal struvite calculi with proteus embedded inside the stones.

These struvite stones, usually 80 percent struvite and about 20 percent apa-

**Table 3 Major factors predisposing to increased morbidity
in females with recurrent bacteriuria**

1 Severe reflux and UTI in infants and children

2 Infection with urea-splitting bacteria which cause struvite renal stones

3 Congenital anomalies that become secondarily infected

4 Bacteriuria in the presence of urinary tract obstruction

5 Analgesic nephropathy, especially with obstruction from papillary necrosis

6 Diabetes, especially with emphysematous pyelonephritis

7 Neurogenic bladder, especially following spinal cord injury

8 Pregnancy

9 Perinephric abscess

SOURCE: Reproduced with permission of publisher from ref. 2.

tite, often contain little calcium and are easily obscured on plain films of the
abdomen unless the kidneys are absolutely free of overlying gas and feces.
Thus, any patient with recurrent *P. mirabilis* infection deserves plain-film tomography of the kidneys. The surgical, bacteriologic, and biochemical consequences of these infection stones are presented in detail elsewhere (2).

Patients with congenital urinary tract anomalies that become secondarily infected

Females with a biologic susceptibility to recurrent bacteriuria and a congenital
anomaly often become secondarily infected. Once the congenital anomaly is
infected, recurrences are characterized by the same organism until the anoma-
lous infected structure is surgically removed. Such anomalies include nonfunctioning duplications of the renal collecting system, pericalyceal diverticula with
stricture of the infundibular connection, unilateral medullary sponge kidneys,
and urachal cysts in the dome of the bladder. In all these instances, the infection of the congenital anomaly is complicated because normal urine containing
antimicrobial agents cannot diffuse into the anomaly. Excision of the congenital anomaly is usually required.

Patients with bacteriuria in the presence of urinary tract obstruction

Sterile calcium oxalate stones obstructing a kidney are occasionally secondarily infected during the course of unsuccessful efforts to extract the calculus
transurethrally. These patients often develop acute infections and require
emergency drainage of the kidney. The child with minimal reflux who develops

ureteral obstruction following unsuccessful ureteral reimplantation is an example of a patient with chronic obstruction and bacteriuria in whom serious loss of renal cortex can occur. In this situation, a benign condition, reflux, is replaced by a serious obstruction in which the infection is driven into the renal tubules, with consequent loss of renal tissue. In the analysis of the causes of renal failure among dialysis candidates in Seattle, 15 of the 22 patients with end-stage renal failure in whom the primary cause was chronic pyelonephritis had "significant obstructive or calculus disease which preceded the initial episode of urinary tract infection in each" (40).

Patients with analgesic nephropathy, especially when complicated by obstruction from papillary necrosis

Approximately 25 percent of patients with analgesic nephropathy have urinary tract infections, and transient attacks of gross hematuria or passage of papillae occur in 14 percent of patients (41). Acute urinary obstruction caused by necrotic papillae, superimposed on urinary infection and occurring in the presence of kidneys already damaged from analgesic abuse, clearly constitutes a urologic emergency if further nephron loss is to be prevented. Since many of these patients are already azotemic, early intervention (by ureteral catheterization to bypass the soft, obstructing papillus or sometimes by percutaneous nephrostomy) is all the more critical. Careful and effective antimicrobial sterilization of the urine, in the presence of azotemia, should accompany immediate relief of the obstruction.

Patients with diabetes, especially those with emphysematous pyelonephritis

An increased prevalence of asymptomatic UTI among diabetic women has been shown by several investigators. In a survey of 333 patients attending a diabetes mellitus outpatient clinic during a 1-year period, 19 percent of the women either had bacteriuria or acquired bacteriuria during the follow-up study; antibody-coated bacteria were initially present in 43 percent of the patients but rose to 79 percent within a mean observation period of 7 weeks (12). This evidence of an increasing immunologic response in diabetic patients who acquire bacteriuria suggests renal parenchymal involvement and a potential increase in morbidity. Papillary necrosis as well as perinephric abscess are also well-recognized hazards in the diabetic patient.

Emphysematous pyelonephritis occurs only in patients with diabetes and is characterized by parenchymal and perirenal infection with gas-forming bacteria in the presence of necrotic renal cortex and medulla. Emphysematous pyelonephritis is a surgical emergency which is usually lethal if treated by medical means only. Our group at Stanford has recently published information on a diabetic patient with nonobstructive, emphysematous pyelonephritis, carefully documented with surgical, radiologic, and histologic photographs (42). The tissue gas was distributed in the parenchymal and perinephric tissues in association with the tissue necrosis. This distribution of gas should not be confused with that seen in cases of pyelonephritis in which the air remains in the collecting system of the kidney (a condition which also occurs in patients who do not have diabetes and is usually not lethal). Every physician should be aware of the characteristic pattern of retroperitoneal air with perinephric and parenchymal gas; recognition of this pattern in a patient with diabetes and with clinically acute pyelonephritis can be lifesaving.

Patients with a neurogenic bladder, especially following spinal cord injury

Nearly all patients with spinal cord injury require catheterization early after their injury because of bladder spasticity or flaccidity; and many of these patients develop ureterectasis, hydronephrosis, reflux, or renal calculi. Introduction of intermittent catheterization or early removal of indwelling urethral catheters, especially when combined with the judicious use of internal sphincterotomy to destroy the pelvic floor obstruction to the urethra from levator muscle spasms, has substantially reduced what used to be major morbidity in this group of patients. Nevertheless, they still require intelligent management, close follow-up, and continuous vigilance to detect the presence of UTI.

Pregnant patients

Probably the only group of females worth screening for asymptomatic bacteriuria are those who are pregnant. There are three reasons, in my view, for screening in this group. First, symptomatic acute pyelonephritis, which will develop in about 25 percent of untreated bacteriuric pregnant women, can be prevented by early detection and treatment of their UTI. While there is little evidence that acute pyelonephritis in the third trimester causes serious or permanent renal damage, this morbidity can be prevented for the pregnant mother. Second, there is an increased incidence of "small babies" and perinatal mortality, but studies to date have not shown that this association with bacteriuria can be prevented by treatment of the urinary tract infection. Nevertheless, the obstetrician with a bacteriuric patient should be aware of the statistical increase in small babies and perinatal mortality. Third, the major renal complication which I have seen in pregnant patients with bacteriuria is the occurrence of proteus infections with struvite stone formation complicating the course of the pregnancy. Early detection of the infection with urea-splitting organisms in the first trimester might prevent struvite renal stone formation.

Patients with perinephric abscess

The mortality rate from perinephric abscess is about 50 percent, with one-third of the cases undiagnosed before necropsy (43). The distinction between acute pyelonephritis and perinephric abscess can often be difficult to make. In the analysis from Parkland Memorial Hospital in Dallas no patient with acute pyelonephritis was febrile for more than 4 days, whereas all patients with perinephric abscess were febrile for a minimum of 5 days with a median febrile period of 7 days (the median febrile period of pyelonephritis was 2 days) (43).

The treatment of perinephric abscess is surgical drainage, and medical procrastination often leads to death. Ultrasonography represents a genuine advance in the early diagnosis of perinephric abscess; any patient with acute pyelonephritis who fails to resolve as expected should have an ultrasound study. On rare occasions, a computerized tomographic scan may be required for diagnosis.

SOME OBSERVATIONS ON THE PATHOGENESIS OF REINFECTIONS

Introital colonization

If longitudinal studies are performed with frequent cultures of the vaginal vestibule and urethra in women with recurrent bacteriuria, colonization of the vaginal vestibule and distal urethral mucosa with Enterobacteriaceae can be shown to precede the occurrence of bacteriuria (44). Since the fecal reservoir is apparently the same in women with and without urinary tract infections (45), these observations suggest that characterization of susceptibility lies in the presence of colonization of the vaginal vestibule with Enterobacteriaceae from the rectal flora. As can be seen in Figure 1, each urinary infection (except for the second infection with an *E. coli* O6) was preceded by colonization of the vaginal vestibule with the specific pathogen causing the bacteriuria. When the vaginal vestibule was continuously colonized with an *E. coli* O75 for nearly a year, three consecutive bacteriuric episodes occurred with the same *E. coli* O75.

The basic observation, then, appears to be that enterobacteria from the rectal reservoir must first colonize the introital mucosa of the vagina before bacteriuria can occur. The implication of the corollary of this observation is clinically important: In the absence of introital colonization with enterobacteria, bacteriuria should not occur. This observation does not mean that introital colonization with enterobacteria invariably leads to bacteriuria. Indeed, although the 29-year-old woman in Figure 1 was colonized for nearly 1 year with *E. coli* O75 on the vaginal mucosa, she experienced only three episodes of bacteriuria; she received antimicrobial agents for 10 days only after the occurrence of each infection. Thus, there are undoubtedly other factors which influence the occurrence of bacteriuria once the introital mucosa is colonized, but our data suggest that without introital colonization, bacteriuria cannot occur.

Bollgren and Winberg have also shown that periurethral colonization precedes bacteriuria in young girls (46).

A second aspect of introital colonization relates to the observation that introital cultures from normal volunteers resistant to UTI are much less commonly colonized with Enterobacteriaceae (47, 48). In two separate analyses we found that the mean percentage incidence of carriage of Enterobacteriaceae on the vaginal introitus in control volunteers is about 20 percent, whereas the carriage incidence in women susceptible to bacteriuria between actual infections is

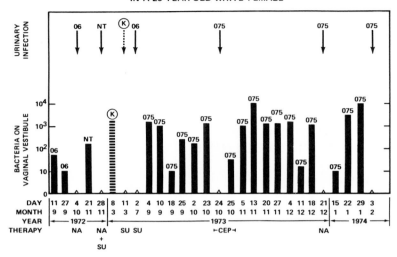

BACTERIOLOGIC COURSE OF RECURRENT BACTERIURIA
IN A 29-YEAR-OLD WHITE FEMALE

Figure 1 Clinical course of a 29-year-old married Caucasian woman followed through multiple urinary tract infections which occurred over 27 months. Bacteriuric episodes are shown, together with every consecutive culture preceding the bacteriuria in which the same strain producing the infection was found on the vaginal vestibule. ▲, without overlying bars, indicates vaginal vestibule cultures with no detectable Enterobacteriaceae. NA, nalidixic acid; SU, sulfonamide; CEP, cephalexin; K, *Klebsiella*; NT, nontypeable *E. coli*. Numbers on the bars and the arrows refer to specific O serogroups of *E. coli*. [*Reproduced with permission of publisher (54).*]

about 50 percent ($p < 0.001$). Some investigators have not confirmed these observations, but in general it is fair to say that their techniques have been substantially different, their frequency of cultures has been much less than in our studies, and there has been little assurance that the susceptible patients maintained their susceptibility to UTI. The issue is obviously an important one because if the observation that introital colonization with Enterobacteriaceae is increased in women susceptible to UTI is correct, the biologic basis of this increased colonization holds the key to the basic cause of recurrent bacteriuria.

Bacterial adherence

In a series of publications in the *Journal of Urology* during 1975 and 1976 we reported our efforts to study a number of factors which determine bacterial survival and growth rates on the vaginal mucosal surface. When healthy volunteers were compared with susceptible women, we were unable to show any significant difference in vaginal pH, vaginal estrogen indices, vaginal glycogen concentration, vaginal leukocytes, vaginal immunoglobulins, or the presence of normal indigenous bacteria. Because of these difficulties, we turned to a study of bacterial adherence and were able to show that a given strain of *E. coli*, an *E. coli* O6, adhered more avidly to washed vaginal mucosal cells from women susceptible to recurrent bacteriuria than to washed cells from control volunteers resistant to UTI (49).

When 20 adult women with a history of at least three documented urinary infections (mean age of 36 years) were compared with 20 volunteer women with no history of urinary infections (mean age 29 years), the mean score of adherent bacteria per vaginal epithelial cell was 42.6 ± 25 in the patient group and 19.4 ± 9 in the control group ($p < 0.001$). The individual adherence data are shown in Figure 2. No correlation was found between the degree of bacterial adherence for each subject in the patient and control groups and the age of the subject, the day of the menstrual cycle on which the cells were obtained, the presence or absence of enterobacteria in the introital culture at the time of cell sampling, the use of birth control pills or intrauterine devices, and whether or not the patient had had a hysterectomy.

The data in Figure 2 represented the first biologic difference we had shown which might explain introital colonization differences between controls and patients. Kallenius and Winberg compared the adherence of periurethral epithelial cells from 20 patients and 20 controls in young girls using an *E. coli* O75 (50). Their data in children were virtually superimposable on Figure 2.

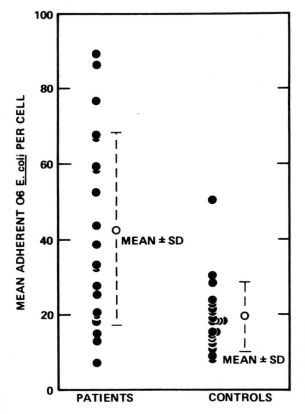

Figure 2 Mean adherent *E. coli* O6 per cell for vaginal epithelial cells from each patient and control subject. [*Reproduced with permission of publisher (49).*]

Using the same adherence model, it was possible to determine whether bacterial strains causing UTI had greater adherence capability than fecal strains from the same patient which had never caused urinary infection. When 18 bacteriuric strains of *E. coli* were compared with 19 strains isolated from anal cultures of the same bacteriuric patients which had neither caused bacteriuria nor colonized the vaginal mucosa, there was no difference in adherence capability between the two groups of *E. coli*. Moreover, when eight strains of *P. mirabilis* which had not only caused UTI but had formed renal struvite calculi were compared with 10 anal isolates of *P. mirabilis* which had never caused urinary infections, bacterial adherence was again similar (51).

We concluded from these two studies that if bacterial adherence is related to UTI, susceptibility lies more with the host than with the pathogenicity of the infecting organism.

Cervicovaginal antibody

Although we had looked at vaginal total immunoglobulins (especially IgG) as well as at vaginal agglutinating antibodies as a measure of antigen-specific antibody early in our studies and found no difference between patients and controls (52), we realized from several studies on the oral cavity and the intestinal tract that local mucosal antibody could strongly influence bacterial adherence. We decided to measure local vaginal antibody again in patients and controls, this time using an antigen-specific antibody technique which would allow assessment of IgG and IgA. We chose the indirect immunofluorescent technique of antibody coating of bacteria whereby rectal and vaginal bacteria were incubated with vaginal antibody before application of the fluorescein-conjugated antisera to human immunoglobulins.

To our surprise, we found that control volunteers who were resistant to UTI and who were not colonized vaginally with Enterobacteriaceae had specific antibody (mainly IgA and IgG) directed against their fecal Enterobacteriaceae. On the other hand, patients who were colonized with Enterobacteriaceae on their vaginal introitus rarely showed such antibodies (53).

In most of our comparisons between healthy controls and susceptible patients we found little difference in total immunoglobulins when measured by Mancini diffusion plates; we did show a substantial difference in IgG when we compared control patients with a subset of susceptible women who were colonized vaginally with more than 100 Enterobacteriaceae per milliliter of vaginal transport fluid. These data are presented in Table 4, which shows that fluorescent-antibody-positive bacteria were found in 45 of 46 collections from four healthy volunteers but in only 6 of 47 collections from 13 susceptible patients. When these controls were compared with this subset of heavily colonized patients, one-tenth the amount of total IgG was found in vaginal fluid of the patients compared with the controls.

In further experiments, we have demonstrated that this vaginal antibody shows wide cross reactivity with different O serogroups of *E. coli*, both common and uncommon, as well as to the galactose-deficient J_5 mutant of *E. coli* O111. Thus, local vaginal antibody shows a wide cross reactivity between different

Table 4   Cervicovaginal antibody (FA+) and IgG concentration in patients with >100 Enterobacteriaceae per milliliter in their introital cultures*

Subjects	No. of subjects	No. of samples	No. of FA+	Samples FA+, %	IgG, mg/dl
Control volunteers	4	46	45	98	20.4 ± 21.9
Susceptible patients†	13	47	6	13	2.1 ± 3.9

* FA+ = fluorescein-conjugated antibody to human globulin; IgG = measured with low-level radial immunodiffusion Endoplates.
† Introitus colonized with >100 Enterobacteriaceae per milliliter of transport broth.
SOURCE: Reproduced with permission of publisher from (2).

species and strains of Enterobacteriaceae. It is also interesting that despite the absence of cervicovaginal antibody in susceptible patients colonized vaginally with *E. coli*, they all had salivary antibody directed against their colonizing organism.

Some of the more obvious reasons for diminished cervicovaginal antibody are (1) antigen-antibody complexing of the available local antibody, (2) failure to produce local vaginal antibody (despite normal salivary antibody), or (3) inactivation of cervicovaginal antibody by means other than antigen-antibody complexing, e.g., by bacterial proteases. Whatever the reason, including the excellent possibility of antigen-antibody complexing of available cervicovaginal antibody by the colonizing Enterobacteriaceae organisms per se, it is difficult to ignore the absence of cervicovaginal antibody in colonized UTI-prone women as an important permissive factor in recurrent bacteriuria.

REFERENCES

1 Stamey TA et al: The localization and treatment of urinary tract infections: The role of bactericidal urine levels as opposed to serum levels. *Medicine* 44:1, 1965.

2 Stamey TA: *The Pathogenesis and Treatment of Urinary Tract Infections.* Baltimore, Williams & Wilkins, 1980.

3 Kraft JK, Stamey TA: The natural history of symptomatic recurrent bacteriuria in women. *Medicine* 56:55, 1977.

4 Messing EM, Stamey TA: The early diagnosis, pathology and treatment of interstitial cystitis. *Urology* 12:381, 1978.

5 Stamey TA, Pfau A: Some functional, pathological, bacteriological and chemotherapeutic characteristics of unilateral pyelonephritis in man: II. Bacteriologic and chemotherapeutic characteristics. *Invest Urol* 1:162, 1963.

6 Fairley KF et al: Simple test to determine the site of urinary tract infection. *Lancet* 2:427, 1967.

7 Thomas V et al: Antibody-coated bacteria in the urine and the site of urinary tract infection. *N Engl J Med* 290:588, 1974.

8 Guttmann D: Follow-up of urinary tract infection in domiciliary patients, *Urinary Tract Infection, Proceedings of the Second National Symposium.* London, Oxford University Press, 1973, chap 8, p 62.

9 Bergstrom T et al: Studies of urinary tract infections in infancy and childhood: VIII. Reinfection versus relapse in recurrent urinary tract infections. Evaluation by means of identification of infecting organisms. *J Pediatr* 71:13, 1967.

10 Kunin CM et al: Urinary tract infection in school children: An epidemiologic, clinical and laboratory study. *Medicine* 43:91, 1964.

11 Mabeck CE: Treatment of uncomplicated urinary tract infection in non-pregnant women. *Post Grad Med J* 48:69, 1972.

12 Forland M et al: Urinary tract infections in patients with diabetes mellitus. Studies on antibody coating of bacteria. *JAMA* 238:1924, 1977.

13 **Harris RE et al:** Asymptomatic bacteriuria in pregnancy: Antibody-coated bacteria, renal function and intrauterine growth retardation. *Am J Obstet Gynecol* 126:20, 1976.

14 **Cattell WR et al:** *The Localization of Urinary Tract Infection and Its Relationship to Relapse, Reinfection and Treatment.* London, Oxford University Press, 1973.

15 **Wientzen RL et al:** Localization and therapy of urinary tract infections of childhood. *Pediatrics* 63:467, 1979.

16 **Stamey TA et al:** Serum versus urinary antimicrobial concentrations in cure of urinary tract infections. *N Engl J Med* 291:1159, 1974.

17 **Forsgren A, Gnarpe H:** Tetracycline interference with the bactericidal effect of serum. *Nature* 244:82, 1973.

18 **Naumann P:** The value of antibiotic levels in tissue and in urine in the treatment of urinary tract infections. *J Antimicrob Chemother* 4:9, 1978.

19 **Kincaid-Smith P, Fairley KF:** Controlled trial comparing effect of two and six weeks' treatment for recurrent urinary tract infection. *Br Med J* 2:145, 1969.

20 **Kincaid-Smith P et al:** Controlled trials of treatment in urinary tract infection, in Kincaid-Smith P, Fairley KF (eds): *Renal Infection and Renal Scarring.* Melbourne, Mercedes 1970, p 165.

21 **Bergstrom T et al:** Studies of urinary tract infections in infancy and childhood: X. Short or long-term treatment in girls with first or second-time urinary tract infections uncomplicated by obstructive urological abnormalities. *Acta Paediat Scand* 57:186, 1968.

22 **Grüneberg RN, Brumfitt W:** Single-dose treatment of acute urinary tract infection: A controlled trial. *Br Med J* 3:649, 1967.

23 **Williams JD, Smith EK:** Single-dose therapy with streptomycin and sulfametopyrazine for bacteriuria during pregnancy. *Br Med J* 4:651, 1970.

24 **Ronald AR et al.:** Bacteriuria localization and response to single-dose therapy in women. *JAMA* 235:1854, 1976.

25 **Fang LST et al:** Efficacy of single-dose and conventional amoxicillin therapy in urinary tract infection localized by the antibody-coated bacteria technique. *N Engl J Med* 298:413, 1978.

26 **Bailey RR, Abbott GD:** Treatment of urinary tract infection with a single dose of amoxycillin. *Nephron* 18:316, 1977.

27 **Bailey RR, Abbott GD:** Treatment of urinary tract infection with a single dose of trimethoprim-sulfamethoxazole. *Can Med Assoc J* 118:551, 1978.

28 **Ludwig P et al:** Single-dose therapy of acute cystitis in adult females: Prospective randomized comparison of four regimens, *Proceedings of the 19th Interscience Conference on Antimicrobial Agents and Chemotherapy, Boston 1979.* Washington, American Society for Microbiology, 1979, abstract 58.

29 **Stamey TA:** *Urinary Infections.* Baltimore, Williams & Wilkins, 1972.

30 **Lincoln K et al:** Resistant urinary infections resulting from changes in the resistance pattern of fecal flora induced by antibiotics and hospital environment. *Br Med J* 3:305, 1970.

31 **Winberg J et al:** Epidemiology of symptomatic urinary tract infection in childhood. *Acta Paediatr Scand Suppl* 252:3, 1974.

32 **Stamey TA, Condy M:** The diffusion and concentration of trimethoprim in human vaginal fluid. *J Infect Dis* 131:261, 1975.

33 **Stamey TA et al:** Prophylactic efficacy of nitrofurantoin macrocrystals and trimethoprim-sulfamethoxazole in urinary infections. *N Engl J Med* 296:780, 1977.

34 **Brooks D, Houston IB:** Symptomatic urinary infection in childhood: Presentation during a four-year study in general practice and significance and outcome at seven years. *J R Coll Gen Pract* 27:678, 1977.

35 **Govan DE et al:** Management of children with urinary tract infections. The Stanford experience. *Urology* 6:273, 1975.

36 **Newcastle Asymptomatic Bacteriuria Research Group:** Asymptomatic bacteriuria in schoolchildren in Newcastle-upon-Tyne. *Arch Dis Child* 50:90, 1975.

37 **Asscher AW et al (Cardiff-Oxford Bacteriuria Study Group):** Sequelae of covert bacteriuria in schoolgirls. A four-year follow-up study. *Lancet* 2:889, 1978.

38 **Rolleston GL et al:** Relationship of infantile vesicoureteric reflux to renal damage. *Br Med J* 1:460, 1970.

39 **Edwards D et al:** Disappearance of vesicoureteric reflux during long-term prophylaxis of urinary tract infection in children. *Br Med J* 2:285, 1977.

40 **Schechter H et al:** Chronic pyelonephritis as a cause of renal failure in dialysis candidates. Analysis of 173 patients. *JAMA* 216:514, 1971.

41 **Bock KD, Nitzsche T:** Analgesic nephropathy—symptomatology and clinical course, in Losse H et al (eds): *4th International Symposium on Pyelonephritis, Munster 1979.* Stuttgart, Thieme, 1980.

42 **Freiha FS et al:** Emphysematous pyelonephritis, *Urol Digest* 18:9, 1979.

43 **Thorley JD et al:** Perinephric abscess. *Medicine* 53:441, 1974.

44 **Stamey TA et al:** Recurrent urinary infections in adult women: The role of introital enterobacteria. *Calif Med* 115:1, July 1971.

45 **Grüneberg RN et al:** *Escherichia coli* serotypes in urinary tract infection: Studies in domiciliary, antenatal and hospital practice, in O'Grady F, Brumfitt W (eds): *Urinary*

Tract Infection. Oxford, Oxford University Press, 1968, p 68.

46 **Bollgren I, Winberg J:** The periurethral aerobic flora in girls highly susceptible to urinary infections. *Acta Paediat Scand* 65:81, 1976.

47 **Stamey TA, Sexton CC:** The role of vaginal colonization with Enterobacteriaceae in recurrent urinary infections. *J Urol* 113:214, 1975.

48 **Schaeffer AJ, Stamey TA:** Studies of introital colonization in women with recurrent urinary infections: IX. The role of antimicrobial therapy. *J Urol* 118:221, 1977.

49 **Fowler JE Jr, Stamey TA:** Studies of introital colonization in women with recurrent urinary infections: VII. The role of bacterial adherence. *J Urol* 117:472, 1977.

50 **Kallenius G, Winberg G:** Bacterial adher-ence to periurethral epithelial cells in girls prone to urinary tract infections. *Lancet* 2:540, 1978.

51 **Fowler JE Jr, Stamey TA:** Studies of introital colonization in women with recurrent urinary infections: X. Adhesive properties of *Escherichia coli* and *Proteus mirabilis:* Lack of correlation with urinary pathogenicity. *J Urol* 120:315, 1978.

52 **Stamey TA, Howell JJ:** Studies of introital colonization in women with recurrent urinary infections: IV. The role of local vaginal antibodies. *J Urol* 115:413, 1976.

53 **Stamey TA et al:** The immunologic basis of recurrent bacteriuria: Role of cervicovaginal antibody in enterobacterial colonization of the introital mucosa. *Medicine* 57:47, 1978.

54 **Harrison JH et al (eds):** *Campbell's Urology*. Philadelphia, Saunders, 1979, p 458.

Treatment of cryptococcal, candidal, and coccidioidal meningitis

JOHN E. BENNETT

The purpose of this series is to update recent developments in specific areas of infectious disease. While that is a laudable goal, the paucity of new developments within the purview of this chapter suggests the necessity of alternatives. The goal chosen was therefore to gather into one place the information a physician needs to treat cryptococcal, candidal, and coccidioidal meningitis. Hence, there will be no discussion of the pathogens themselves, laboratory or clinical diagnosis, or treatment of infection beyond the meninges. To prevent repetition, discussion begins with generalities about antifungal therapy relevant to the three fungal meningitides and then proceeds to details specific for each.

ANTIFUNGAL AGENTS

Intravenous amphotericin B (Fungizone for infusion[1])

Effective use of this drug requires a substantial fund of information. Detailed references can be found in an earlier review (1).

Contraindications   Preexisting azotemia is not, as commonly supposed, a contraindication. Azotemic patients require the same amphotericin B dose as patients with normal renal function because drug elimination is unchanged by azotemia (2). Naturally, the added burden of amphotericin B–induced nephrotoxicity makes the patient with prior azotemia more difficult to manage. Still, the nephrotoxicity is dose-dependent and largely reversible. The permanent element of the drug-induced renal damage is unrelated to the level of azotemia during therapy but is correlated with the total dose given in a course (3). Permanent renal damage becomes an important consideration as a rule only in patients receiving a total of over 4 g. It is rarely wise to assume that

[1] Brand name of E. R. Squibb & Sons.

54

preexisting renal disease negates the chance of using amphotericin B success-fully. History of an anaphylactic reaction to amphotericin B may or may not contraindicate further use of the drug. As discussed below, many of these reac-tions do not have a clear allergic basis. Rash during amphotericin B therapy is usually attributable to other causes. Safety of amphotericin B during pregnancy is not well established. Treatment during the third trimester has not damaged the fetus in a half dozen instances known to the author.

Initiating therapy   Amphotericin B is administered intravenously in 5% dex-trose in water (D_5W). Heparin and hydrocortisone hemisuccinate can be added to the bottle without harming amphotericin B (4), but electrolyte addi-tives will cause the bottle to become cloudy with aggregated drug. Cloudy amphotericin B solutions also result with some lots of D_5W and are not recom-mended for infusion. The infusion bottle need not be covered during infusion because light causes no drug destruction under normal conditions of use (4). Adults generally receive the drug in 500 ml of D_5W. The volume of D_5W used to dilute the drug is not important, despite what the package insert says, but the infusion duration is important. Many physicians are reluctant to administer full doses of the drug in less than 1 h because of the theoretical potential of fatal cardiac arrhythmias. Cardiac toxicity can be induced in dogs or rabbits with rapid infusions of 4.5 mg/kg, a dose never given intentionally to humans. Infu-sion durations of 2 or 3 h are common. More prolonged infusions do not seem to decrease any of the toxic reactions. Patients not receiving other intravenous therapy should have the needle removed after the infusion to decrease phlebitis. A 21- or 23-gauge needle moved to a different site with each infusion also preserves venous access.

The very first one or two amphotericin B infusions require special attention because the physiologic effects may frighten the patient and alarm the nursing staff. Patients should be warned they may have a violent chill, followed by sweat-ing and prostration. Ambulatory patients should be instructed to stay in bed and use blankets as necessary to keep warm if they feel chilly. Severity of the reaction is variable but is generally worse in the presence of preexisting fever, cardiac or pulmonary disease, and, perhaps, leukocyte transfusions. A sudden rise in body temperature occurs roughly 30 to 120 min after onset of the am-photericin B infusion. This may be accompanied by a rigor of variable severity. Before or during the fever there may be dyspnea, cyanosis, hypotension, or delirium. Patients with obstructive lung disease may wheeze, but edema of mucous membranes does not occur. The mechanism of these untoward effects is unknown, but pretreatment with adrenal corticosteroids blunts the severity of the reaction. Reactions decrease with continued infusions of a given dose of the same lot of amphotericin B. Because there is some dose dependence in the reaction, a test dose of 1 mg is often given to adults. This can be given over 10 to 15 min. Blood pressure, pulse, and temperature are monitored every 15 to 30 minutes for 2 to 3 h from the start of infusion. The size of the next dose and the decision whether to add hydrocortisone hemisuccinate to the bottle depends on the severity of the reaction to the test dose, rapidity of disease progression, and the patient's cardiopulmonary status. Patients already receiving systemic adrenal corticosteroids equivalent to prednisone 20 mg (adult dose) probably will not benefit from additional hydrocortisone in the infusion. Other patients will show a reduction in fever and the associated acute reactions with the addition of 25 to 50 mg hydrocortisone to the intravenous infusion. This amount can be decreased gradually to zero as the patient develops tolerance to amphotericin B. The beneficial effect of hydrocortisone probably is reduced when excessively long infusion intervals are used, such as 8 to 12 h, because of the drug's short half-life in the body. Oral prednisone and other long-acting steroids should not be used for this purpose because of their potential for decreasing host resistance to infection. Mild febrile reactions to amphotericin B can be controlled by preinfusion aspirin. Administration of aspirin or hydrocortisone once the fever or chills begin accomplishes nothing, as the fever peaks in 30 to 60 min and declines over 1 or 2 h whether antipyretics are given or not. Discontinuing the amphotericin B infusion because of a chill similarly has no observable effect on the severity or duration of the reaction.

Almost all patients can and should have the dose advanced to 0.3 to 0.5 mg/kg over the first 3 days. Patients with fulminant mycoses and severe febrile reactions can be given incremental doses every 8 h until the desired dosage is achieved. One convenient way to start therapy is to place amphotericin B (0.3 mg/kg) and heparin (1000 units) in 500 ml of D_5W and infuse 25 ml (1.0 mg) over 10 to 15 min. A "piggyback" of D_5W is used to maintain the infusion over 2 h while vital signs are obtained. Hydrocortisone is added to the amphotericin B remaining in the bottle if dictated by the severity of the reaction, and then the remaining amount is infused. If the physician elects to give only a fraction of the dose, hydrocortisone can be given through the side arm when amphotericin B is restarted.

Maintaining therapy When amphotericin B is used alone in cryptococcal and candidal meningitis, a dose of 0.5 to 0.6 mg/kg daily is recommended. Hemodialysis, peritoneal dialysis, and liver disease do not alter the recommended dose. Patients whose febrile reactions have largely abated will appreciate being changed to double-dose alternate-day therapy. Phlebitis is less; ambulation and appetite improve. The chemotherapeutic effect is unaltered. This change to alternate-day therapy can be made in increments to test for increased febrile reactions, e.g., to give on consecutive days 30, 0, 45, 0, and 60 mg. The potential for nephrotoxicity is not reduced with alternate-day double-dose therapy.

Toxicity should be monitored by twice-a-week determination of body weight, serum creatinine, serum potassium and bicarbonate levels, and hematocrit or hemoglobin levels. Nausea, vomiting, and anorexia (with attendant dehydration and hypokalemia) may increase azotemia and weakness unless fluid and potassium intake is increased. Normally, a dose of 0.5 mg/kg daily or 1.0 mg/kg on alternate days leads gradually to a steady level of azotemia and anemia. The serum creatinine in patients with no prior azotemia reaches a plateau at around 2.5 to 3.0 mg/dl; the hematocrit levels off at about 25 percent. Blood transfusions should be avoided. The normocytic, normochromic anemia is due to decreased erythrocyte production. This drug effect disappears over the first 3 months after treatment. Thrombocytopenia is a rare, idiosyncratic side effect. Other reversible side effects rarely interfere with therapy but include cylindruria, renal tubular acidosis, and mild leukopenia. Mannitol was once advocated to minimize nephrotoxicity but failed to prove useful.

Intrathecal amphotericin B

Amphotericin B has been injected by needle into the cerebrospinal fluid (CSF) in the lumbar sac and the cisterna magna CSF. Subcutaneous reservoirs with tubes extending into the lateral cerebral ventricles or cisterna magna have also been used. Complications vary with the site, but dosage regimens are the same. Treatment is often begun on a schedule of three times a week, beginning with 0.1 mg and increasing in 0.1-mg increments to 0.5 mg. Treatment frequency is reduced to twice weekly after a few weeks. Patients with coccidioidal meningitis, who are often treated for one or more years, are given the drug every week or two during the latter phases of therapy.

Lumbar intrathecal injections are often followed by radicular pain. Transient but occasionally profound asymmetrical leg weakness, with or without urinary retention and fecal incontinence, may appear a few hours after the injection. There are theoretical reasons to believe that radiculitis is less if the drug is diluted in 10% instead of 5% dextrose and the patient is placed in a head-down position, 30° below horizontal, during the procedure or right after it (5). If the asymmetry of radiculitis can be interpreted to mean that extradural leakage of drug causes the reaction, movement of hyperbaric drug away from the puncture site could be helpful. This technique is difficult without moving the patient to a sigmoidoscopy table for the lumbar puncture. Whether administration of amphotericin B in hyperbaric solution is actually useful is unknown. Patients with meningitis-induced headache may have excruciating headache when tilted head downward. Addition of hydrocortisone hemisuccinate (10 to 25 mg) to the injection decreases radicular pain and can be used with either isobaric or hyperbaric injections. Prolonged treatment via the lumbar route leads to increasing difficulty in withdrawing CSF and with rising CSF protein, both problems presumably resulting from chemical arachnoiditis. Bacterial meningitis resulting from any one lumbar puncture is unlikely, but this complication is not rare among patients receiving many months of injections.

Needle injections into the cisterna magna require a cooperative patient and an experienced operator. The novice should practice on cadavers and be supervised by an expert. Absence of a single experienced operator who will perform all the patient's injections is a strong contraindication to this mode of treatment. Subarachnoid hemorrhage is the most common major complication of cisternal punctures, resulting in over 30 reported fatalities (6). Progressive obtundation following the procedure requires urgent neurosurgical consultation concerning posterior fossa exploration. Puncture of the medulla causes immediate reactions that may include respiratory arrest. Needle puncture injury is less common than hemorrhage but may be hard to avoid when the cisterna magna is all but ablated by dense basal meningitis. Much less serious but more frequent complications are due to the chemical irritation by amphotericin B.

Small bleeds may cause some of these reactions also. The patient develops occipital, cervical, and sometimes interscapular pain within an hour or two of the injection, accompanied by nausea. Transitory fever and emesis may occur. Narcotic analgesics bring relief, but the addictive potential of chronic narcotic administration makes this undesirable.

Implantation of a siliconized-rubber subcutaneous reservoir connected by tubing to the CSF allows nearly painless, simple access to the CSF, but implantation is far from simple. Lumbar implantation is unpopular because a laminectomy is required and progressive arachnoiditis gradually makes the device unusable. Cisternal implantation offers the promise of putting drug where meningitis is most apparent at autopsy, i.e., the basal meninges. Suboccipital craniotomies are formidable procedures, and too little is known of the problems with reservoirs in this site for this procedure to be recommended. Much more is known about implanting the tubing into the lateral cerebral ventricle. A single burr hole over the nondominant frontal lobe provides access. Insertion into a normal-sized ventricle is not easy, and the presence of cerebral edema further complicates the procedure. In one series (7) of 31 procedures, 21 encountered such complications as hemiparesis, quadrantanopia, improperly positioned or nonfunctioning tubing, bacterial meningitis, wound infection, subcutaneous CSF leak, and intracranial hemorrhage. Adverse reactions to injecting amphotericin B into the third ventricle should prompt an anteroposterior skull film before using a newly placed reservoir to ensure that the radiopaque tip of the tubing is not in the midline. Complications with the reservoir occurred in 11 of 16 patients in the above-mentioned series (7). In these 16 patients 8 of 22 reservoirs had to be removed or became unusable because of leaking or clogging. CSF infection occurred in 8 patients, *Staphylococcus epidermidis* being the most common pathogen. Even injections of amphotericin B into properly placed, uninfected reservoirs cause headache, nausea, and fever. Mixing amphotericin B with hydrocortisone (10 to 25 mg) decreases the reactions. Infection of the reservoir may present in an indolent fashion with exaggerated and prolonged reactions to amphotericin B injections. Ventricular CSF may show only a mild pleocytosis, unlike more conventional cases of bacterial meningitis. Lumbar CSF cultures may not contain the bacterial pathogen, but cultures of the reservoir are positive. Of course, more severe and extensive infections also occur. If the reservoir does not become clogged with fibrinous exudate, parenteral antibiotics may clear the infection and obviate replacement (7).

Special problems are encountered when intraventricular amphotericin B is administered to patients with hydrocephalus and CSF shunts. Drug flows out of the ventricle into the shunt, rather than downward into the basilar meninges. Placement of a multiple-puncture reservoir proximally in the shunt with an on-off device distal to it allows one to inject the drug and close the shunt for about 4 h, in the hope of allowing downward flow. When hydrocephalus is caused by obstruction of the outlets of the fourth ventricle, intraventricular drug fails to treat the basilar meninges. Intraventricular injection of radioisotope with scintillation camera views can document patency of the pathway into the basilar meninges.

Amphotericin B methyl ester

This water-soluble derivative of amphotericin B has been available in small quantities for experimental use only. Hydrochloride, ascorbate, and aspartate salts have been used. In chemotherapy of experimental animals the drug was less nephrotoxic than the parent compound but also less effective. Studies in human beings have been halted, at least temporarily, because of the occurrence of deafness and perhaps other signs of neurotoxicity.

Flucytosine (5-fluorocytosine, Ancobon[1])

This synthetic agent is commercially available in 250- and 500-mg capsules. The usual dose is 37.5 mg/kg orally every 6 hours. Relatively low efficacy and drug resistance arising during therapy have diminished use of flucytosine as a single agent (8). Combination with amphotericin B has been increasingly popular in cryptococcal and candidal meningitis. Addition of flucytosine is thought to permit a lower dosage of amphotericin B, lessening toxicity due to the latter agent. Amphotericin B may decrease secondary flucytosine resistance. Toxicity to flucytosine is uncommon when the drug is used alone but quite common during combination therapy. These reactions include leukopenia, thrombocytopenia, colitis, hepatitis, and rash. There is evidence that bone marrow toxicity and perhaps diarrhea are associated with flucytosine blood levels above 100 to 125 μg/ml (9, 10). Documentation of this relationship is obfuscated by the lag of up to 8 to 13 days between elevated blood level and peak toxicity (10). Some patients maintain high blood levels and experience no toxicity. At doses of 37.5 mg/kg every 6 h, flucytosine blood levels do not usually exceed 100 μg/ml except in azotemic patients. Flucytosine is excreted almost entirely in the urine as unchanged drug. A dosage reduction is usually required when the serum creatinine exceeds about 1.5 to 1.7 mg/dl. According to one commonly used nomogram, the dose interval is doubled at creatinine clearances of 20 to 40 ml/min and increased fourfold at clearances of 10 to 20 ml/min (11). The author's practice is to reduce the dosage by the stated amount and leave the interval constant. With severe or changing azotemia, the nomogram is useless, and blood levels must be measured. Patients receiving hemodialysis may be given a single dose of 37.5 mg/kg after hemodialysis, but periodic determination of blood levels must be done to ascertain subsequent doses. The price of gross miscalculation may be death. Flucytosine-induced neutropenia, thrombocytopenia, and colitis have caused fatalities from sepsis, hemorrhage, and intestinal perforation, respectively (8).

When patients with fungal meningitis deteriorate despite treatment with flucytosine–amphotericin B, there is superficial logic in raising the amphotericin B dosage to 0.5 mg/kg daily or higher. This, of course, negates one of the principal advantages of the combination, which is to decrease amphotericin B toxicity. There is currently no evidence from clinical or experimental animal

---

[1] Brand name of Roche Laboratories.

studies that flucytosine increases the efficacy of amphotericin B when the latter is used in doses of 0.5 mg/kg daily or more. In the author's unpublished experience with 12 patients treated with such a regimen, 9 developed flucytosine toxicity. The high and variable azotemia made adjustment of flucytosine dosage difficult.

Patients receiving flucytosine should have their leukocyte and platelet count, serum transaminase, and alkaline phosphatase measured twice a week. They should be questioned often for abdominal pain and diarrhea. A prompt decrease in dosage may reverse bone marrow or intestinal toxicity and prevent temporary discontinuation of the drug. Abnormal liver function has occurred in about 4 percent of patients receiving flucytosine but to date has been reversible and nonlethal. Once hepatoxicity has occurred, the drug has been discontinued and not reinstituted. It is not known whether rechallenge is safe.

Flucytosine is teratogenic for rats. Use during pregnancy, particularly in the first trimester, is not advised.

Intrathecal flucytosine is never indicated because systemic administration results in excellent CSF levels. Intravenous flucytosine sometimes can be obtained from the manufacturer on an investigational basis. The capsules can be made into a shake suspension for administration by nasogastric tube.

Miconazole

This synthetic agent is commercially available in vials containing 200 mg of the drug dissolved in polyethoxylated castor oil, together with antibacterial preservatives. Intravenous miconazole has not been shown to be useful in fungal meningitis. The data are fragmentary but not encouraging. The package insert is quite misleading. Intrathecal miconazole has been employed in occasional cases of coccidioidal meningitis and, rarely, in cryptococcal meningitis, but the relative merits of this drug and intrathecal amphotericin B are unknown.

CRYPTOCOCCAL MENINGITIS

Anatomy of the infection

Disease of the central nervous system is both the most common presenting manifestation and the most common cause of death in cryptococcosis. Despite the name *cryptococcal meningitis*, patients with cryptococcosis of the central nervous system (who reach autopsy) have not only meningitis but often clusters of cryptococci in the brain, particularly in the basal ganglia and in perivascular areas of the cortical gray matter (12). Occasionally, these masses are large enough to be detected by computerized axial tomography. Cultures often reveal asymptomatic infection of extracranial organs. In one series of patients with cryptococcal meningitis, positive cultures were found in the urine of 10 out of 27 patients and in the blood of 5 out of 20 (13). Not rarely, sputum culture is positive in the absence of radiologically demonstrable disease. Considering the anatomy of the infection, chemotherapeutic activity is required in far more areas than the CSF. In fact, complete cures are often obtained with one regimen that usually gives no detectable antifungal activity in the CSF, namely, intravenous amphotericin B.

Cryptococcal meningitis can cause either cerebral edema or hydrocephalus. The clinical manifestations are similar, but management is considerably different. Computerized axial tomography reveals normal or small ventricles in the presence of edema but ventricular dilatation and sometimes periventricular edema in hydrocephalus. In acute hydrocephalus, ventricular dilatation may not be detected for a week or two after onset of symptoms. The patient who has rapidly progressive symptoms, very high opening pressure on lumbar puncture, and strongly positive India ink smear of CSF and who has received less than a month of therapy is more likely to have cerebral edema than hydrocephalus. Communicating or noncommunicating hydrocephalus can occur any time before, during, or in the few weeks following therapy. Patients presenting with hydrocephalus at time of diagnosis have an indolent onset of symptoms, often extending over a few months.

Management

Underlying disease Approximately one-third of patients with cryptococcal meningitis are receiving adrenal corticosteroids at the onset of the mycosis. The correlation of a poorer prognosis with corticosteroid use during therapy suggests that every effort should be made to reduce the corticosteroid dose to as low a level as possible during antifungal therapy (14). Abrupt discontinuation of dexamethasone given in doses adequate to treat cerebral edema (16 to 24 mg/day in an adult) may precipitate death from brainstem compression. Renal transplant recipients with cryptococcal meningitis present a distressing dilemma. The cure rate from their cryptococcosis is about 20 percent when azathioprine and prednisone are maintained during antifungal therapy (10). Yet the problems inherent in homograft rejection, hemodialysis during antifungal therapy, and later retransplantation are also formidable. No strong recommendation is possible, but it seems reasonable to sacrifice a poorly functioning homograft and in other cases to reduce the prednisone and azathioprine dosage as much as possible. In contrast to daily corticosteroid therapy, administration of a few days of high-dose corticosteroids to patients with Hodgkin's disease or acute leukemia does not seem to result in decided impairment of the response to antifungal therapy. The chance of remission of the neoplasm warrants any small risk of worsening the cryptococcosis. The presence of neutropenia, per se, does not seem to weight the prognosis of cryptococcosis heavily. Similarly, there has been no enthusiasm for leukocyte transfusion therapy of neutropenic patients with cryptococcosis.

Antifungal therapy Combined flucytosine–amphotericin B therapy is currently the most popular regimen. Because this popularity stems at least in part from results of a multicenter clinical trial (10), the study deserves close scrutiny. Patients were randomly assigned to one of two regimens: amphotericin B (0.3 mg/kg) plus flucytosine (150 mg/kg) each day for 6 weeks and amphotericin B 0.4

mg/kg) for 10 weeks. The former regimen had been employed successfully before (15). The latter was chosen to approximate the regimen used at Vanderbilt (16), seventy-eight patients were enrolled; 9 did not meet the diagnostic criteria and 3 were lost by death before treatment or signing out at onset of therapy. Of the remaining 66 patients 15 did not receive therapy according to protocol. Flucytosine toxicity caused 7 of the 15 deviant courses of therapy. As shown in Table 1, the combination was more effective in every category than amphotericin B alone. None of the differences in the table was significant at the 5 percent level. It may be important that the eventual outcome, including results of retreatment, was death because of or with active cryptococcosis in 8 of 34 (24 percent) initially treated with the combination compared with 15 of 32 (47 percent) initially treated with amphotericin B alone. If this difference is real, it may be related to the more rapid culture conversion seen in study patients begun on the combination.

The cryptococcal collaborative study unequivocally showed that 6 weeks of the combination was as good as the amphotericin B regimen chosen. The study was not designed to show that the combination was superior and, in fact, did not prove that. It was the collaborative study group's opinion, however, that taking all facts into consideration, the combination was superior. In the same breath, one must note that flucytosine toxicity occurred in a third of patients and resulted in premature discontinuation of the drug in 7 of 34 patients. This event was much more frequent at the start of the study, suggesting that experience with the drug helped avoid this problem.

An important criticism of the study was that the dose of amphotericin B used, 0.4 mg/kg daily, may have been too low. Many clinicians, including the author, prefer to use 0.5 to 0.6 mg/kg daily or 1.0 to 1.2 mg/kg every other day for

Table 1 Results of cryptococcal meningitis collaborative trial

	Flucytosine–amphotericin B			Amphotericin B		
		Cured or improved*			Cured or improved*	
	Treated	No.	%	Treated	No.	%
Protocol adherent	24	16	67	27	11	41
No immunosuppressive drugs	14	10		11	6	
Prednisone <10 mg/day	5	4		3	2	
Tumor chemotherapy	2	1		6	2	
Azathioprine-prednisone	3	1		7	1	
All protocol courses	34	23	68	32	15	47
All courses	34	26	76	32	17	53

* Cured meant no evidence of active cryptococcosis on complete examination, including lumbar puncture, at least 12 months after end of therapy. Cases considered improved were discharged with negative cultures and had no evidence of cryptococcosis when last seen, but complete examination was not done 1 year after therapy or patient died of other causes in the year after treatment.

cryptococcal meningitis. Another criticism is that the duration of combination therapy should have been longer than 6 weeks, perhaps the 10 weeks used for amphotericin B alone. Further experience with the combination will be necessary to determine whether either criticism is valid. In the meantime, it is important for clinicians to understand that no patient should have therapy terminated at an arbitrary time just to match the duration used by the study group. It is more logical to collect prognostic data before starting therapy, to evaluate the patient's rate of response during therapy, and to adjust the duration of therapy to the patient's situation. Patients with positive blood cultures (14) or receiving azathioprine and prednisone (Table 1) are extremely difficult to cure with any regimen. Other poor prognostic factors are hematologic malignancies, adrenal corticosteroid therapy, positive CSF India ink smears, high initial CSF opening pressures, low CSF glucose, and positive extraneural cultures at two or more sites (including urine, sputum, stool, and blood) (14). Weekly CSF examinations are extremely valuable in estimating appropriate duration of therapy. Persistent hypoglycorrhachia and positive CSF cultures or smears indicate incomplete response (14). It is the author's practice to require the following criteria to be met at the time of discharge: fasting CSF glucose in nondiabetics of at least 40 mg/dl; no growth in the last four CSF specimens, with the proviso that at least 3 ml was cultured for fungus each time; and a minimum of 12 weeks' therapy before discharging a patient with a persistently positive India ink smear. This last policy stems from observing a relapse rate of 50 percent among patients discharged with a positive India ink smear of the CSF.

The CSF antigen titer has been valuable in this institution in determining length of therapy, but in the hands of others, including the collaborative study group (10), it has not been as useful. The major problem has been laboratory-to-laboratory and run-to-run variability in titer. This problem can be overcome if the physician freezes a specimen of CSF from the onset of therapy and sends it for testing when other evidence suggests that therapy should be terminated. A fourfold fall in titer between the two specimens supports the decision to end therapy (14).

The physician's decision to use amphotericin B alone or with flucytosine is far less important than the physician's knowledge about the chosen regimen. Therapy should be given at accepted dosages and without interruption until careful monitoring dictates cessation of treatment.

There are a few situations in which amphotericin B alone appears preferable to the combination: patients receiving hemodialysis or peritoneal dialysis; patients with neutropenia, thrombocytopenia, or changing liver disease; and patients with frequent emesis or other conditions prohibiting oral medications.

Drug susceptibility must be considered in selecting therapy. Fortunately, *Cryptococcus neoformans* remains uniformly susceptible to amphotericin B, even when isolated from unsuccessfully treated patients. The author found 1 out of 101 pretreatment isolates to be resistant to flucytosine, i.e., to have a minimum inhibitory concentration exceeding 15 μg/ml. Isolates obtained during or after flucytosine therapy should be tested for flucytosine susceptibility, and the drug should be avoided when resistance occurs. True secondary drug resistance causes the isolate to grow well in all dissolvable concentrations of the drug. Intermediate values (25 to 100 μg/ml) for the MIC are suspect and may be an artifact created by improper testing procedures.

Intrathecal amphotericin B is advocated by some people in the treatment of cryptococcal meningitis. In the author's experience, complications of this procedure are far more impressive than therapeutic effects. Without better evidence of efficacy, it seems reasonable to reserve intrathecal therapy for patients relapsing after a seemingly adequate course of amphotericin B or flucytosine–amphotericin B and patients unable to tolerate even 0.3 mg of amphotericin B per kilogram of body weight daily.

Follow-up   Thorough posttreatment examinations are necessary to detect relapse before sequelae occur. These examinations should be done 3, 6, and 12 months after therapy. Subsequent relapse is rare. Each examination should include routine examination of the CSF, including fungal culture of 3 to 5 ml, India ink smear, and antigen titer. Urine and sputum should also be cultured for *Cryptococcus*. CSF antigen is usually undetectable 3 months after treatment in patients cured of the infection.

Surgical excision of mass lesions   Computerized axial tomography is now detecting mass lesions in the brain of occasional patients with cryptococcal meningitis. These lesions have rarely been detected by radioisotope scans, EEG, and other older procedures. It is not known whether drainage or excision of such masses expedites cure. There are patients who have responded to drugs alone despite mass lesions. In two cases followed by the author, the mass persisted several years despite cure.

Hydrocephalus   As mentioned above, communicating or noncommunicating hydrocephalus can complicate the course of cryptococcal meningitis. Symptoms are difficult to distinguish from those of the meningitis and secondary cerebral edema. Nausea and vomiting may be attributed incorrectly to amphotericin B. Frequent computerized axial tomographs in patients not doing well are extremely valuable. Appearance of hydrocephalus in the presence of appropriate symptoms should prompt placement of a shunt. Active meningitis is not a contraindication because the shunt does not act like a foreign body and does not impair cure. Uncontrolled cryptococcal meningitis does seem to make clogging of the shunt more likely. Shunt valves not readily clogged with fibrinous debris should be selected. Two tandem reservoirs or other devices which allow testing shunt patency by palpation should be inserted on the tubing. If intraventricular therapy is elected in the future, a reservoir for injection and an on-off valve should be included.

Cerebral edema   Patients with severe meningitis who are early in therapy, have normal-sized cerebral ventricles, and develop signs of brainstem compression should be suspected of having cerebral edema. This condition responds poorly to such osmotic agents as mannitol and oral glycerol. Dexamethasone in adult dose of about 24 mg per day can reverse signs of brainstem compression in hours, providing the patient is not already decorticate. The maximum beneficial effect is achieved within 24 h. Abrupt tapering of dexamethasone can lead to rapid reappearance of brainstem compression. Administration of dexamethasone can be lifesaving but is not undertaken lightly. The drug makes cryptococcosis difficult to control. The fungus fails to disappear or may even reappear in cultures of various body fluids despite appropriate antifungal therapy. Repeated efforts must be made to taper dexamethasone dosage slowly until the patient can tolerate discontinuance of the corticosteroid. Only then can substantial progress be made in eradicating the infection.

CANDIDAL MENINGITIS

Candida albicans and occasionally other *Candida* species may reach the meninges via the bloodstream or by direct extension (17). Management of hematogenous *Candida* meningitis resembles that of cryptococcal meningitis, with a few exceptions. Rarity of the disease and occurrence of occasional cures with nonspecific therapy has impaired the evaluation of drug therapy. Intravenous amphotericin B with (18, 19) or without (20) flucytosine has resulted in many cures, relapse being rare. Intrathecal amphotericin B does not appear to be needed. Use of flucytosine alone is controversial (21). Estimates of the incidence of flucytosine resistance in pretreatment cultures vary with geographic area and technique, ranging from roughly 5 to 40 percent (8). Isolates with intermediate levels of resistance usually are synergistic with amphotericin B in vitro. Flucytosine minimum inhibitory concentrations of 100 μg/ml or less are probably no contraindication to combined flucytosine–amphotericin B therapy, using the same dose and duration as in cryptococcal meningitis. If the flucytosine susceptibility cannot be determined, use of amphotericin B alone appears preferable.

Treatment of *Candida* meningitis is more complex when infection occurs by direct extension. Neurosurgery or meningomyelocele can predispose to this infection. The neurosurgery is usually extensive, such as that following radical cancer excision or massive trauma. Alternatively, surgery is not extensive, but a piece of siliconized rubber is implanted as a shunt or missing dura mater is replaced with plastic or fascia. Cure of direct extension *Candida* meningitis is difficult unless infected foreign bodies are removed and dural leaks are closed. If an infected shunt is functioning and cannot be removed, one could try oral flucytosine and amphotericin B given both intravenously and directly into the shunt. Amphotericin B given only by the intravenous route does not reach adequate CSF concentrations to sterilize the shunt.

COCCIDIOIDAL MENINGITIS

This dreaded disease can be controlled, but cures are rare. Patients in whom the meningitis is controlled may relapse in bone, lung, or subcutaneous tissue. Necessarily, this chapter must focus on meningitis alone.

Anatomy of the infection

Patients presenting with chronic meningitis due to *Coccidioides immitis* and who come to autopsy usually have infection confined to the meninges, principally at the base of the brain (22, 23). Perhaps because of the location, infection often leads to hydrocephalus. The location may also explain why intrathecal amphotericin B has been the mainstay of treatment.

Management

Antifungal therapy   All isolates of *C. immitis* have nearly the same susceptibility to amphotericin B by any one method, regardless of prior therapy (24). Intravenous amphotericin B results in a therapeutic response, but the repeated retreatments necessary to control the infection eventually destroy the kidneys. Despite all the problems of administration, intrathecal amphotericin B has been more effective in achieving long-term control and, on occasion, cure (25, 26). Patients who are ill from extraneural coccidioidomycosis as well as meningitis clearly benefit from intravenous amphotericin B. The role of intravenous drug is much less clear when only meningitis is detected. A short course of intravenous amphotericin B may hasten relief of meningeal symptoms, but long-term therapy is by the intrathecal route. Lumbar hyperbaric amphotericin B is a reasonable way to begin (5). Patients who experience increasing difficulty with these injections and who do not have obstructive hydrocephalus can be treated intraventricularly, using a subcutaneous reservoir. In experienced hands, cisternal therapy can be used. Techniques and complications are given elsewhere in this chapter. Intrathecal therapy is continued for at least 3 months after the lumbar CSF no longer gives a positive complement-fixation test for antibody to *C. immitis* (25, 26). This is rarely less than a year. Ventricular CSF is unreliable for purposes of serology because the titer is lower than in the lumbar area (27). Lumbar CSF protein is an unreliable guide in that either intrathecal therapy or hydrocephalus may elevate the protein. The usual intrathecal regimens do not cause hypoglycorrhachia. Patients tolerating intrathecal amphotericin B poorly have limited alternatives at present. Very little is known about intrathecal miconazole, and intravenous miconazole does not control coccidioidal meningitis.

Hydrocephalus   A major goal in treating coccidioidal meningitis is to keep the infection so well controlled that hydrocephalus does not develop. The shunt does not act as a nidus of infection or lead to serious spread of the disease, but the advent of hydrocephalus signals impediments to CSF circulation that complicate intrathecal therapy. Drug injected into the lumbar theca may remain in the spinal meninges. Intraventricular drug will flow out the shunt unless an on-off valve is in place. If the outlet of the fourth ventricle is blocked, intraventricular drug can never reach the basilar meninges. In selecting a route for injection, intrathecal radioisotope and rapid scintillation camera scanning can reveal a great deal about where drug is likely to go. When there is no reasonable route to give intrathecal drug, intravenous therapy can be used as long as the patient's kidneys, veins, and stamina permit.

REFERENCES

1 **Bennett JE:** Chemotherapy of systemic mycoses. *N Engl J Med* 290:30, 1974.

2 **Bindschadler DD, Bennett JE:** A pharmacologic guide to the clinical use of amphotericin B. *J Infect Dis* 120:427, 1969.

3 **Butler WT et al:** Nephrotoxicity of amphotericin B. *Ann Intern Med* 61:175, 1964.

4 **Block ER, Bennett JE:** Stability of amphotericin B in infusion bottles. *Antimicrob Agents Chemother* 4:648, 1973.

5 **Alazraki NP et al:** Use of a hyperbaric solution for the administration of intrathecal amphotericin B. *N Engl J Med* 290:641, 1974.

6 **Keane JR:** Cisternal puncture complications. Treatment of coccidioidal meningitis with amphotericin B. *Calif Med* 119:10, 1973.

7 **Diamond RD, Bennett JE:** Intrathecal therapy of fungal meningitis using a subcutaneous reservoir. *N Engl J Med* 288:186, 1973.

8 **Bennett JE:** Drugs five years later: Flucytosine. *Ann Intern Med* 86:319, 1977.

9 **Kauffman CA et al:** Simple assay for 5-fluorocytosine in the presence of amphotericin B. *Antimicrob Agents Chemother* 9:381, 1976.

10 **Bennett JE et al:** A comparison of amphotericin B alone and combined with flucytosine in the treatment of cryptococcal meningitis. *N Engl J Med* 301:126, 1979.

11 **Schönebeck J et al:** Pharmacokinetic studies on the oral antimycotic agent 5-fluorocytosine in individuals with normal and impaired renal function. *Chemotherapy* 18:321, 1973.

12 **Salfelder K:** Cryptococcosis, in Baker RD (ed): *Human Infection with Fungi, Actinomycetes and Algae.* New York, Springer, 1971, p 383.

13 **Butler WT et al:** Diagnostic and prognostic value of clinical and laboratory findings in cryptococcal meningitis. *N Engl J Med* 270:59, 1964.

14 **Diamond RD, Bennett JE:** Prognostic factors in cryptococcal meningitis. A study of 111 cases. *Ann Intern Med* 80:176, 1974.

15 **Utz JP et al:** Therapy of cryptococcosis with a combination of flucytosine and amphotericin B. *J Infect Dis* 132:368, 1975.

16 **Drutz DJ et al:** Treatment of disseminated mycotic infections: A new approach to amphotericin B therapy. *Am J Med* 45:405, 1968.

17 **Bayer AS et al:** Candida meningitis. Report of seven cases and review of the literature. *Medicine* 55:477, 1976.

18 **Lillien LD et al:** *Candida albicans* meningitis in a premature neonate treated with 5-fluorocytosine and amphotericin B: A case report and review of the literature. *Pediatrics* 61:57, 1978.

19 **Chesney JP et al:** Candida meningitis in newborn infants: A review and report of combined amphotericin B–flucytosine therapy. *Johns Hopkins Med J* 142:155, 1978.

20 **Roe DC, Haynes RE:** *Candida albicans* meningitis successfully treated with amphotericin B. *Am J Dis Child* 124:926, 1972.

21 **Nordström L et al:** Candida meningoencephalitis treated with 5-fluorocytosine. *Scand J Infect Dis* 9:63, 1977.

22 **Forbus WD, Bestebreurtje AM:** Coccidioidomycosis: A study of 95 cases of the disseminated type with special reference to the pathogenesis of the disease. *Milit Surg* 99:653, 1946.

23 **Fiese MJ:** *Coccidioidomycosis.* Springfield, Ill, Charles C Thomas, 1958, p 117.

24 **Collins MS, Pappagianis D:** Uniform susceptibility of various strains of *Coccidioides immitis* to amphotericin B. *Antimicrob Agents Chemother* 11:1049, 1977.

25 **Winn WA:** The treatment of coccidioidal meningitis. *Calif Med* 101:78, 1964.

26 **Winn WA:** Coccidioidal meningitis: A follow-up report, in Ajello L (ed): *Coccidioidomycosis.* Tucson, University of Arizona Press, 1967, p 55.

27 **Goldstein E et al:** Ventricular fluid and the management of coccidioidal meningitis. *Ann Intern Med* 77:243, 1972.

ADDITIONAL REFERENCES

Ajello L (ed): *Coccidioidomycosis.* Miami, Symposia Specialists, 1977.

Drutz D, Catanzaro A: Coccidioidomycosis. *Am Rev Respir Dis* 117:559, 727, 1978.

Emmons CW et al: *Medical Mycology.* Philadelphia, Lea & Febiger, 1977.

Fetter BF et al: *Mycoses of the Central Nervous System.* Baltimore, Williams & Wilkins, 1967.

Mandell GL et al: *Principles and Practice of Infectious Diseases.* New York, Wiley, 1979.

Odds FC: *Candida and Candidosis.* Baltimore, University Park Press, 1979.

Bacteriology, clinical spectrum of disease, and therapeutic aspects in coryneform bacterial infection

JOHN A. WASHINGTON II

GENERAL DESCRIPTION

The term *diphtheroid* or, more precisely, *coryneform* is used to describe a group of asporogenous, gram-positive, rod-shaped bacteria which resemble but do not include *Corynebacterium diphtheriae*. Although there is general agreement that the group includes other species of *Corynebacterium*, there is little consensus on what other genera should be included. To *Corynebacterium*, Cowan (1) added *Listeria* and *Kurthia*, while Rogosa et al. (2) added *Arthrobacter, Cellulomonas*, and *Kurthia*. Neither *Arthrobacter* nor *Cellulomonas* is pathogenic in human beings and will therefore be omitted from this discussion. Often referred to as a diphtheroid or *Corynebacterium*, *Propionibacterium acnes* is anaerobic to aerotolerant, forms major amounts of propionic and acetic acids as end products of carbohydrate fermentation, and properly belongs to the family Propionibacteriaceae. Further complicating the picture is the rather confusing taxonomy of the genus *Corynebacterium* itself.

With no intent of slighting anyone's preferences, I have arbitrarily elected to limit my discussion of the coryneform group of bacteria to the genera *Corynebacterium* (excluding *C. diphtheriae*), *Propionibacterium*, and *Kurthia*.

Taxonomy

The coryneform group of bacteria are nonsporeforming, non-acid-fast, oxidase-negative, gram-positive, rod-shaped bacteria. The genera *Corynebacterium* and *Kurthia* are aerobic to facultatively anaerobic, while the genus *Propionibacterium* is anaerobic. Carbohydrates are used fermentatively or not at all by *Corynebacterium* species other than *C. aquaticum*, which uses carbohydrates oxidatively. Carbohydrates are not used by *Kurthia*. All members of the group are catalase-positive except for *Kurthia*, *C. vaginale*, *C. pyogenes*, and *C. haemolyticum*; the latter two species, however, may be weakly catalase-positive. Motility is exhibited only by *C. aquaticum* and *Kurthia*.

The taxonomic positions of the following species of *Corynebacterium* are in question because their cell wall compositions differ substantially from those of other corynebacteria: *C. pyogenes*, *C. haemolyticum*, *C. equi*, *C. aquaticum*, and *C. vaginale* (*Haemophilus vaginalis*). The differential characteristics of species of *Corynebacterium* are listed in Table 1. The validity of most of the generally accepted corynebacterial species has been supported by studies demonstrating that each of these species produces distinctive volatile and nonvolatile acid metabolic products (3). Except for *Propionibacterium acnes*, which can be identified on the basis of positive catalase and indole reactions, all other nonsporeforming anaerobic gram-positive bacilli require analysis of fatty acid end products from peptone-yeast extract–glucose (PYG) cultures for identification (4, 5).

Ecology

Corynebacteria and propionibacteria are the dominant organisms on the skin of adults and are often present in concentrations exceeding 100 per square centimeter (6). Corynebacteria and propionibacteria are present in the conjunctiva of approximately 25 and 50 percent, respectively, of normal, healthy eyes (7, 8). Corynebacteria are seldom listed among isolates from the human gastrointestinal tract, and studies of nonsporeforming anaerobic bacteria in human feces have shown the propionibacteria to be but minor components of this flora (9). Excluding *C. vaginale*, corynebacteria are present in the vagina of approximately 80 percent of children (10) and 20 percent of adults (11–13). Propionibacteria are present in the vagina of approximately 25 percent of adults (12) but infrequently in children (10). Complicating the issue of its pathogenic role in causing vaginitis, *C. vaginale* has been isolated from the vagina of 12 percent of children (10) and from that of 20 to 40 percent of asymptomatic adults (11, 12). Corynebacteria are frequently present in "urethral" urine (13, 14), while propionibacteria are absent from this site (13). Both corynebacteria and propionibacteria are abundant in the oral cavity. Little is known of the normal distribution of *Kurthia* in human beings, although it has been isolated without apparent pathogenic significance from sputum and the eye (15, 16).

Many corynebacterial species occur as indigenous flora or cause infections in animals (17). For example, *C. pseudotuberculosis* is found predominantly in sheep, as well as in the soil of sheds and corrals in many parts of the world where sheep are housed and sheared. It can cause local or disseminated disease in sheep, horses, and (rarely) cattle. *C. equi* causes equine pneumonia, while *C. pyogenes* causes localized, purulent, and occasionally disseminated infections in domestic animals.

Because of the widespread distribution of the coryneform bacteria on the skin and mucous membranes, they are frequently isolated from a variety of clinical specimens and pose a considerable problem in interpretation. For example, they have been isolated from 17 to 34 percent of patients with positive blood cultures at the Mayo Clinic and affiliated hospitals between 1968 and 1975 (18), but these isolates have rarely been of any importance and have only rarely reflected the presence of endocarditis (19, 20), the major disease entity in which

Table 1 Differential characteristics of corynebacterial species (1–4)

			Acid from				Nitrate	
	Catalase	Motility	Glucose	Maltose	Sucrose	Lactose	reduced	Urease
C. diphtheriae	+	–	+	+	–	–	+	–
C. pseudotuberculosis	+	–	+	+	d*	–	d	+
C. xerosis	+	–	+	+	+	–	+	–
C. renale	+	–	+	–	–	d	–	+
C. kutscheri	+	–	+	+	+	–	+	+
C. pseudodiphtheriticum†	+	–	–	–	–	–	+	+
C. bovis	+	–	+	d	–	–	–	–
Group JK	+	–	+	–(+)*	–	–	–	–
C. pyogenes‡	–(+^{w})	–	+	+	+	+	–	–
C. haemolyticum‡	–(+^{w})	–	+	+	+	+	–	–
C. aquaticum	+	+	+	+	+	–	–(+)	–
C. vaginale¶	–	–	+	+	d	–	–	–

* Reactions in parentheses indicate reactions by a minority of isolates; d = different reactions reported; w = weak.
† Often referred to as C. hofmannii.
‡ C. pyogenes and C. haemolyticum are differentiated by the former's proteolytic activity, e.g., gelatin hydrolysis.
¶ Often referred to as Haemophilus vaginalis.

they are repeatedly isolated from cultures of blood. Other problems posed by this group of bacteria can be illustrated by the frequency (approximately 20 percent) of their isolation from cultures taken of the operative site at the time of total hip arthroplasty (21, 22). For these reasons, extreme care must be taken in obtaining specimens for cultures and in the interpretation of the isolation of coryneform bacteria in the laboratory. The validity of such findings is often established by repeated isolation of the organism from multiple specimens (e.g., three or more separate sites in the operative wound or three separate phlebotomies per febrile episode).

INFECTIONS

Two major reviews by Kaplan and Weinstein (23) and by Johnson and Kaye (24) have certainly substantiated the diversity of diseases associated with diphtheroids in human beings. Johnson and Kaye (24) added to their own cases those reported and reviewed by Kaplan and Weinstein (23) and found the spectrum of diseases to include endocarditis (31 cases), bacteremia (5 cases), meningitis and/or brain abscess (6 cases), osteomyelitis (2 cases), suppurative adenitis (3 cases), pneumonia (1 case), lung abscess (1 case), wound infection (2 cases), and bacterial hepatitis (1 case). They also reported that the majority of isolates from cases other than endocarditis (12 of 21) were microaerophilic or anaerobic while the converse was true of isolates from cases with endocarditis (4 of 31). The spectrum of diseases associated with propionibacteria was thoroughly covered by Finegold (25) in 1977 and included infections of the paranasal sinuses, meninges and/or brain, head and neck, endocardium, pleuropulmonary tree, biliary tract, urinary tract, bones and joints, and soft tissues.

In approaching the areas of clinical manifestations and treatment of coryneform infections, I have elected to focus on cases reported in the past decade instead of reviewing exhaustively all reported in history. My intent has not been to neglect historical precedent but to review the subject contemporaneously.

Ocular infections

Coryneform bacterial infection of the eye is rare (7), despite the frequency of isolation of corynebacteria and propionibacteria from the conjunctivae of normal healthy eyes (7, 8). Hanscom and Maxwell (26) isolated a *Corynebacterium*, CDC group A4, on two separate occasions from the vitreous humor of a patient with endophthalmitis secondary to a penetrating injury with a metallic foreign object. The eye retained functional visual acuity following removal of the lens, anterior vitreous, and foreign body, as well as intravitreous and intravenous therapy with methicillin, gentamicin, and steroids. Of particular interest was the production of endophthalmitis in rabbits following intravitreous inoculation of the same organism.

Endophthalmitis related to propionibacteria (seven *P. acnes*, one *P. avidum*) has been reported in five cases by Jones and Robinson (27), in two cases by

Forster (28), and in one case by Friedman et al. (29). Trauma and/or surgery preceded the infection in all cases. The infections in four of the five cases reported by Jones and Robinson (27) were mixed and were respectively associated with *Bacterionema* and *Micrococcus*, *Fusobacterium nucleatum* and *Pseudomonas aeruginosa*, *Actinomyces naeslundii* and *Staphylococcus epidermidis*, and *Micrococcus*. No details were given regarding antimicrobial therapy of these five infections, except that none received intraocular antibiotics, one eye required enucleation, two achieved good visual acuity, and two were left with impaired visual acuity. All authors stressed the point that endophthalmitis due to *P. acnes* was initially thought on clinical grounds to be fungal in origin.

Jones and Robinson (27) also reported propionibacteria in association with four cases of keratitis (one *P. avidum*, three *P. acnes*) in pure (two cases) or mixed (two cases) culture; one case of preseptal cellulitis (*P. acnes*) in mixed culture; and two cases of canaliculitis (*P. acnes*) in mixed culture.

Central nervous system infections

Abscess   In their review in 1970, Johnson and Kaye (24) listed 6 cases (12 percent) of meningitis and/or brain abscess among the 52 cases with infections caused by diphtheroids. Subsequently, Finegold (25) identified a total of seven reported cases of brain abscess from which *Propionibacterium* was isolated in pure or mixed culture. These abscesses were preceded in three instances by otitis media and/or mastoiditis, in one instance each by pulmonary infection and congenital heart disease, and in two instances by no known precipitating event or underlying condition. Of 60 patients with brain abscess seen at the Mayo Clinic between 1961 and 1973, there were 5 from whose abscesses *P. acnes* was isolated as part of a mixed infection; all but 1 (who died) of these 5 recovered without major neurological residua (30). Underlying conditions or antecedent events in these five cases were otic or paranasal sinus infection, oral infection, pulmonary infection, or congenital heart disease. Brain abscess has been associated with *C. haemolyticum* in two cases, a fatal mixed infection with *Fusobacterium necrophorum* (31) and one which was merely mentioned in a letter to the editor (32).

Meningitis   Vale and Scott (33) described a case of meningitis due to *C. bovis*, treated successfully with ampicillin, and a case with an epidural abscess from which *Staphylococcus aureus* was cultured. Two subsequent cerebrospinal fluid cultures from this patient yielded *C. bovis*. While the authors speculated that the second patient had a relatively mild meningitis due to *C. bovis*, they provided no other laboratory data to substantiate this impression and their patient responded to surgical drainage of the abscess and treatment with cloxacillin.

P. acnes was reported as the cause of acute meningitis in a previously normal adult; the meningitis was successfully treated with penicillin G intravenously (34). It has also been reported as the cause of chronic meningitis in three cases; two of them recovered, one with and one without penicillin therapy, and the third failed to recover following penicillin and then tetracycline therapy (35). In their report of chronic meningitis, French et al. (35) cited 13 cases with acute diphtheroid (including two due to *P. acnes*) meningitis. Seven of the nine cases reported between 1917 and 1935 died, while only one of four reported between 1954 and 1968 died. Various antimicrobial regimens (including aureomycin and streptomycin; penicillin; and cephalothin, chloramphenicol, and penicillin, respectively) were used in the surviving cases in the latter group.

Shunt infections   *P. acnes*, *C. xerosis*, and *C. bovis* have caused central nervous system shunt (36–40) and postneurosurgical infections (40), including immune complex glomerulonephritis (38–40).

The therapy in these cases usually included both antibiotics and surgery with removal or replacement of the infected shunt or drainage of infected fluid. Infected shunts were removed from two of the three patients with glomerulonephritis (39, 40). The third patient failed to respond to 6 weeks of intravenous penicillin but responded to therapy with erythromycin and rifampin (38).

Upper respiratory infections

Otitis   *Corynebacterium* and *Propionibacterium* are not infrequently isolated, often in mixed cultures, from middle ear fluid in children with acute and chronic otitis media (41–44) and from sinus aspirates in patients with sinusitis (25). Because of the polymicrobial nature of most of these infections, the clinical significance of coryneform bacteria in such cases remains obscure.

Pharyngitis   MacLean et al. (45) were the first to report the isolation of *C. haemolyticum* from large numbers of soldiers with pharyngitis in the South and West Pacific. Similar reports of the isolation of this species from patients with upper respiratory infections have been made by Ryan (46) and Fell et al. (47). A maculopapular or scarlatiniform rash was a common feature in the patients reported by Ryan and Fell et al. but was rarely seen in those reported by MacLean et al. MacLean et al. were unable to reproduce the disease following inoculation of the organism into normal volunteers. The significance of *C. haemolyticum* in causing upper respiratory infections remains obscure since neither mycoplasmal nor viral studies were performed in any of the series reported.

Lower respiratory infections

In their 1970 review, Johnson and Kaye (24) cited one case each of pneumonia and lung abscess caused by diphtheroids. Since then a considerable number of such cases have been added to the literature.

Reported cases of corynebacterial pneumonia and/or lung abscess have been summarized in Table 2. It is striking that pleuropulmonary infections due to *C. equi* predominate in the immunosuppressed host. All but one of the patients with *C. equi* infection had recent or remote histories of proximity to, or contact

Table 2 Corynebacterial pleuropulmonary infections

Case	Ref.	Age	Species	Underlying condition or antecedent events	Source of isolate	Type of infection	Antimicrobial therapy	Course and outcome
1	48	29	C. equi	Plasma cell hepatitis; receiving steroids, 6-mercaptopurine	Bronchoscopic aspirate	Abscess, lung (RUL)	Erythromycin 250 mg every 6 h for 8 weeks	Abscess cavity disappeared
					Abscess fluid	Abscess subcutaneous, abdominal wall; appeared 6 weeks after cessation of erythromycin	Erythromycin	Abscess incised and drained
2	49	45	C. equi	Renal transplant; receiving prednisone and azathioprine	Bronchial brush biopsy; postmortem lung (LUL)	Abscess, lung (LUL)	Erythromycin 2 g daily and gentamicin 80 mg IM every other day for 14 days; flucytosine and amphotericin B	Died in renal failure following myocardial infarction; autopsy confirmed presence of culture-positive lung abscess
3	50	39	C. equi	Lymphoma, received chemo- and radiation therapy	Blood culture, bronchial brushings	Abscess lung (LUL)	Ampicillin, 4 g then 2 g daily for 2 weeks and again with gentamicin with septi-	Abscess resolved and patient discharged; readmitted with fever, lymphadenopathy,

				Underlying disease	Source of isolate	Diagnosis	Therapy	Outcome
							cemic episode (serum bactericidal titer of 1:4 to 1:8; erythromycin added	clear lungs; C. equi recovered from blood; died of disseminated aspergillosis
4	51	13	C. equi	Leukemia; received chemotherapy	Sputum	Pneumonia (LLL)	Oxacillin IV for 48 h, then clindamycin 1.9 g daily and chloramphenicol 2 g daily IV for 10 days	Discharged with resolving pneumonia, then readmitted for relapse of LLL pneumonia
					Bronchial washings	Pneumonia, recurrent (LLL)	Chloramphenicol for 10 days	Pneumonia resolved
5	52	26	C. equi	Hodgkin's disease	Lung (RML), thoracentesis fluid, bronchial washings	Abscess lung (RML), progressing to empyema, LUL cavity, LLL and RUL infiltrates	Penicillin 5 million units every 6 h IV for 10 days, followed by erythromycin 1 g every 6 h IV for 14 weeks	Chemo- and radiation therapy given for 1 to 3 weeks, respectively; stopped because of neutropenia; resumed when neutropenia reversed; pneumonia slowly resolved while receiving chemo- and radiation therapy
6	53	52	C. equi	Reticuluhm cell sarcoma; received chemo- and radiation therapy	Blood, thoracentesis fluid	Pneumonia (LLL), empyema	Cephalothin 12 g IV daily, gentamicin 5 mg/kg IM daily	Died, deteriorating pulmonary, cardiac, and renal status; no autopsy; serum bactericidal titer of 1:8 while on therapy

Table 2 Corynebacterial pleuropulmonary infections (Continued)

Case	Ref.	Age	Species	Underlying condition or antecedent events	Source of isolate	Type of infection	Antimicrobial therapy	Course and outcome
7	53	47	C. equi	Hodgkin's disease; treated with chemo- and radiation therapy	Transthoracic lung biopsy, blood, skin lesion; lung tissue removed surgically	Pneumonia and abscess (RUL), pustules	Erythromycin, 2 g daily during initial and second episodes; during second episode, also received tetracycline, 2 g daily for 7 days and gentamicin 4 mg/kg IM daily for 14 days	Underwent right upper lobectomy, became afebrile, discharged; readmitted in 2 weeks with recurrent skin pustules, pneumonia, and pharyngitis which resolved with antimicrobial therapy; serum bactericidal titer while on erythromycin of 1:16 to 1:32
8	54	39	C. pyogenes	Inoperable breast carcinoma	Thoracentesis fluid	Empyema	Sulfadiazine, followed by penicillin G, 20 million units IV daily for 15(?) days	Pleural fluid continued to accumulate but cultures remained negative after fifteenth day of penicillin therapy
9	55	57	C. pyogenes	None known	Postmortem lung	Pneumonia (RLL, LLL), lipid pneumonitis (?)	Not identified	Died 19 days after admission; bacilli and cocci seen in strains of lung postmortem
10	56	67	C. pyogenes	Asthmatic bronchitis	Sputum (pure culture)	Pneumonia (RLL, LLL)	Cotrimoxazole, ampicillin	Pneumonia resolved following several weeks of therapy

11	57	68	Undefined	Chronic obstructive pulmonary disease; dental extractions 3–4 months PTA	—	Pneumonia (RLL)	Procaine penicillin G 600,000 units IM every 6 h for 3 weeks	Pneumonia resolved; patient was readmitted in 2 months with recurrent pneumonia and with empyema; resolved with prolonged penicillin therapy
					Thoracentesis fluid	Pneumonia, recurrent with empyema	Penicillin G 1 million units IV every 4 h for 1 month; then 800,000 units PO every 6 h for 2 months	
12	58	72	CDC group D2	Chronic obstructive pulmonary disease, arteriosclerotic heart disease with congestive failure; *Haemophilus influenzae* pneumonia 3 weeks PTA	Transtracheal aspirate	Pneumonia (LLL)	Oxacillin 2 g IV every 6 h and gentamicin 80 mg IV every 8 h for 3 days, then penicillin G 1 million units IV every 4 h for 7 days	Pneumonia resolved
13	59	28	*C. pseudotuberculosis*	Exposure to sick horses 2 months PTA and to microorganism in laboratory 5 weeks PTA	Transtracheal aspirate	Pneumonia (LLL)	Erythromycin 500 mg every 6 h for 2 weeks	Pneumonia resolved; eosinophilia noted in peripheral blood and sputum smears

with, horses, cattle, sheep, or swine. One patient (Case no. 13) with *C. pseudotuberculosis* pneumonia was a veterinary student with a history of exposure both to horses ill with a cough and to a culture of the organism in the microbiology laboratory. While the possibility of opportunistic infection following prolonged asymptomatic carriage of these organisms cannot be ruled out, it is interesting to note the observation made by Gardner et al. (51) that except for the case they reported, *C. equi* was not isolated in a 5-year period from cultures of sputum from other children with leukemia and other forms of malignancy.

A variety of antibiotic regimens was used for treating corynebacterial pleuropulmonary infections (Table 2); 6 of the 13 patients received one or more courses of erythromycin, alone or in combination with another antimicrobial agent, presumably on the basis of in vitro susceptibility test results. Where stated, the MICs of erythromycin were between 0.12 and 0.4 μg/ml, while those of penicillins were variable (three of seven strains tested were resistant). Resolution of the corynebacterial infection ultimately occurred in 11 of the 13 patients, although 3 patients required additional therapy for recurrent infections with the same organism.

Propionibacteria are infrequently associated with anaerobic bacterial pneumonia, empyema, or lung abscess and seldom, if ever, in pure culture (25).

Kurthia has been isolated from the sputum of a patient with lobar pneumonia, but no details of the case were given and the organism was assumed not to be related to the patient's illness (15).

Bacteremia

Although corynebacteria and propionibacteria are frequently isolated from blood cultures (18), clinically significant coryneform bacteremia unrelated to endocardial or intravascular infection remains rare and occurs most often in immunosuppressed hosts. Of special interest are three reports covering 48 patients, most of whom had leukemia or marrow transplants and all of whom had bacteremia due to a previously unrecognized *Corynebacterium* species [subsequently designated group JK by Riley et al. at the Center for Disease Control (4)], characterized principally by resistance to virtually all antimicrobials except vancomycin (60–62). Because of the nature of these patients' underlying diseases and the fact that many were leukopenic, the effects of antimicrobial therapy are difficult to assess. Pearson et al. (61) found that the infection was cleared in five of six patients receiving erythromycin or vancomycin and that other antibiotics to which the organism was resistant were ineffective clinically. Stamm et al. (62) divided their patients into three groups: (1) five (four granulocytopenic) of seven patients receiving no antimicrobial therapy because the organism was thought to be a contaminant died; (2) five (four granulocytopenic) of nine patients receiving at least 48 h of an antibiotic to which the organism was susceptible died; and (3) none of eight patients who had hyperalimentation lines removed and received appropriate antimicrobial therapy died, despite the fact that five patients were granulocytopenic. Of the four patients reported by Hande et al. (60), two died too rapidly for evaluation of therapy to be made, one responded to vancomycin but died subsequently of

P. aeruginosa sepsis, and one responded to vancomycin and erythromycin along with replacement of a central nervous system shunt. Stamm et al. (62) found that 40 percent of marrow transplant patients were colonized at one or more sites with group JK corynebacteria and that the incidence of colonization correlated significantly with prolonged hospitalization and prior antibiotic exposure.

Other cases include an 85-year-old diabetic with ketoacidosis who had *C. aquaticum* septicemia and who responded to cephalothin, 8 g daily for 10 days (63), and a 15-year-old girl who developed *C. haemolyticum* septicemia in association with appendicitis and who apparently recovered following a 10-day course of penicillin and an appendectomy (64). Irwin et al. (65) described a 70-year-old man with a chronic febrile illness of unknown etiology from whose blood a cell-wall-defective variant of *Corynebacterium* was isolated and who responded clinically to a 4-week course of erythromycin (1 g every 6 h) and a 10-day course of streptomycin (1 g daily).

Although coryneform bacteria can be recovered occasionally from intravenous catheters, they do not appear to cause catheter-related bacteremia (66, 67).

Endocarditis

Of reported cases with diseases caused by diphtheroids, 60 percent (31 out of 52) had endocarditis, according to Johnson and Kaye's 1970 review (24). By 1977, Van Scoy et al. (68) were able to review 64 reported cases and added 3 of their own to the literature. The organisms from the latter group of 3 cases belonged to group JK (4), were all resistant to penicillin, and were uniformly inhibited and killed only by vancomycin. Of the total of 67 cases reviewed, 37 had prosthetic valves and 28 did not. The mortality rates in the groups with and without prosthetic valves were 50 and 48 percent, respectively, but these figures are misleading in that 8 patients in the latter group died in the preantibiotic era (mortality in the antibiotic era was 5 out of 19, or 26 percent) and the diagnosis or cure of 5 patients who were reported as cured without surgery in the former group was questionable. Cure, at any rate, was difficult to ascribe exclusively to antibiotics or surgery and was often related to a combination of both these treatment modalities. Of the three cases reported by Van Scoy et al. (68) one died with recurrent endocarditis following replacement of an infected prosthetic aortic valve and treatment initially with penicillin and gentamicin and later with a 42-day course of vancomycin; the second died with no evidence of infection following 5 weeks of erythromycin and a second replacement of a dehisced mitral valve; and the third survived following initial prosthetic valve replacement and a 46-day course of erythromycin.

The documentation of coryneform bacterial endocarditis is difficult because blood cultures may remain negative or require prolonged incubation to become positive and because corynebacteria or propionibacteria are such frequent contaminants of blood cultures.

The first recognized case of endocarditis, if not the first recognized case of disease, due to *Kurthia bessonii* was reported in 1979 by Pancoast et al. (69). The patient was treated with oxacillin and gentamicin and underwent valve replacement for a cusp abscess, fistula, and markedly destroyed aortic valve. No details were given regarding the duration of antimicrobial therapy or eventual outcome for the patient.

Intraabdominal infections

Corynebacteria and propionibacteria play a very minor role in intraabdominal infections with the possible exception of those involving the liver.

Kaplan and Weinstein (23) described what probably remains the sole reported case of "bacterial hepatitis" due to anaerobic diphtheroids. The organisms were isolated from the bone marrow and an open liver biopsy in a patient with fever of unknown origin, slightly elevated liver enzymes, and a mild inflammatory reaction in the hepatic portal areas. Because the organism was not specifically noted to be present in stained tissue sections and because of the reported frequency of contamination by *P. acnes* of surgically removed gallbladder stones, bile, and tissue (70), the significance of the anaerobic diphtheroids in Kaplan and Weinstein's patient with hepatitis is highly questionable.

Liver abscesses associated with anaerobic and facultatively anaerobic diphtheroids have been reported by Balfour and Minken in a 4-year-old child with a recent history of trauma (71) and by Muangmanee and Jaroonvesama in a 40-year-old diabetic (72), respectively. The organisms were seen in a gram-stained smear of and cultured from pus removed at the time of surgery in the first case and were cultured from seven separate aspirates from the abscess and from pus in the pleural cavity in the second case. The first case responded to incision and drainage and to systemic penicillin and kanamycin for 10 and 7 days, respectively. The second case responded to chloramphenicol, 1.5 g daily for 14 days.

Genitourinary infections

Bacteriuria Coryneform bacterial infection of the urinary tract is rare, despite the frequency with which such bacteria are present in urethral urine (13, 14). Segura et al. (73) reported a case of mixed corynebacterial-propionibacterial bladder infection, confirmed by suprapubic aspiration, in an elderly male with carcinoma of the prostate and urinary retention.

Vaginitis Acute, self-limited, ulcerative vulvovaginitis without regional lymphadenopathy was found by Laufe in eleven cases to be associated with *C. pyogenes* (74). Three of the cases had other *Corynebacterium* species isolated from vaginal cultures. Since no viral studies were performed, the precise significance of *C. pyogenes* in these cases remains uncertain.

The clinical significance of *C. vaginale* (*Haemophilus vaginalis*) remains as controversial as its taxonomic position. The organism has been isolated from the vagina of approximately 20 to 40 percent of asymptomatic women (11, 12). In a quantitative bacteriological study of vaginal flora, Levison et al. (75) could find no significant difference in the frequency of isolation or numbers of *C. vaginale* between patients with or without vaginitis. In contrast, Pheifer et al. (76) isolated *C. vaginale* from 17 of 18 women with signs of vaginitis but only 1 of 18 normal matched controls ($p < 0.002$). On the basis of clinical improvement and eradication of *C. vaginale* with metronidazole, they speculated that *C. vaginale* played an etiologic role in nonspecific vaginitis, possibly together with vaginal anaerobic bacteria. These differences may be due to the findings by Pheifer et al. (76) of objective signs and laboratory features of nonspecific vaginitis in many asymptomatic women studied. Persistence of *C. vaginale* was associated with recurrence of signs of nonspecific vaginitis in the majority of patients treated with sulfonamide vaginal cream, doxycycline, or ampicillin, whereas all but one of the women given metronidazole had negative cultures for *C. vaginale* and clearing of vaginal discharge. Levison et al. (75) found only 70 percent of strains of *C. vaginale* to be inhibited by 12.5 μg of metronidazole per milliliter under anaerobic conditions, whereas Pheifer et al. (76) reported that all their strains were inhibited by 8 μg/ml of the compound under similar conditions.

Obviously, more studies are needed to elucidate further the role of *C. vaginale* in causing vaginitis. Of interest are reports of *C. vaginale* bacteremia, usually in association with septic abortion and postcesarean or postpartum endometritis but also occasionally in newborn babies (77–79). In most instances, there was prompt clinical response to ampicillin, penicillin, or cephalosporin (with or without aminoglycoside) therapy. Since Pheifer et al. (76) did find *C. vaginale* in the urethra of 79 percent of male partners of infected women, it is interesting to note a case report by Patrick and Garnett (80) of *C. vaginale* bacteremia which followed transurethral prostatectomy and which responded promptly to trimethoprim-sulfamethoxazole.

Urethritis   Another group of uncertain and controversial taxonomic and clinical status is the so-called NSU corynebacteria ("*Corynebacterium genitalium*"), believed by Furness and coworkers (81) to cause many episodes of nonspecific urethritis and epididymitis, as well as some cases of bacteriuria, cervicitis, conjunctivitis, pericarditis, bacteremia, osteomyelitis, and wound infections.

Skin and soft tissue infections

Skin   Although *P. acnes* is a prominent member of the indigenous cutaneous microflora, several lines of evidence suggest that this organism plays an important role in the pathogenesis of acne:

1   Adolescents with acne are more heavily colonized with *P. acnes* than those without.

2   Clinical improvement is directly related to the administration of antibiotics which decrease colonization with *P. acnes*.

3   *P. acnes* can activate complement.

4   *P. acnes* and extracts thereof, as well as lipase it produces, are chemotactic for neutrophils (82).

C. minutissimum is one of several species classified by Noble and Somerville (6) as fluorescent diphtheroids, i.e., porphyrin-producing, which are normally present on the skin and which multiply under certain conditions to produce a disease called *erythrasma*. The circumscribed, scaling, and red-fluorescing lesions associated with this disease occur in the intertriginous areas, especially the axilla, groin, and toewebs. Mild forms of the disease respond to antibacterial soap, while erythromycin is the drug of choice in severe cases (6).

Soft tissue infections *C. bovis* has been reported to be involved in an infected posttraumatic leg ulcer which cleared slowly with ampicillin and local measures (33), while *C. pyogenes* was involved in an infection of the foot with osteomyelitis and sinus tract formation following frostbite (83). In the latter case, the organism was also isolated from blood, and surgical drainage and sulfanilamide both failed to clear the foot infection.

Despite the frequency of their occurrence in the skin and upper respiratory tract, corynebacteria are seldom involved in wound infections following head and neck cancer surgery (84). Corynebacteria and propionibacteria accounted for 3 and 15 percent, respectively, of isolates from 33 scalp abscesses related to intrapartum direct fetal heart rate monitoring with a spiral electrode (85). Coryneform bacteria were infrequent isolates in a study of foot ulcers in diabetics by Louie et al. (86).

Henderson reported a case and reviewed six previously reported cases of suppurative lymphadenitis due to *C. pseudotuberculosis* (87). Histologically, the disease is characterized by tuberculoid granulomas with clusters of coryneform bacteria. The lesions may be acute or insidious in onset, and recovery usually follows excision of the involved nodes.

Bone and joint infections

Postoperative infections Although corynebacteria and propionibacteria can be isolated from approximately 20 percent of cultures taken of the operative wound during total hip arthroplasty (21, 22), these organisms rarely cause deep wound sepsis following this operation. In an analysis of 2694 patients who had 3215 total hip arthroplasties at the Mayo Clinic and who were followed for 2 to 5 years, deep wound sepsis occurred in 42 hips, 1 involved *P. acnes*, and none involved corynebacteria (88). Moggio et al. (22) and Petrini et al. (89) each reported one case with *P. acnes* infection following total hip or knee arthroplasty. In two cases the infections were late in onset (22, 89) while one occurred within 3 months of surgery (88).

Osteomyelitis According to two recent reviews, *P. acnes* is rarely involved in bone infections (90, 91). Two cases of osteomyelitis due to a microaerophilic diphtheroid and to *C. pyogenes*, respectively, were cited by Johnson and Kaye (24). Both were cured with antibiotic therapy. Newman and Mitchell (92) reported a case with osteomyelitis of the cervical spine due to *Propionibacterium* which responded to 15 weeks of benzylpenicillin, 2 g daily. Ceilley (93) reported a diabetic woman with a foot ulcer and lumbar vertebral osteomyelitis. *C. haemolyticum* was isolated from cultures of blood and a needle biopsy of the infected vertebra, which gradually responded to ampicillin (12 g intravenously daily for 6 weeks), followed by orally administered ampicillin with probenecid. Morrey et al. (94) reported three cases of osteomyelitis: one of the femur due to *P. acnes* and two of the elbow due to *Corynebacterium*; both of the latter were mixed infections (*Staph. epidermidis* in one case and group D streptococci in the other). In each case the coryneform bacteria were isolated from multiple operative sites. The patient with *P. acnes* infection underwent total hip arthroplasty and received penicillin G intravenously (20 million units daily) for 4 weeks, followed by 3 months of penicillin orally (500 mg daily), and was doing well at the time of follow-up 15 months later. The infection in the patient with the mixed *S. epidermidis–Corynebacterium* infection cleared with intravenous clindamycin (2.4 g daily) for 7 days, followed by 4 weeks of oral clindamycin (1.8 g daily). The third patient received multiple antibiotics without success and eventually underwent a shoulder disarticulation for an epithelioid sarcoma.

Septic arthritis   *C. pyogenes* was found to cause septic arthritis in the knee of a patient with a benign monoclonal gammopathy and localized plasmacytic reaction (95). The infection cleared following 4 months of oral penicillin G (800,000 units four times daily).

Rheumatoid arthritis   Whether coryneform bacteria play any role in rheumatoid arthritis remains unsettled. Several studies have demonstrated significantly higher isolation rates of various corynebacteria or propionibacteria from synovial fluids and membranes from patients with rheumatoid arthritis than from controls (96, 97). Since specimens from both groups of patients were apparently collected and processed in the same manner, it seems reasonable to conclude that some or most of the coryneform bacteria recovered were endogenous, rather than exogenous, in origin. Unfortunately, no epidemiological data were presented in any of the studies, and it would certainly be important to determine whether there was any correlation between a positive culture and a history of prior joint aspiration or injection or of prior surgery. Positive cultures of the operative wound during total hip arthroplasty, for example, were found by Fitzgerald et al. (21) to occur more frequently in hips which had undergone prior surgery than in those which had not. Attempts to link coryneform bacteria with rheumatoid arthritis by serological or immunological means remain inconclusive. As summarized by Marmion (98), the isolation of coryneform bacteria from synovial fluids and membranes from patients with rheumatoid arthritis may simply be a consequence of a deficiency in their reticuloendothelial system rather than a cause of their disease.

ANTIMICROBIAL SUSCEPTIBILITY

The majority (≥98 percent) of 118 strains of *Corynebacterium* from skin were found by Heczko et al. (99) to be susceptible to benzylpenicillin, ampicillin, amoxycillin, cephalosporins, tetracycline, gentamicin, kanamycin, neomycin,

Table 3   Antimicrobial susceptibility of group JK corynebacteria (4)

Antimicrobial	Cumulative % inhibited at increasing concentration, $\mu g/ml$					
	<1	2	4	8	16	32
Amikacin	51	61	62	63	63	64
Ampicillin	28	34	43	49	51	52
Cephalothin	25	30	42	47	48	48
Chloramphenicol	0	2	27	49	55	73
Clindamycin	26	31	38	45	45	47
Erythromycin	59	60	74	80	89	93
Gentamicin	57	58	59	60	60	60
Methicillin	8	74	24	25	27	40
Penicillin	28	36	44	46	48	48
Tetracycline	24	43	49	54	68	73
Vancomycin	100					

and erythromycin. All strains tested were susceptible to ≤12.5 $\mu g/ml$ of vancomycin and ≤0.04 $\mu g/ml$ of rifampin. Approximately 20 percent of strains required more than 3.1 $\mu g/ml$ of methicillin or cloxacillin for inhibition. Significantly less susceptible are the group JK corynebacteria (4, 60–62, 68), 85 strains of which were studied by Riley et al. (4) (Table 3).

Hoeffler et al. (100) determined the susceptibility of 73 strains of *P. acnes* and four related species (*P. granulosum*, *P. avidum*, *C. minutissimum*, and *C. parvum*) to 32 antimicrobial agents. Benzylpenicillin, ampicillin, cephalothin,

Table 4   Minimum inhibitory concentrations (MICs) of antibiotics for *Kurthia*

Antibiotic	MIC, $\mu g/ml$	Antibiotic	MIC, $\mu g/ml$
Penicillin	3.1	Erythromycin	0.78
Ampicillin	3.1	Chloramphenicol	3.13
Carbenicillin	100	Oxacillin	26
Cephalothin	25	Clindamycin	6.25
Gentamicin	6.25	Kanamycin	25
Amikacin	3.13		

minocycline, clindamycin, and erythromycin inhibited all strains at concentrations of ≤0.8 μg/ml. Rifampin inhibited all strains except *C. minutissimum* at concentrations of ≤0.2 μg/ml. Gentamicin was the most active aminoglycoside, inhibiting all strains at concentrations of ≤6.25 μg/ml. According to Finegold (25), vancomycin is quite active against most gram-positive anaerobic bacteria, including *Propionibacterium*.

In vitro susceptibility data for *Kurthia bessonii* are limited to those published by Faoagali (16) and Pancoast et al. (69). The former reported susceptibility to penicillin, ampicillin, sulfonamides, and tetracycline; the latter reported the following MICs in Table 4.

CONCLUSIONS

Coryneform bacteria have assumed increasing importance as a cause of opportunistic infections, especially in immunosuppressed hosts and those with implanted prosthetic material or devices. Therapy with penicillins, with or without an aminoglycoside, or erythromycin has generally proved effective, except in patients with granulocytopenia or implanted prosthetic materials or devices and in those infected with resistant (group JK) strains. Infected prosthetic materials or devices generally require removal or replacement. Because of the apparently increasing prevalence of resistant corynebacteria, it is necessary to determine the susceptibility of clinically significant coryneform bacteria to penicillins, cephalosporins, erythromycin, tetracycline, and vancomycin. As of this writing, all strains are uniformly susceptible to vancomycin.

REFERENCES

1 Cowan ST: *Manual for the Identification of Medical Bacteria*, ed 2. New York, Cambridge University Press, 1974, p 57.

2 Rogosa M et al: Coryneform group of bacteria, in *Bergey's Manual of Determinative Bacteriology*, ed 8. Baltimore, Williams & Wilkins, 1974, p 599.

3 Reddy CA, Kao M: Value of acid metabolic products in identification of certain corynebacteria. *J Clin Microbiol* 7:428, 1978.

4 Riley PS et al: Characterization and identification of 95 diphtheroid (group JK) cultures isolated from clinical specimens. *J Clin Microbiol* 9:418, 1979.

5 Holdeman LV et al: *Anaerobe Laboratory Manual*, ed 4. Blacksburg Va, Virginia Polytechnic Institute and State University, 1977, p 57.

6 Noble WC, Somerville DA: *Microbiology of Human Skin*. Philadelphia, Saunders, 1974.

7 Locatcher-Khorazo D, Seegal BC: *Microbiology of the Eye*. St. Louis, Mosby, 1972, p 13.

8 McNatt J et al: Anaerobic flora of the normal human conjunctival sac. *Arch Ophthalmol* 96:1448, 1978.

9 Peach S et al: The non-sporing anaerobic bacteria in human feces. *J Med Microbiol* 7:213, 1974.

10 Hammerschlag MR et al: Anaerobic microflora of the vagina in children. *Am J Obstet Gynecol* 131:853, 1978.

11 Tashjian JH et al: Vaginal flora in asymptomatic women. *Mayo Clin Proc* 51:557, 1976.

12 Levison ME et al: Quantitative microflora of the vagina. *Am J Obstet Gynecol* 127:80, 1977.

13 Finegold SM et al: Significance of anaerobic and capnophilic bacteria isolated from the urinary tract, in Kass EH (ed): *Progress in Pyelonephritis*. Philadelphia, Davis, 1965, p 159.

14 Pfan A, Sacks T: The bacterial flora of the vaginal vestibule, urethra and vagina in the normal premenopausal woman. *J Urol* 118:292, 1977.

15 Elston HR: *Kurthia bessonii* isolated from clinical material. *J Pathol Bacteriol* 81:245, 1961.

16 Faoagali JL: Kurthia, an unusual isolate. *Am J Clin Pathol* 62:604, 1974.

17 Knight HD: Corynebacterial infections, in Hubbert WT et al (eds): *Diseases Transmitted from Animals to Man*, ed 6. Springfield, Ill, Charles C Thomas, 1975, p 263.

18 **Ilstrup DM:** Organisms from blood cultures at the Mayo Clinic: 1968 to 1975, in Washington JA II (ed): *The Detection of Septicemia.* West Palm Beach, Fla, CRC Press, 1978, p 23.

19 **Wilson WR et al:** Prosthetic valve endocarditis. *Ann Intern Med* 82:751, 1975.

20 **Johnson WD:** Prosthetic valve endocarditis, in Kaye D (ed): *Infective Endocarditis.* Baltimore, University Park Press, 1976, p 129.

21 **Fitzgerald RH Jr et al:** Bacterial colonization of wounds and sepsis in total hip arthroplasty. *J Bone Joint Surg* 55-A: 1242, 1973.

22 **Moggio M et al:** Wound infections in patients undergoing total hip arthroplasty. *Arch Surg* 114:815, 1979.

23 **Kaplan K, Weinstein L:** Diphtheroid infections of man. *Ann Intern Med* 70:919, 1969.

24 **Johnson WD, Kaye D:** Serious infections caused by diphtheroids. *Ann NY Acad Sci* 174:568, 1970.

25 **Finegold SM:** *Anaerobic Bacteria in Human Disease.* New York, Academic, 1977.

26 **Hanscom T, Maxwell WA:** *Corynebacterium* endophthalmitis: Laboratory studies and report of a case treated by vitrectomy. *Arch Ophthalmol* 97:500, 1979.

27 **Jones DB, Robinson NM:** Anaerobic ocular infections. *Trans Am Acad Ophthalmol Otolaryngol* 83:309, 1977.

28 **Forster RK:** Etiology and diagnosis of bacterial postoperative endophthalmitis. *Trans Am Acad Ophthalmol Otolaryngol* 85:320, 1978.

29 **Friedman E et al:** Endophthalmitis caused by *Propionibacterium acnes. Can J Ophthalmol* 13:50, 1978.

30 **Brewer NS et al:** Brain abscess: A review of recent experience. *Ann Intern Med* 82:571, 1975.

31 **Washington JA II et al:** Brain abscess with *Corynebacterium haemolyticum:* Report of a case. *Am J Clin Pathol* 56:212, 1971.

32 **Altmann G, Bogokovsky B:** Brain abscess due to *Corynebacterium haemolyticum. Lancet* 1:378, 1973.

33 **Vale JA, Scott GW:** *Corynebacterium bovis* as a cause of human disease. *Lancet* 2:682, 1977.

34 **Schlesinger JJ, Ross AL:** *Propionibacterium acnes* meningitis in a previously normal adult. *Arch Intern Med* 137:921, 1977.

35 **French RS et al:** Chronic meningitis caused by *Propionibacterium acnes. Neurology* 24:624, 1974.

36 **Nastasi G et al:** Colonization of Spitz-Holter valves by rare bacterial flora. *Acta Neurochir (Vienna)* 26:173, 1972.

37 **Schoenbaum SC et al:** Infections of cerebrospinal fluid shunts: Epidemiology, clinical manifestations, and therapy. *J Infect Dis* 131:543, 1975.

38 **Bolton WK et al:** Ventriculojugular shunt nephritis with *Corynebacterium bovis. Am J Med* 59:417, 1975.

39 **Beeler BA et al:** *Propionibacterium acnes:* Pathogen in central nervous system shunt infection: Report of three cases including immune complex glomerulonephritis. *Am J Med* 61:935, 1976.

40 **Skinner PR et al:** Propionibacteria as a cause of shunt and postneurosurgical infections. *J Clin Pathol* 31:1085, 1978.

41 **Fulghum RS et al:** Anaerobic bacteria in otitis media. *Ann Otol* 86:196, 1977.

42 **Brook I et al:** Aerobic and anaerobic bacteriology of acute otitis media in children. *J Pediatr* 92:13, 1978.

43 **Brook I et al:** Bacteriology of chronic otitis media. *JAMA* 241:487, 1979.

44 **Giebink GS et al:** The microbiology of serous and mucoid otitis media. *Pediatrics* 63:915, 1979.

45 **MacLean PD et al:** A hemolytic corynebacterium resembling *Corynebacterium ovis* and *Corynebacterium pyogenes* in man. *J Infect Dis* 79:69, 1946.

46 **Ryan WJ:** Throat infection and rash associated with an unusual corynebacterium. *Lancet* 2:1345, 1972.

47 **Fell HWK et al:** *Corynebacterium haemolyticum* infections in Cambridgeshire. *J Hyg* 79:269, 1977.

48 **Golub B et al:** Lung abscess due to *Corynebacterium equi:* Report of first human infection. *Ann Intern Med* 66:1174, 1967.

49 **Savdie E et al:** Lung abscess due to *Corynebacterium equi* in a renal transplant recipient. *Med J Aust* 1:817, 1977.

50 **Marsh JC, von Graevenitz A:** Recurrent *Corynebacterium equi* infection with lymphoma. *Cancer* 32:147, 1973.

51 **Gardner SE et al:** Pneumonitis due to *Corynebacterium equi. Chest* 70:92, 1976.

52 **Carpenter JL, Blom J:** *Corynebacterium equi* pneumonia in a patient with Hodgkin's disease. *Am Rev Respir Dis* 114:235, 1976.

53 **Berg R et al:** *Corynebacterium equi* infection complicating neoplastic disease. *Am J Clin Pathol* 68:73, 1977.

54 **Chlosta EM et al:** An opportunistic infection with *Corynebacterium pyogenes* producing empyema. *Am J Clin Pathol* 53:167, 1970.

55 **Vega LE, Gavan TL:** *Corynebacterium pyogenes*—a pathogen in man. Report of a case. *Cleve Clin Q* 37:207, 1970.

56 **Hajickova V, Hajicek V:** *Corynebacterium pyogenes* varietas *hominis* als Ursache

einer fibrosierenden Bronchopneumo-
pathie. *Schweiz Med Wochenschr* 102:142,
1972.

57 **Nazemi MM, Musher DM:** Empyema due
to aerobic diphtheroids following dental
extraction. *Am Rev Respir Dis* 108:1221,
1973.

58 **Jacobs NF, Perlino CA:** "Diphtheroid"
pneumonia. *South Med J* 72:475, 1979.

59 **Keslin MH et al:** Corynebacterium
pseudotuberculosis: A new cause of infectious and eosinophilic pneumonia. *Am J
Med* 67:228, 1979.

60 **Hande KR et al:** Sepsis with a new species
of *Corynebacterium. Ann Intern Med*
85:423, 1976.

61 **Pearson TA et al:** *Corynebacterium* sepsis
in oncology patients: Predisposing factors,
diagnosis, and treatment. *JAMA* 238:1739,
1977.

62 **Stamm WE et al:** Infection due to
Corynebacterium species in marrow transplant patients. *Ann Intern Med* 91:167,
1979.

63 **Weiner M, Werthamer S:** *Corynebacterium aquaticum* septicemia. *Am J Clin
Pathol* 64:378, 1975.

64 **Jobanputra RS, Swain CP:** Septicaemia
due to *Corynebacterium haemolyticum. J
Clin Pathol* 28:798, 1975.

65 **Irwin RS et al:** Cell wall–deficient bacterial cultural surveillance: A useful
laboratory aid. *Am J Med* 59:129, 1975.

66 **Collins RN et al:** Risk of local and systemic infection with polyethylene intravenous catheters: A prospective study
of 213 catheterizations. *N Engl J Med*
279:340, 1968.

67 **Maki DG et al:** A semi-quantitative culture method for identifying intravenous-
catheter-related infection. *N Engl J Med*
296:1305, 1977.

68 **Van Scoy RE et al:** Coryneform bacterial
endocarditis: Difficulties in diagnosis and
treatment, presentation of three cases, and
review of literature. *Mayo Clin Proc*
52:216, 1977.

69 **Pancoast SJ et al:** Endocarditis due to
Kurthia bessonii. Ann Intern Med 90:936,
1979.

70 **Goodhart GL et al:** Pigment vs. choles-
terol cholelithiasis: Bacteriology of gallbladder stone, bile, and tissue correlated
with biliary lipid analysis. *Digestive Dis*
23:877, 1978.

71 **Balfour HH, Minken SL:** Liver abscess
due to *Corynebacterium acnes:* Diphtheroid as a pathogen. *Clin Pediatr* 10:55,
1971.

72 **Muangmanee L, Jaroonvesama N:** Diphtheroid liver abscess: Report of a case. *J
Med Ass Thail* 57:207, 1974.

73 **Segura JW et al:** Anaerobic bacteria in the
urinary tract. *Mayo Clin Proc* 47:30, 1972.

74 **Laufe LE:** Acute ulcerative vulvovaginitis
due to *Corynebacterium pyogenes. Obstet
Gynecol* 3:46, 1954.

75 **Levison ME et al:** Quantitative bacteriology of the vaginal flora in vaginitis. *Am J
Obstet Gynecol* 133:139, 1979.

76 **Pheifer TA et al:** Nonspecific vaginitis:
Role of *Haemophilus vaginalis* and treatment with metronidazole. *N Engl J Med*
298:1429, 1978.

77 **Regamey C, Schoenknecht FD:** Puerperal
fever with *Haemophilus vaginalis* septicemia. *JAMA* 225:1621, 1973.

78 **Monif GRG, Baer H:** *Haemophilus
(Corynebacterium) vaginalis* septicemia.
Am J Obstet Gynecol 120:1041, 1974.

79 **Venkataramani TK, Rathbun HK:**
*Corynebacterium vaginale (Hemophilus
vaginalis)* bacteremia: Clinical study of 29
cases. *Johns Hopkins Med J* 139:93, 1976.

80 **Patrick S, Garnett PA:** *Corynebacterium
vaginale* bacteraemia in a man. *Lancet*
1:987, 1978.

81 **Furness G, Evangelista AT:** A diagnostic
key employing biological reactions for dif-
ferentiating pathogenic *Corynebacterium
genitalium* (NSU corynebacteria) from
commensals of the urogenital tract. *Invest
Urol* 16:1, 1978.

82 **Esterly NB, Furey NL:** Acne: Current
concepts. *Pediatrics* 62:1044, 1978.

83 **Ballard DO et al:** Infection due to
Corynebacterium pyogenes in man. *Am J
Clin Pathol* 17:209, 1947.

84 **Becker GD et al:** Anaerobic and aerobic
bacteriology in head and neck cancer surgery. *Arch Otolaryngol* 104:591, 1978.

85 **Okada DM et al:** Neonatal scalp abscess
and fetal monitoring: Factors associated
with infections. *Am J Obstet Gynecol*
129:185, 1977.

86 **Louie TJ et al:** Aerobic and anaerobic bacteria in diabetic foot ulcers. *Ann Intern
Med* 85:461, 1976.

87 **Henderson A:** Pseudotuberculous adenitis
caused by *Corynebacterium pseudotuberculosis. J Med Microbiol* 12:147, 1979.

88 **Fitzgerald RH Jr et al:** Deep wound sepsis
following total hip arthroplasty. *J Bone
Joint Surg* 59-A:847, 1977.

89 **Petrini B et al:** Anaerobic bacteria in late
infections following orthopedic surgery.
Med Microbiol Immunol 167:155, 1979.

90 **Raff MJ, Melo JC:** Anaerobic osteomyelitis.
Medicine 57:83, 1978.

91 **Lewis RP et al:** Bone infections involving
anaerobic bacteria. *Medicine* 57:279, 1978.

92 **Newman JH, Mitchell RG:** Diphtheroid
infection of the cervical spine. *Acta Or-
thop Scand* 46:67, 1975.

93 **Ceilley RI:** Foot ulceration and vertebral osteomyelitis with *Corynebacterium*

88 Current clinical topics in infectious diseases

haemolyticum. Arch Dermatol 113:646, 1977.

94 **Morrey BF et al:** Diphtheroid osteomyelitis. *J Bone Joint Surg* 59-A:527, 1977.

95 **Norenberg DD et al:** *Corynebacterium pyogenes* septic arthritis with plasma cell synovial infiltrate and monoclonal gammopathy. *Arch Intern Med* 138:810, 1978.

96 **Bartholomew LE, Nelson FR:** *Corynebacterium acnes* in rheumatoid arthritis: I. Isolation and antibody studies. *Ann Rheum Dis* 31:22, 1972.

97 **Duthie JJR et al:** Do diphtheroids cause rheumatoid arthritis? In Dumonde DC

(ed): *Infection and Immunology in the Rheumatic Diseases*. Oxford, Blackwell, 1976, p 171.

98 **Marmion BP:** A microbiologist's view of investigative rheumatology, in Dumonde DC (ed): *Infection and Immunology in the Rheumatic Diseases*. Oxford, Blackwell, 1976, p 245.

99 **Heczko PB et al:** Susceptibility of human skin aerobic diphtheroids to antimicrobial agents in vitro. *J Antimicrob Chemother* 3:141, 1977.

100 **Hoeffler U et al:** Antimicrobial susceptibility of *Propionibacterium acnes* and related microbial species. *Antimicrob Agents Chemother* 10:387, 1976.

Rocky Mountain spotted fever: a clinical dilemma

LISA G. KAPLOWITZ
JANET J. FISCHER
P. FREDERICK SPARLING

INTRODUCTION

Rocky Mountain spotted fever (RMSF, tick-borne typhus fever) is the most prevalent rickettsial disease in the United States, and its reported incidence has been gradually increasing since 1959. For the past 30 years, most cases of RMSF have occurred in the southeastern United States, with smaller endemic foci scattered throughout the country (1–6). The biology, ecology, and epidemiology of the causative organism, *Rickettsia rickettsii*, and its major tick vectors (the dog ticks and wood ticks) are well understood and discussed elsewhere (4, 6–10). The purpose of this review is to discuss the spectrum of clinical presentations of RMSF and to summarize new developments in diagnosis and disease prevention.

In spite of the availability of effective antibiotic therapy (11–13), mortality from this disease has remained in the range of 5 to 8 percent, compared with mortality in the preantibiotic era of approximately 20 percent (6, 14). Most deaths can be attributed to a delay in diagnosis of rickettsial disease and in institution of appropriate therapy by the physician and not to a delay by patients in seeking treatment (6, 15, 16). Difficulties in diagnosis are due in part to lack of a widely available laboratory test that is sensitive and reactive early in the disease. Therefore, a presumptive diagnosis must be made, and therapy begun, based on the clinical presentation of the patient and a history of possible tick exposure. RMSF is a systemic illness with protean manifestations, and in our experience, serious errors can sometimes be made if one waits for "typical" illness to develop before instituting therapy.

We reviewed the experience with this disease at the North Carolina Memorial Hospital over a 10-year period (1970–1979) and found 131 cases that were clinically and serologically consistent with Rocky Mountain spotted fever; 60

L.G.K. was supported in part by Public Health Service grant AI07151-01 from the National Institute of Allergy and Infectious Diseases. We gratefully acknowledge the assistance of Suzanne Edwards in the computer analysis of our RMSF data and David Walker for his helpful discussions other cases with a consistent clinical course lacked adequate serologic documentation and are excluded from this discussion. Our cases spanned all ages and included outpatients as well as inpatients; all occurred between April and early October. Of the 131 patients, 54 were classified as definite on the basis of a positive immunofluorescent stain of tissue for rickettsiae, a positive rickettsial isolation, or a fourfold rise in complement-fixing antibody to the spotted fever group of antigens. The remaining 77 were classified as probable on the basis of compatible clinical illness (fever plus headache and/or rash) plus any one of the following criteria: (1) autopsy findings of a diffuse small vessel vasculitis consistent with RMSF; (2) positive convalescent complement-fixation antibody titer (single titer greater than or equal to 1:8); (3) fourfold rise or fall in Weil-Felix agglutinins (OX19 or OX2); or (4) single reciprocal titer OX19 or OX2 ≥ 320 with classic clinical course including a typical distribution of the rash. The definite and probable cases were similar in most respects, but patients with definite RMSF generally had more severe disease. Analysis of the illness suffered by these patients forms the basis for much of this report. Comparisons with other series are limited to those with some serologic documentation or rickettsial isolation.

PATHOGENESIS

Rickettsemia occurs early in the course of infection, followed by rickettsial invasion of vascular endothelium (17). The organisms then proliferate within the nucleus and cytoplasm of endothelial and smooth muscle cells of the capillary bed, leading eventually to a diffuse necrotizing vasculitis (17). Although the existence of a toxin has been postulated, there is at present no firm evidence for the production of a clinically significant toxic substance by R. *rickettsii*. Cellular damage appears to result directly from rickettsial parasitization (17). Vasculitis and thrombosis resulting from localized rickettsial proliferation can occur in any organ system, accounting for the systemic nature of the disease.

CLINICAL PRESENTATIONS

The prodrome

After an incubation period of 2 to 14 days, the disease usually begins with fever, malaise, headache, and myalgias. Table 1 summarizes the incidence of each of the major presenting complaints from recent well-documented clinical series. Fever has been present in all the cases studied, often greater than 102°F. Morning remission of fever is not uncommon, with maximum febrile response occurring in the afternoon and evening (18). The reported incidence of headache varies from 53 to 92 percent. Series with large numbers of young children have a lower incidence of this symptom, since children under 5 years old often do not complain of headache. For older children and adults, the incidence of headache is greater than 80 percent. Myalgias have been noted in 45 to 83 percent of patients. These symptoms are nonspecific; it is the rash of RMSF, usually occurring 3 to 4 days after the onset of symptoms, that is considered the

Table 1   Early clinical manifestations of RMSF

	Present series* (N = 131)		Other series, %	Ref.
	No.	%		
Fever	131	100	100	1, 3, 5, 6, 19
>102°F	115	88		
Headache	104	79	53–92	3, 5, 6, 19
Myalgias	94	72	45–83	3, 5, 6

* North Carolina Memorial Hospital 1970–1979.

hallmark of the disease and the usual indication for institution of specific therapy.

Rash

The presence of a rash has been accepted by many as essential for the diagnosis of Rocky Mountain spotted fever. Since a significant number of clinical series require the presence of a rash for inclusion in their study, it is difficult to determine the true incidence of this sign in RMSF. In the large epidemiologic review by Hattwick et al. (6) 92 percent of 778 laboratory-confirmed cases had a rash. This correlates well with our series, in which 90 percent of the cases had a rash at some time during the illness (Table 2). Of the 13 patients without rash, 6 were black and 7 white.

The onset of rash can be quite variable. In our series, 14 percent developed the rash on the first day of symptoms, and 77 percent of those with rash developed it by the fifth day of clinical illness. In contrast, 24 patients (20 percent of those with rash) had no rash until the sixth day of illness or later; 6 of these patients developed the rash after day 10. In 4 patients the day of onset of rash was unknown. Late onset of rash may result in fatal delay in diagnosis and institution of therapy (24). One case from our series illustrates this point.

H.W., a 68-year-old white male, noted a tick attached to his neck in late July; 3 days later he had the onset of fever of 102°F, nausea, diarrhea, and malaise. He presented to the medical clinic on the first day of illness and was diagnosed as having a viral

Table 2   Rash in RMSF

	Present series		Other series, %	Ref.
	No. of patients No. tested	%		
Any rash	118/131	90	92	6
Palms or soles distribution	97/118	82	23–77	1, 3, 5
Petechial rash	53/118	45	35–60	6, 19

syndrome. He returned 2 days later with a temperature of 104°F and continued malaise; serum sodium level and platelet count were normal. Aside from a tachycardia and minimal lymphadenopathy, his physical examination was unremarkable. The diagnosis of RMSF was considered, but no therapy was instituted because of the lack of rash. On the sixth day of illness, a punctate rash was noted on the lower extremities. The rash became more diffuse and the patient became lethargic throughout the day. By the time he returned to the hospital early on the seventh day of illness, he was comatose and hypotensive; the rash had become ecchymotic. A skin biopsy revealed large numbers of rickettsiae by immunofluorescent stain. He expired later in the day in spite of institution of chloramphenicol and intensive supportive care.

Most often the rash of RMSF begins on the extremities, often around the wrists and ankles, and spreads centripetally to the trunk, with relative sparing of the face. It may start with a truncal or diffuse distribution, however. In Vianna's series, 13 percent had the rash begin on the abdomen and 10 percent had a diffuse onset of rash (3).

The rash often involves the palms and/or soles as it progresses. In our study, 82 percent of those with rash had involvement of the palms or soles at some point in their illness. In other series where this has been noted, between 23 and 77 percent of cases had a rash involving palms or soles (1, 3, 5). It is important to note that the distribution of the rash on the palms and soles may not occur until late in the course of the disease. Almost half (43 percent) of our patients with palm and sole involvement developed this distribution after the fifth day of disease.

The rash of RMSF not only changes distribution with time but often changes character as well (14, 18, 19). It usually begins as maculopapular lesions that may progress to become petechial or ecchymotic. In our series 45 percent of those with a rash had petechial or hemorrhagic lesions some time in their course; most of these (39 out of 53, or 74 percent) developed the petechial lesions on or after the sixth day of disease. Other series have reported from 35 to 60 percent incidence of petechial rash (6, 19). Very rarely, the rash may be urticarial or pruritic, as noted in two of our patients.

While the character of the rash of RMSF can help differentiate this disease from other acute infectious exanthems, one should not require the presence of a classic rash to consider the diagnosis. Up to 10 percent of patients with RMSF do not have rash, and the exanthem may occur too late for therapy to be effective.

Gastrointestinal and hepatic manifestations

The frequency of gastrointestinal signs and symptoms in RMSF (Table 3) has not been appreciated by most physicians. Of our patients, 82 of 131 (63 percent) had nausea, vomiting, or diarrhea before therapy was started. In most the onset of gastrointestinal symptoms occurred in the first 3 days of illness (56 out of 82 or 68 percent); 7 percent (9 out of 131) of our patients reported gastrointestinal distress as their chief complaint, and many were initially diagnosed as having viral gastroenteritis. Middleton recently discussed the importance of gastroin-

Table 3 Gastrointestinal symptoms and signs in RMSF

	Present series* (N = 131)		Other series†	
	No.	%	%	Ref.
Nausea or vomiting	73	56	30–66	3, 5
Diarrhea	26	20	1–13	3, 5
Abdominal pain	44	34	6–33	3, 5
Hepatomegaly	20	15	20–25	3, 19
Splenomegaly	18	14	15–44	1, 3, 5, 19
Jaundice	10	8		

* On presentation.
† Time of occurrence in illness not specified.

testinal symptoms in 66 patients from this institution seen between 1970 and 1974 (20).

Abdominal pain is a relatively common symptom in this disease. Many with this symptom actually have severe myalgias of the abdominal wall musculature; in others the pain is of gastrointestinal or hepatic origin. Those with severe abdominal pain may be mistakenly thought to have an acute surgical abdomen (5).

W.E., a 17-year-old black female, noted the onset of malaise in mid-May and 4 days later noted lower abdominal pain which gradually increased, with associated nausea and vomiting. She was admitted on the seventh day of illness with a fever of 103.6°F and diffuse abdominal pain with rebound tenderness. She was treated with chloramphenicol for presumed bacterial peritonitis. The pain localized to the right upper quadrant, and the day after admission she had surgery for presumed cholecystitis. The gallbladder and biliary tree were normal at surgery, but the liver was diffusely enlarged; a liver biopsy showed minimal inflammation. Transaminase values were normal throughout her hospitalization. Two days after surgery, macular lesions were noted on her forearms and abdomen. She did well with continuation of chloramphenicol therapy. Convalescent serum showed a diagnostic rise in complement-fixation antibodies to RMSF.

Hepatomegaly and splenomegaly occur in a significant percentage of patients. In our series 16 patients had elevated serum bilirubin values at the time of diagnosis, reaching a maximum of 12 mg/dl (Table 4); 26 patients had elevation of SGPT. Elevations in hepatic transaminases have also been noted in the literature (21, 22). The SGOT was consistently higher than the SGPT in those patients in whom both were measured, possibly reflecting the presence of myositis rather than hepatitis. Unfortunately, not enough concurrent CPK or aldolase values were available to confirm this hypothesis. Of 62 patients with alkaline phosphatase levels measured before therapy, 22 had mildly to moder-

Table 4   Serum bilirubin and transaminases before therapy in RMSF (present series)

	No. of patients
	No. tested
Bilirubin, mg/dl:	
1.5–4.9	10/53
5.0–9.9	3/53
10–12	3/53
SGOT (normal 7–29 units/liter)	
60–99	10/71
100–500	25/71
>500	9/71
SGPT (normal 12–29 units/liter)	
60–99	11/66
100–500	15/66

ately elevated values; no fractionation of this enzyme was done. Five patients with elevated bilirubin or transaminase values died; two of the five had mild vasculitis of the portal triads at autopsy.

In summary, gastrointestinal symptoms are common in RMSF. Abdominal pain is also not infrequent and may be due to myositis of the abdominal muscles. The incidence of hepatitis is difficult to determine but when present is usually mild.

Skeletal muscle involvement

Myalgias are common in RMSF and occurred in 72 percent of our patients (94 out of 131). Of these, 22 had severe myalgias (17 percent), most with marked muscle tenderness on physical examination. Skeletal muscle involvement has been noted in isolated case reports, associated with marked elevation in CPK and aldolase values (21, 23). Severe muscle weakness was also noted in one case (23). Of the 24 in our series who had CPK measured, it was elevated in 10, often to very high levels (100 times normal levels). Myositis is probably more common in RMSF than is generally realized. Most of the patients with markedly elevated CPK values had involvement of several other organ systems as well.

Central nervous system manifestations

It has been realized for many years that a significant number of patients with RMSF have central nervous system abnormalities as part of their illness (24–26). The incidence of neurologic dysfunction varies according to the severity of illness in the patients reported and the specific definition of neurologic abnormalities but has varied from 21 to 77 percent in series of serologically documented cases (1, 3, 5, 6, 19).

Headache, the most common neurologic symptom, may be diffuse and is often bifrontal and frequently severe. Of the 104 patients in our series with headache, 28 percent described it as severe. Since young children often do not complain of headache, it is an unreliable symptom in those under 5 years old. Lethargy is frequently noted and, less commonly, confusion or disorientation. In our series 37 patients (28 percent) were noted to be confused during their illness. These patients may be unable to provide an adequate history of exposure to ticks initially, making diagnosis more difficult.

Thirty patients (23 percent) had more serious neurologic complications, including stupor or delirium, seizures, ataxia, papilledema, focal neurologic deficits, and coma (Table 5). Specific localizing signs were uncommon, although a few patients did have focal signs on neurologic examination, as has been reported by others (26). Transient hearing loss has been reported to occur in RMSF but was not found in our series (3, 19, 27). Cranial and peripheral nerve abnormalities may also occur but are extremely rare (24).

When neurologic signs are prominent, the diagnosis of RMSF may be overlooked, especially in the absence of rash, as illustrated with the following case.

K.B., a 6-year-old black girl, presented with a 2-week history of fever and lethargy, progressing to ataxia and seizures. A transient rash had been present about a week into her illness but none was present on admission. The initial diagnosis was viral meningoencephalitis. A markedly positive OX19 titer was obtained on the fifteenth day of illness and chloramphenicol begun. In spite of the late institution of therapy, she did well, with apparent recovery of full neurologic function except for possible residual cognitive dysfunction. Convalescent complement-fixation titer was 1:32 compared with an acute titer of 0.

The diagnosis may not be considered in the elderly with neurologic dysfunction since RMSF is primarily a disease of children and young adults. Four patients in our series were elderly women who presented primarily with abnor-

Table 5 Neurologic complications of RMSF (present series, $N = 131$)

	No.	%
Any severe neurologic complication	30	23
Stupor or delirium	28	21
Coma	13	10
Seizures	11	8
Ataxia	7	5
Focal neurologic signs	3	2
Papilledema	2	1.5

mal mental status. All were febrile, but two had no rash initially. Therapy was delayed in only one patient and all did well after appropriate therapy.

Neck stiffness is a relatively common complaint, occurring in 32 of our patients (24 percent). Often this is due to myalgias of the neck musculature. A total of 23 patients (17.5 percent) were felt to have true meningismus; 36 patients (27 percent) complained of photophobia. The incidence of meningeal signs has ranged from 13 to 25 percent when this sign has been noted (1, 3, 5). Meningitis, bacterial or viral, is often considered in the differential diagnosis in these patients.

Many authors claim that the cerebrospinal fluid is invariably normal in RMSF. Our results (Table 6) support others who have documented increased protein and pleocytosis in some patients (27–29). Since only the sickest patients generally had a lumbar puncture, it is probable that the frequencies of abnormal values reported in Table 6 are higher than would be found in unselected patients with RMSF. Cerebrospinal fluid pleocytosis (>5 WBC per cubic millimeter) occurred in 24 out of 63 patients (38 percent); 9 patients had CSF white blood cell counts over 100 per cubic millimeter. All patients with total CSF white blood cell counts greater than 100 had between 70 and 95 percent polymorphonuclear leukocytes; 5 patients had modest depression of CSF glucose (<50 mg/dl) without evidence for concomitant bacterial meningitis; all of these had very serious disease, and 4 died.

Brain scans were done in a few patients and were all normal. EEGs done on

Table 6   Cerebrospinal fluid findings in RMSF* (present series)

	No. of patients No. tested
Elevated opening pressure, $\geq$250 mmH$_2$O	5/35
Elevated protein, mg/dl	22/62
50–99	16
100–300	6
Decreased glucose, <50 mg/dl	5/62
Elevated white blood cell count, WBC/mm³	24/63
5–9	9
10–99	8
$\geq$100	7
Differential white blood cell count, among those with $\geq$5 WBC/mm³	
Lymphocyte predominance	11/24
Polymorphonuclear predominance	12/24
Unknown	1/24

* Of 131 patients in the North Carolina Memorial Hospital series, a lumbar puncture was performed in 63 before therapy.

those with marked neurologic abnormalities showed diffuse cortical dysfunction; one patient showed some localization of EEG abnormalities. This is in agreement with EEG abnormalities found by others (24).

Of the 30 patients with marked neurologic dysfunction, 10 died. Of the 20 who survived, all eventually recovered neurologic function; one patient required months to recover fully, and the child discussed above may have residual cognitive dysfunction. No formal psychometric testing was done on any patients after recovery. Few have studied the extent of permanent neurologic damage in patients with RMSF. Rosenblum et al. studied 37 patients 1 to 8 years after the episode of RMSF and reported that 21 had residual neurologic abnormalities detected by history, physical examinations, or EEG (30). Many of these findings were subjective, however, including headache, emotional lability, nervousness, and overactivity; no control group was studied. Abnormal EEGs were reported for 12 patients. There was some correlation between residual neurologic damage and severity of initial disease, including duration of fever. Those treated early had a low incidence of residual damage. A recent study attempted to measure the intellectual sequelae of RMSF in 12 children (31). Compared with matched controls, those with prior RMSF had mild but consistent defects in intellectual functioning. No correlation was attempted between the severity of RMSF and subsequent levels of intelligence. In summary, neurologic dysfunction is relatively common in RMSF, and although prompt therapy often appears to prevent serious sequelae in survivors, permanent impairment may occur.

Ocular manifestations

Conjunctivitis occurs relatively frequently in RMSF (1, 5) and was noted in 40 of our patients (30 percent) and in 15 to 45 percent of cases elsewhere. Conjunctival petechiae have also been noted by others (19) and were seen in at least one of our patients. Other ocular involvement is not usually reported, but in the past 10 years there have been reports of funduscopic changes in RMSF and one report of anterior nongranulomatous uveitis (32–35). Retinal abnormalities have included retinal vein engorgement, retinal edema, flame-shaped hemorrhages, papilledema, cytoid bodies, and arterial occlusion (33). Fluorescein angiography may show focal areas of capillary nonperfusion with perivascular staining adjacent to infarcted areas (35). Patients with papilledema had normal spinal fluid pressure (33). The optic fundus findings are quite compatible with a small vessel vasculitis, with associated vessel thrombosis and microinfarcts, similar to pathologic findings in other organs. All the retinal abnormalities resolved with appropriate treatment of RMSF.

Cardiovascular manifestations

Direct invasion of vascular endothelium by rickettsiae results in a necrotizing vasculitis, with increased capillary permeability and extravasation of fluid from the vasculature. Edema was noted in 26 of our patients (20 percent) and was often periorbital; other series have had an incidence of edema of from 4 to 33 percent

(1, 3, 5). Of 60 patients in whom albumen was measured, 24 had a level less than 3 g/dl. Hypoalbuminemia and edema were correlated with increased severity of disease as determined by the number of complications present.

Hypotension and shock can result from increased capillary permeability; 22 of our patients (17 percent) had significant hypotension before therapy was instituted. The incidence of hypotension is poorly documented in other series. Often, the correction of hypotension by intravenous administration of saline or colloid solutions results in the development or exacerbation of edema; the edema resolves once vascular integrity has been restored.

Direct myocardial involvement can also occur in this disease, with exacerbation of hypotension in some cases (3, 27, 28). Of 70 patients who had ECGs in our series, 18 (26 percent) had abnormalities consistent with myocarditis and 11 had arrhythmias, including nodal rhythm, atrial fibrillation, and terminal arrhythmias. Congestive heart failure may occur as a result of myocarditis, but it is often difficult to differentiate cardiac failure from the pneumonitis and pulmonary edema that are a direct result of rickettsial vasculitis. Bradford and Hackel reported myocardial lesions in all fatal cases (36). Five of their patients had ECG evidence of myocarditis before death, and two had enzymatic evidence of myocardial damage. Autopsy series are obviously a highly biased sample, however, and clinically evident myocarditis is relatively uncommon in patients less severely affected by RMSF.

Renal involvement

While renal failure in RMSF has been noted in isolated case reports (16, 37), it has received relatively little attention compared with other complications of the disease. In our series, 18 patients (14 percent) had renal insufficiency with BUN values greater than 50 mg/dl before therapy; no patient had known prior renal disease. Urinalyses revealed mild to moderate proteinuria in many and mild pyuria in a few patients but did not reveal more specific abnormalities. A few patients responded rapidly to intravenous hydration with increased urine output and a fall in BUN and creatinine; three required peritoneal dialysis. Of the 18 patients with renal failure, 10 died, including the 3 who were dialyzed. Patients with renal insufficiency who survived had complete recovery of renal function without obvious permanent renal damage. The long-term effects on the kidneys are unknown, however.

In most cases, the acute renal failure of RMSF is a consequence of hypovolemia, hypotension, and subsequent acute tubular necrosis. Rhabdomyolysis with myoglobinuria has been postulated as a possible cause of renal failure but has not been documented to date (37). Similarly, there is little evidence for immunologic renal or vascular damage. Walker and Mattern recently reviewed the clinical and pathologic aspects of renal failure in RMSF in 10 fatal cases from this hospital (37). The major renal lesion was a focal perivascular nephritis similar to the small vessel vasculitis seen in other organs; no clinical or pathologic evidence of acute glomerulonephritis was found. They did not feel this renal lesion could be implicated in the pathogenesis of acute renal failure, in agreement with other studies (38).

Pulmonary involvement

Twenty-two patients in our series (17 percent) had pneumonitis before treatment, as evidenced by an abnormal physical examination or chest radiograph. Five patients were initially diagnosed as having pneumonia or bronchitis because of prominent respiratory symptoms. Sixteen patients developed severe respiratory difficulties in the course of their disease. In most, respiratory decompensation was due to an exacerbation of pneumonitis and the development of noncardiogenic pulmonary edema. Two patients acquired pulmonary superinfections, with one case each of proteus and mucor pneumonia. The patient with mucor pneumonia died on the twelfth day of RMSF and at autopsy had evidence of both systemic mucormycosis and rickettsial disease by appropriate fungal and fluorescent rickettsial stains. Ten patients required support with a mechanical respirator; nine of these died.

Donohue has recently discussed in greater detail pulmonary involvement in 33 patients hospitalized with RMSF at this hospital and summarized previous reports of pneumonitis in the literature (39). Cough was a prominent symptom in one-third of the patients he studied. Radiographic changes included interstitial and alveolar infiltrates, consolidation, and pleural effusions, in agreement with other reports (40). Pleural effusions, present in five patients in Donohue's series, were small and in two patients were bilateral. Thoracenteses were performed in two patients, one of whom had a transudate, the other an exudate.

Noncardiogenic pulmonary edema, secondary to fluid extravasation from the pulmonary vasculature, is usually responsible for pulmonary infiltrates and impaired gas exchange. Retrospective analysis of lung tissue from autopsied cases has revealed rickettsiae in pulmonary capillary endothelium by immunofluorescent staining, supporting the role of direct capillary damage as the cause of pneumonitis (41). Since pulmonary edema is often initiated or exacerbated by the administration of large amounts of intravenous fluids, care should be taken with fluid management so that blood pressure and cardiac output will be maintained while pulmonary capillary hydrostatic pressure is minimized (39). Cardiac dysfunction may contribute to the development of pulmonary edema but usually is of secondary importance.

Coagulopathy and bleeding complications

Coagulopathies associated with RMSF have been noted in many published case reports (42–47). In our series 20 patients (15 percent) had a coagulopathy or clinical bleeding; 14 (11 percent) had a circulating anticoagulant, elevated fibrin split products, or low fibrinogen levels. Two other patients had a coagulopathy that was probably the result of hepatic dysfunction. Of six patients with bleeding, only two had coagulopathies, but all had thrombocytopenia. Four patients with severe coagulopathy died, and two who survived developed skin necrosis. In those who survived, the coagulopathy resolved with appropriate therapy of RMSF; only one of these patients received heparin.

While thrombocytopenia is common, the basis for the coagulopathy in RMSF is somewhat uncertain. Although the laboratory findings are in many cases typical of disseminated intravascular coagulation (DIC), Walker feels that true DIC, defined as deposition of fibrin in healthy portions of the microcirculation, does not occur in RMSF (17). Consumption of clotting factors may occur in the foci of vascular injury, and hepatic injury may contribute to decreased serum concentrations of coagulation factors. Whatever the mechanism of the coagulopathy, it usually resolves with treatment of the infection; specific therapy for DIC is rarely indicated.

Skin necrosis and gangrene

Five patients (4 percent) had skin necrosis or peripheral gangrene as a complication of their disease. Two patients had distal gangrene of the digits, and both died. One patient had extensive peripheral gangrene of all extremities; he survived a stormy course and eventually required amputation of multiple digits, a Syme's amputation, and a BK amputation as well. One 8-year-old child had diffuse sloughing of purpuric lesions, with eventual full recovery. Massive skin necrosis has been previously reported in RMSF (48). The fifth patient had ischemic toe lesions, but these eventually resolved completely. Only two of the five patients had evidence of coagulopathy. Skin necrosis and distal gangrene are probably due primarily to localized vasculitis and resulting small vessel thrombosis and not to disseminated intravascular coagulation.

Morbidity and mortality

Forty-nine patients (37 percent) in our series had at least one of the following complications: severe neurologic dysfunction, coagulopathy, renal failure, pulmonary insufficiency, cardiovascular dysfunction, hepatic disease, or skin necrosis. Many had multiple complications. Thirty (23 percent) had more than two, and fourteen (11 percent) had more than four complications. Among many variables analyzed, the single factor which correlated best with development of complications was age: 18 of 22 persons (82 percent) over 40 years old developed at least one complication. Ten patients (7.6 percent) died, and multiple complications (neurologic, renal, and others) were present in these patients before effective treatment was instituted.

Mild disease

The discussion to this point has emphasized the clinical patterns of RMSF mainly in hospitalized patients with disease of moderate to marked severity, in keeping with other reports (1, 7, 13, 15, 19, 28, 29, 49–52). We therefore wish to stress that fully one-third of the patients in our series had mild disease and were managed as outpatients; all had serologic confirmation of RMSF. The incidence of milder forms of RMSF is uncertain, for several reasons. Reports from tertiary care centers, including ours, undoubtedly are heavily biased toward more severe disease. Moreover, patients treated early in the course of RMSF often do not develop positive convalescent Weil-Felix or complement-fixation titers (64), and those treated as outpatients frequently do not have convalescent serologies measured. Underreporting of the disease by physicians also occurs to a significant degree. A serologic survey to determine the prevalence of milder forms of RMSF is now being conducted in the Piedmont plateau region of North Carolina (the area of the United States with the highest reported incidence of RMSF), and the results are awaited with interest.

Familial cases

Familial cases of RMSF have been noted by others (5, 6, 52–56) and occur more frequently than many physicians realize. We encountered four pairs of familial cases over a 10-year period, all well documented by serologies or positive immunofluorescent rickettsial stain of tissue. There were three pairs of mother-child cases and one sibling pair. In two other cases, siblings were hospitalized elsewhere simultaneously with presumptive RMSF, making the incidence of familial cases 6 to 8 percent in our series. While aerosol transmission of disease has been postulated in cases of laboratory-acquired RMSF (57, 58) and possible transmission by needle or blood transfusion has been reported (59, 60) there is no evidence for person-to-person transmission in familial cases. The diagnosis of RMSF must be considered in familial cases of febrile exanthematous illness.

Hyperendemic foci of disease

Within an endemic focus of RMSF, there may be relatively small areas where the incidence of disease is extremely high (4). One such area, a small town in North Carolina, has been studied by one of us (J.J.F.). Along a ½-mi stretch of road, 12 cases have occurred in about 40 households over a 10-year period. It has been postulated that a large population of infected ticks took refuge in the nearby woods and fields after an adjacent farm was converted into a golf course. Such changes in ecology may account for variations in local prevalence of RMSF.

LABORATORY DATA

Many of the laboratory abnormalities seen in RMSF have been discussed in the sections on the complications of the illness. Certain other laboratory findings are extensively used by the clinician in deciding whether a patient has RMSF, especially hematological values and serum sodium levels.

Table 7 summarizes certain hematologic data from our patients with RMSF. While the total white blood cell count is usually normal in this disease (3, 5, 14), 36 patients (28 percent) had a leukocytosis (>10,000 per cubic millimeter) without evidence of a concomitant bacterial infection. Of those with a differential cell count 69 percent had greater than 10 percent band-form granulocytes, while 10 percent had greater than 50 percent bands. The number of bands reached a maximum between the fourth and tenth days of disease, with a mean percentage of bands of 20 to 30 percent. Toxic granules and Döhle bodies may occur as well. Hall and Schwartz recently noted similar findings (61) and concluded that an increased percentage of immature granulocytes in the absence of

**Table 7 Hematologic data before
therapy of RMSF (present series)**

Laboratory test	No. tested	No.	%
WBC/mm³	129		
<10,000		93	72
10,000–15,000		19	15
>15,000		17	13
Percent bands	121		
>10%		83	69
>25%		48	40
>50%		12	10
Platelet count per mm³	117		
<150,000		61	52
50,000–99,000		21	18
<50,000		17	14.5

leukocytosis should help differentiate RMSF from meningococcal disease (in which a leukocytosis is usually present) and viral meningitis (in which the percentage of bands is usually less than 10 percent).

Anemia is unusual in RMSF, though six of our patients had hematocrits less than 30. Five patients with normal red blood cell counts initially had a significant fall in hematocrit after therapy was begun, without obvious hemorrhage. Two of these patients had evidence of microangiopathic hemolytic anemia on peripheral smear. Two others had possible hemolysis on the basis of glucose 6-phosphate dehydrogenase deficiency. Seven patients required blood transfusions some time in the course of their disease. After recovery all had complete resolution of anemia.

Thrombocytopenia is the best-documented hematologic abnormality in RMSF (53, 62–64). A low platelet count did not necessarily indicate severe disease in our series; 27 patients with clinically uncomplicated disease had platelet counts less than 150,000. Those with more than four complications, however, all had thrombocytopenia (<150,000 per cubic millimeter). Thrombocytopenia is apparently caused by consumption of platelets in areas of localized vascular injury (17), and few of these patients have evidence of diffuse coagulopathy. The platelet count often decreases during the first few days of therapy before returning to normal, despite appropriate antibiotic use. Hemorrhage rarely occurs in RMSF, and platelet transfusions are seldom necessary.

Hyponatremia has been widely reported in RMSF (19, 27, 28, 52). Hyponatremia (serum sodium <132 meq/liter) was present in 56 percent of our patients, and was marked (<120 meq/liter) in 8 percent. Inappropriate antidiuretic hormone secretion has been postulated as a cause of hyponatremia but not definitively proved (65). Presence of hyponatremia is not necessarily an indication of severe disease. Thirty-seven patients with low sodium levels in our series had no complications of their disease. In contrast, two patients who died had normal serum sodium levels on presentation shortly before death.

We conclude that the presence of increased numbers of immature granulocytes, decrease in platelet count, or decrease in serum sodium may be of some help in deciding whether a patient with a febrile illness might have RMSF, but absence of these findings does not exclude the diagnosis.

DIFFERENTIAL DIAGNOSIS

The differential diagnosis of RMSF is extensive, and a full discussion is beyond the scope and intent of this review. A few diseases are considered most frequently, and often the most difficult to distinguish on a clinical basis is meningococcemia. Myalgias, petechial or hemorrhagic rash, increase in immature granulocytes in the peripheral blood, cardiovascular collapse, and meningoencephalitis may occur with either disease. The clinical course of meningococcal disease is usually more rapid than that of RMSF, and meningococcal skin lesions tend to occur most frequently on the trunk and lower extremities. Attempts should be made to visualize gram-negative diplococci in skin lesion aspirates, buffy coat smears, or cerebrospinal fluid, but these examinations are frequently negative. It may be impossible to differentiate the two diseases at first, necessitating initiation of treatment for both (chloramphenicol or penicillin and tetracycline) pending bacterial culture results.

Measles may closely resemble RMSF, especially atypical measles, where the rash may exactly mimic that of RMSF (66). Many other illnesses may simulate RMSF, including enteroviral infections, leptospirosis, and murine typhus. When there is a high suspicion of RMSF, empiric therapy for rickettsial disease should be given pending serologic results.

SEROLOGIC DIAGNOSIS

Serologic tests have been the major means of making the diagnosis of RMSF. Unfortunately, these tests are rarely positive early in the course of disease and many tests suffer from a relative lack of specificity and sensitivity.

The Weil-Felix test, most frequently used to diagnose RMSF, measures antibodies which agglutinate *Proteus vulgaris* strains OX19 or OX2 rather than specific rickettsial antibodies and thus is relatively nonspecific. Elevated titers have been reported in proteus infections, leptospirosis, and acute liver disease, as well as in other rickettsial infections (6). In reviewing results from our serology laboratory from 1973 through 1979, elevated OX19 or OX2 titers (reciprocal of highest positive dilution ≥ 320) were found in patients with hepatitis, carcinoma, sickle-cell disease, and sarcoidosis but without evidence of RMSF. Weil-Felix agglutinins usually become elevated 10 to 14 days after the onset of symptoms but may not reach maximum levels for over 3 weeks. Clearly, this response is too slow for most clinical decisions about institution of therapy. While most patients with RMSF develop reciprocal titers of 320 or greater, early therapy may suppress or delay the eventual titer rise (67). As with most serologic tests, a fourfold or greater rise in titer is more meaningful than a single elevated titer.

The complement-fixation test for RMSF with R. *rickettsii* antigen is highly specific for the spotted fever group of organisms. The major disadvantage of this test is the long time before it becomes positive (68). The antibody measured is usually not present until the second week of illness and may not appear until 4 to 6 weeks after onset of disease. Early antibiotic therapy may completely prevent the development of complement-fixing antibodies (67).

Recently developed serologic tests that are not widely available include microagglutination (69), microimmunofluorescence (70), and indirect hemagglutination (71, 72) techniques. In comparative studies by Philip et al., these tests appeared to be more sensitive than the complement-fixation and Weil-Felix tests (73). None of the tests was positive before the sixth day of illness, but all resulted in a more pronounced increase in titer compared with the complement-fixation test. Once again, patients treated very early in their disease were least likely to be seropositive for RMSF by any test. Hechemy et al. confirmed that the microimmunofluorescent method was more sensitive than the Weil-Felix agglutinins (74). Newhouse et al. compared the immunofluorescent, complement-fixation, and microagglutination tests using somewhat different techniques and found that the fluorescent antibody test was the most sensitive and the microagglutination test the least sensitive (75). Available data on specificity of the above tests are scanty (73, 75). Further studies are necessary before these tests can be used with confidence.

OTHER LABORATORY DIAGNOSTIC METHODS

Direct isolation of rickettsiae from blood and tissue samples is rarely attempted. The techniques used for rickettsial isolation are time-consuming, dangerous to laboratory personnel, and not readily available to most physicians. Other means of identifying rickettsiae in patients with suspected RMSF have been reported recently. DeShazo et al. describe a monocyte culture technique that enabled them to diagnose disease in monkeys as early as the fourth day of febrile illness (76). Monocytes from infected monkeys were maintained in cell culture, and the intracellular organisms were identified by immunofluorescence. The technique was not sensitive enough to detect organisms in freshly isolated monocytes, however, and required a few days of cell multiplication before organisms could be seen. While the procedure is promising, experience with human patients has not been reported.

At present, the only definitive means available for early, rapid diagnosis of RMSF is direct immunofluorescent staining of tissue for rickettsiae (77, 78). Organisms can be found in skin lesions as early as the third or fourth day of disease. Causes for false negative results include therapy with tetracycline or chloramphenicol for over 24 h before biopsy and failure to obtain a section through a focus of vasculitis (78). At present the procedure is not used on patients without a rash. While the technique so far is not highly sensitive, it does appear to be specific. In the series of Walker et al. 9 of 17 patients biopsied with serologically documented RMSF had positive immunofluorescent examination of skin biopsies for rickettsiae; no false positive result was documented in 10 patients with other exanthems (78). The sensitivity of the procedure has increased since that published report. Biopsies are obtained before therapy whenever possible, and skin lesions are marked with India ink to guarantee sectioning through the area of most severe vasculitis (D. Walker, personal communication). Unfortunately direct immunofluorescent staining for rickettsiae is available only at a limited number of medical centers.

TREATMENT AND PREVENTION

Therapy for RMSF has not changed significantly for nearly 30 years. While chloramphenicol is often preferred for the treatment of patients who are more severely ill, limited in vitro data indicate that tetracycline may actually be more active against *R. rickettsiae* (79). No controlled studies are available comparing the efficacy of tetracycline and chloramphenicol in RMSF, but clinical experience indicates that each is effective. Since both are rickettsiostatic, they should be continued for 2 to 3 days after fever resolves, for an average course of 5 to 7 days. There is no role for prophylactic antibiotics in RMSF. Smadel showed in scrub typhus that administration of prophylactic antibiotics to human volunteers only postponed the onset of illness (80). Kenyon et al. studied prophylactic treatment of RMSF in guinea pigs with similar results (81). When treatment preceded expected disease onset by over 48 h, the onset of illness was delayed but not prevented. RMSF was prevented in guinea pigs by administration of a single dose of oxytetracycline 24 to 48 h before expected onset of disease (81). Since the incubation period of RMSF is variable in human beings, it is impossible to predict the onset of symptoms after an infected tick bite. Also, since only a small percentage of ticks in endemic areas are infected (10, 82, 83), it is best to observe an individual after tick exposure and institute therapy only at the first sign of clinical disease. While corticosteroids have been used in patients with severe disease (84), there is no objective evidence that they are necessary or efficacious.

At present, there is no commercial vaccine available for RMSF. The first inactivated vaccine, derived from tissues of infected ticks in the 1920s (85), was felt to be effective on the basis of decreased severity of disease and decreased mortality in retrospective studies (86). The next inactivated vaccine was prepared from infected embryonated chick eggs in the 1930s and was presumed to be effective for human beings based on animal studies (87). This vaccine was eventually made commercially available. In 1973, DuPont et al. reported human volunteer studies of both vaccines (88). While both vaccines prolonged the incubation period and decreased the frequency of clinical relapse, neither conferred significant protection against the development of RMSF. This study further showed that solid immunity occurred after prior illness with RMSF. Because of these results, the commercial vaccine was withdrawn by the Food and Drug Administration. A new formalin-inactivated vaccine prepared from rickettsiae grown in chick embryo cell tissue culture is presently under study by Kenyon's group (89–92). Preliminary studies in human subjects show improved induction of humoral and cell-mediated immunity to rickettsiae compared with previously available vaccines (91). The vaccine has been administered to monkeys with resulting protection against rickettsial challenge (92). While no direct-challenge study in human beings has been reported to date, this vaccine shows promise of being safe, effective, and quite useful in endemic areas.

THE CLINICAL DILEMMA

RMSF is a highly variable disease, and patients often present without typical signs and symptoms, including a classical rash. It may be either a mild illness or exceedingly severe, with multiple complications and significant mortality. A history of tick exposure can be helpful but is absent in 20 to 30 percent of patients (6, unpublished data). Thus, the physician who sees a patient with RMSF early in the course of disease is faced with a dilemma.

The majority of febrile illnesses seen in primary care medicine are self-limited and should not be treated with antibiotics. Watchful waiting is often practiced in patients with undiagnosed febrile illnesses and can be undertaken with close observation in patients with possible RMSF if they are not severely ill, have had fever for 3 days or less, and lack rash, thrombocytopenia, and neurologic symptoms. One must be aware that such patients sometimes are lost to follow-up and may later return moribund. In view of the well-documented relationship between delayed institution of therapy and increased morbidity and mortality in RMSF, it is our opinion that in endemic areas between April and October it is often proper to treat febrile patients with suspected RMSF with tetracycline in the absence of a definitive diagnosis. We hope this review will help make such decisions more rational.

REFERENCES

1 Hazard GW et al: Rocky Mountain spotted fever in the Eastern United States. N Engl J Med 280:57, 1969.

2 Rothenberg R, Sonenshine DE: Rocky Mountain spotted fever in Virginia: Clinical and epidemiologic features. J Med Entomol 7:663, 1970.

3 Vianna N, Hinman, A: Rocky Mountain spotted fever on Long Island: Epidemiologic and clinical aspects. Am J Med 51:725, 1971.

4 Linnemann C et al: Rocky Mountain spotted fever in Clermont County, Ohio: Description of an endemic focus. Am J Epidemiol 97:125, 1973.

5 Sexton DJ, Burgdorfer W: Clinical and epidemiologic features of Rocky Mountain spotted fever in Mississippi, 1933–1973. South Med J 68:1529, 1975.

6 Hattwick MA et al: Rocky Mountain spotted fever: Epidemiology of an increasing problem. Ann Intern Med 84:732, 1976.

7 Sonenshine DE et al: Rocky Mountain spotted fever in relation to vegetation in the Eastern United States 1951–1971. Am J Epidemiol 96:59, 1972.

8 Weiss E: Growth and physiology of Rickettsiae. Bacteriol Rev 37:259, 1973.

9 Burgdorfer W: A review of Rocky Mountain spotted fever (tick-borne typhus), its agent and its tick vectors in the United States. J Med Entomol 12:269, 1975.

10 Loving SM et al: Distribution and prevalence of spotted fever group Rickettsiae in ticks from South Carolina, with an epidemiological survey of persons bitten by infected ticks. Am J Trop Med Hyg 27:1255, 1978.

11 Pincoffs MC et al: The treatment of Rocky Mountain spotted fever with chloromycetin. Ann Intern Med 29:656, 1948.

12 Harrell AT et al: Aureomycin, a new orally effective antibiotic: Clinical trial in Rocky Mountain spotted fever, results of susceptibility tests and blood assays using a turbidimetric method. South Med J 42:4, 1949.

13 Ley HL Jr, Smadel JE: Antibiotic therapy of rickettsial diseases. Antibiot Chemother 4:792, 1954.

14 Harrell GT: Rocky Mountain spotted fever. Medicine 28: 333, 1949.

15 Hattwick M et al: Fatal Rocky Mountain spotted fever. JAMA 240:1499, 1978.

16 Green W et al: Fatal viscerotropic Rocky Mountain spotted fever: Report of a case diagnosed by immunofluorescence. Am J Med 64:523, 1978.

17 Walker DH, Bradford WD: The current status of Rocky Mountain spotted fever in childhood, in Rosenberg EH (ed): Perspectives in Pediatric Pathology; New York, Masson, 1981.

18 Parker RR: Rocky Mountain spotted fever. JAMA 110:1185, 1273, 1938.

19 Feigin RD et al: Rocky Mountain spotted fever: Successful application of new insights into physiologic changes during acute infections to successful management of a severely ill patient. Clin Pediat 8:331, 1969.

20 Middleton DB: Rocky Mountain spotted

fever: Gastrointestinal and laboratory manifestations. *South Med J* 61:629, 1978.

21 **Sexton DJ et al:** Late appearance of skin rash and abnormal serum enzymes in Rocky Mountain spotted fever. *J Pediatr* 87:580, 1975.

22 **Ramphal R et al:** Rocky Mountain spotted fever and jaundice. *Arch Int Med* 138:260, 1978.

23 **Krober MS:** Skeletal muscle involvement in Rocky Mountain spotted fever. *South Med J* 71:1575, 1978.

24 **Harrell GT:** Rickettsial involvement of the nervous system. *Med Clin N Am* 37:395, 1953.

25 **Bell W, Lascari A:** Rocky Mountain spotted fever: Neurological symptoms in the acute phase. *Neurology* 20:841, 1970.

26 **Miller JQ, Price TR:** The nervous system in Rocky Mountain spotted fever. *Neurology* 22:561, 1972.

27 **Linnemann CC, Janson PJ:** The clinical presentation of Rocky Mountain spotted fever. *Clin Pediatr* 17:673, 1978.

28 **McReynolds EW, Ray S:** An epidemic of tick-borne typhus in children. *Am J Dis Child* 126:779, 1973.

29 **Torres J et al:** Rocky Mountain spotted fever in the Mid-South. *Arch Int Med* 132:340, 1973.

30 **Rosenblum MJ et al:** Residual effects of rickettsial disease on the central nervous system. *Arch Int Med* 90:444, 1952.

31 **Wright L:** Intellectual sequelae of Rocky Mountain spotted fever. *J Abnorm Psychol* 80:315, 1972.

32 **Cherubini TD, Spaeth GL:** Anterior nongranulomatous uveitis associated with Rocky Mountain spotted fever. *Arch Ophthal* 81:363, 1969.

33 **Presley GD:** Fundus changes in Rocky Mountain spotted fever. *Am J Ophthal* 67:263, 1969.

34 **Raab EL et al:** Retinopathy in Rocky Mountain spotted fever. *Am J Ophthal* 68:42, 1969.

35 **Smith TW, Burton TC:** The retinal manifestations of Rocky Mountain spotted fever. *Am J Ophthal* 84:259, 1977.

36 **Bradford WD, Hackel DB:** Myocardial involvement in Rocky Mountain spotted fever. *Arch Path Lab Med* 102:357, 1978.

37 **Walker DH, Mattern WD:** Acute renal failure in Rocky Mountain spotted fever. *Arch Int Med* 139:443, 1979.

38 **de Brito T et al:** Glomerular response in human and experimental rickettsial disease. *Pathol Microbiol* 31:365, 1968.

39 **Donohue JF:** Pulmonary manifestations of Rocky Mountain spotted fever. *Arch Int Med* 140:223, 1980.

40 **Lees RF et al:** Radiographic findings in Rocky Mountain spotted fever. *Radiology* 129:17, 1978.

41 **Walker DH et al:** Rickettsial infection of the pulmonary microcirculation, the basis of interstitial pneumonitis of Rocky Mountain spotted fever. *Human Pathol* 2:263, 1980.

42 **Trigg JW:** Hypofibrinogenemia in Rocky Mountain spotted fever. *N Engl J Med* 270:1042, 1964.

43 **Atkin MD et al:** A case report of "Cape Cod" Rocky Mountain spotted fever with multiple coagulation disturbances. *Pediatrics* 36:627, 1965.

44 **Deep W et al:** Defibrination syndrome in Rocky Mountain spotted fever. *Va Med Mon* 96:92, 1969.

45 **Graybill JR et al:** Complement and coagulation in Rocky Mountain spotted fever. *South Med J* 66:410, 1973.

46 **Kurnick JE et al:** Disseminated intravascular coagulation in Rocky Mountain spotted fever. *South Med J* 67:623, 1974.

47 **Fine D et al:** Coagulation and complement studies in Rocky Mountain spotted fever. *Arch Int Med* 138:735, 1978.

48 **Griffith GL, Luce EA:** Massive skin necrosis in Rocky Mountain spotted fever. *South Med J* 71:1337, 1978.

49 **Hand WL et al:** Rocky Mountain spotted fever: A vascular disease. *Arch Int Med* 125:879, 1970.

50 **Haynes RE et al:** Rocky Mountain spotted fever in children. *J Pediatr* 76:685, 1970.

51 **Snape PS:** Rocky Mountain spotted fever in Southeastern United States: A review of eighteen cases from Greenville, South Carolina. *South Med J* 66:765, 1973.

52 **Bradford WD, Hawkins HK:** Rocky Mountain spotted fever in childhood. *Am J Dis Child* 131:1228, 1977.

53 **Schaffner W et al:** Thrombocytopenic Rocky Mountain spotted fever. *Arch Int Med* 116:857, 1965.

54 **Sanders DY, Smithson WA:** Rocky Mountain spotted fever in three brothers. *NC Med J* 34:276, 1973.

55 **Jacobs WM, Chusid MJ:** Rocky Mountain spotted fever in an infant: Diagnosis in siblings. *Am J Dis Child* 132:928, 1978.

56 **Bradford WD:** Rocky Mountain spotted fever: A family affair. *Clin Pediatr* 18:634, 1979.

57 **Johnson J, Kadull PJ:** Rocky Mountain spotted fever acquired in a laboratory. *N Engl J Med* 277:842, 1967.

58 **Oster C et al:** Laboratory-acquired Rocky Mountain spotted fever: The hazard of aerosol transmission. *N Engl J Med* 297:859, 1977.

59 **Sexton D et al:** Possible needle-associated Rocky Mountain spotted fever (letter). *N Engl J Med* 292:645, 1975.

60 Wells GM et al: Rocky Mountain spotted fever caused by blood transfusion. *JAMA* 239:2763, 1978.

61 Hall GW, Schwartz RP: White blood cell count and differential in Rocky Mountain spotted fever. *NC Med J* 40:212, 1979.

62 Phillips CW et al: Rocky Mountain spotted fever with thrombocytopenia. *South Med J* 53:867, 1960.

63 Mengel CE, Trygstad C: Thrombocytopenia in Rocky Mountain spotted fever. *JAMA* 183:886, 1963.

64 Rubio T et al: Thrombocytopenia in Rocky Mountain spotted fever. *Am J Dis Child* 116:88, 1968.

65 Sexton DJ, Clapp J: Inappropriate antidiuretic hormone secretion: Occurrence in a patient with Rocky Mountain spotted fever. *Arch Int Med* 137:362, 1977.

66 Horwitz MS et al: Atypical measles rash mimicking Rocky Mountain spotted fever (letter). *N Engl J Med* 289:1203, 1973.

67 Schubert JH: Serologic titers in rickettsial infection as affected by antibiotic treatment. *Public Health Lab* 10:38, 1952.

68 Shepard CC et al: Recent experience with the complement fixation test in the laboratory diagnosis of rickettsial diseases in the United States. *J Clin Microbiol* 4:277, 1976.

69 Fiset P et al: A microagglutination technique for detection and measurement of rickettsial antibodies. *Acta Virol* 13:60, 1969.

70 Philip RN et al: Microimmunofluorescence test for the serological study of Rocky Mountain spotted fever and typhus. *J Clin Microbiol* 3:51, 1976.

71 Shirai A et al: Indirect hemagglutination test for human antibody to typhus and spotted fever group Rickettsiae. *J Clin Microbiol* 2:430, 1975.

72 Anacker RL et al: Indirect hemagglutination test for detection of antibody to *Rickettsia rickettsii* in sera from humans and common laboratory animals. *J Clin Microbiol* 10:677, 1979.

73 Philip RN et al: A comparison of serologic methods for diagnosis of Rocky Mountain spotted fever. *Am J Epidemiol* 105:56, 1977.

74 Hechemy KE et al: Discrepancies in Weil-Felix and microimmunofluorescence test results for Rocky Mountain spotted fever. *J Clin Microbiol* 9:292, 1979.

75 Newhouse VF et al: A comparison of the complement fixation, indirect fluorescent antibody and microagglutination tests for the serologic diagnosis of rickettsial diseases. *Am J Trop Hyg* 28:387, 1979.

76 DeShazo RD et al: Early diagnosis of Rocky Mountain spotted fever: Use of primary monocyte culture technique. *JAMA* 235:1353, 1976.

77 Woodward TE et al: Prompt confirmation of Rocky Mountain spotted fever: Identification of Rickettsiae in skin tissues. *J Infect Dis* 134:297, 1976.

78 Walker DH et al: Laboratory diagnosis of Rocky Mountain spotted fever by immunofluorescent demonstration of *Rickettsia rickettsii* in cutaneous lesions. *Am J Clin Pathol* 69:619, 1978.

79 Ormsbee RA: The comparative effectiveness of aureomycin, terramycin, chloramphenicol, erythromycin and thiocymetin in suppressing experimental rickettsial infections in chick embryos. *J Infect Dis* 96:162, 1955.

80 Smadel JE: Influence of antibiotics on immunologic responses in scrub typhus. *Am J Med* 17:246, 1954.

81 Kenyon RH et al: Prophylactic treatment of Rocky Mountain spotted fever. *J Clin Microbiol* 8:102, 1978.

82 Sexton DJ et al: Rocky Mountain spotted fever in Mississippi: Survey for spotted fever antibodies in dogs and for spotted fever group Rickettsiae in dog ticks. *Am J Epidemiol* 103:192, 1976.

83 Magnarelli LA et al: Rocky Mountain spotted fever in Connecticut: Human cases, spotted fever group Rickettsiae in ticks and antibodies in mammals. *Am J Epidemiol* 110:148, 1979.

84 Workman JB et al: Cortisone as an adjunct to chloramphenicol in the treatment of Rocky Mountain spotted fever. *N Engl J Med* 246:962, 1952.

85 Spencer RR, Parker RR: Rocky Mountain spotted fever: Vaccination of monkeys and man. *Public Health Rep* 40:2159, 1925.

86 Parker RR: Rocky Mountain spotted fever; results of fifteen years' prophylactic vaccination. *Am J Trop Med Hyg* 21:369, 1941.

87 Cox HR: Rocky Mountain spotted fever. Protective value for guinea pigs of vaccine prepared from Rickettsiae cultivated in embryonic chick tissues. *Public Health Rep* 54:1070, 1939.

88 DuPont HL et al: Rocky Mountain spotted fever: A comparative study of the active immunity induced by inactivated and viable pathogenic *Rickettsia rickettsii*. *J Infect Dis* 128:340, 1973.

89 Kenyon RH et al: Preparation of vaccines for Rocky Mountain spotted fever from Rickettsiae propagated in cell culture. *J Infect Dis* 125:146, 1972.

90 Kenyon RH et al: Comparison of three Rocky Mountain spotted fever vaccines. *J Clin Microbiol* 2:300, 1975.

91 Ascher MS et al: Initial clinical evaluation of a new Rocky Mountain spotted fever vaccine of tissue culture origin. *J Infect Dis* 138:217, 1978.

92 Gander JC et al: Evaluation of a killed Rocky Mountain spotted fever vaccine in cynomolgus monkeys. *J Clin Microbiol* 10:719, 1979.

The doctor's dilemma
Have I chosen the right drug? An adequate dose regimen? Can laboratory tests help in my decision?

ERNEST JAWETZ

The person representing Sir Almroth Wright in Shaw's play *The Doctor's Dilemma* insists "Stimulate the phagocytes—drugs are a delusion." Sir Almroth, then director of the inoculation department at St. Mary's Hospital, almost succeeded in blocking Sir Alexander Fleming's interest in soluble products as a possible method of treating infections. Luckily for posterity, Fleming pursued his observations and just half a century ago published his initial studies on penicillin. Today the stimulation of phagocytes remains elusive while innumerable antimicrobial drugs provide the physician with powerful tools in the control of infection. Regrettably, the microbial world has shown remarkable ability to adapt to antimicrobial drugs; consequently, the selection of optimal treatment often remains difficult and the doctor's dilemma is often great.

In most seriously ill patients with probable infections, the physician will formulate an etiologic diagnosis on clinical grounds and will obtain suitable specimens for laboratory diagnosis before starting drugs aimed at the "best guess." If a significant microorganism is isolated, it may be submitted for antimicrobial susceptibility tests and drug activity in the patient's serum may be estimated. This paper reviews some changing aspects of antibiotic susceptibility tests, including determinations of minimal inhibitory concentrations (MIC) and minimal bactericidal concentrations (MBC) and the possible role of serum bactericidal activity test (SBT) as a guide in the selection of antimicrobial drug regimens.

ANTIMICROBIAL SUSCEPTIBILITY TESTS

From the early years of the antibiotic era onward, drugs were assayed by the ability to diffuse from cups or disks in standardized solid media and produce defined growth-inhibition zones of reference strains. Such assay results formed the basis of the dosage labeling of drugs.

Based, in part, on work supported by donations from the Burroughs Wellcome Fund.

Clinical isolates were often tested for drug susceptibility by tube or plate dilution tests. The results of such tests provided the ranges of concentrations of a given drug necessary to inhibit different strains of the same microbial species. This was correlated with estimates of drug levels achieved in different body fluids or organs with various dosage regimens. It formed the basis of generalizations of the susceptibility or insusceptibility of specific infections to a given drug, as judged by laboratory results. If possible, clinical experience was correlated with these predictions.

Tube or plate dilution tests were cumbersome, time-consuming, and expensive, but they had the advantage of providing quantitative results which could be expressed either as MIC or MBC if suitable subcultures were employed. By contrast, disk diffusion tests were simple and cheap but subject to many variables. The inhibition zone around a disk was far more dependent on molecular size, electric charge, and mobility of the drug molecule than on susceptibility of the organism. The zone sizes around disks of two different drugs could not be compared. Disks of several drug strengths had to be employed to provide an estimate of the degree of susceptibility of a clinical isolate.

In spite of these apparent limitations, the convenience of single-disk tests for rapid evaluation of clinical isolates prompted an international study on the many factors which influenced test results. A summary by Ericsson and Sherris (1) concluded that if rigorous test conditions were maintained linear regression lines could express for any drug the relationship between the logarithm of MIC and the diameter of inhibition zones in diffusion tests. With this scientific basis, Bauer et al. (2) introduced the single-disk method for clinical laboratory tests. Standards of zone diameter for susceptibility or resistance of an isolate were established for each drug with rigorous controls. The so-called Kirby-Bauer technique has been widely accepted since the mid-1960s (3, 4).

Several problems were associated with the single-disk method, of which the following deserve mention:

1   The amount of drug contained in the disk used for measuring "susceptibility" cannot in any way be equated with the concentration of the same drug found during therapy in a tissue or body fluid.

2   The single-disk concentration was selected on the basis of bimodal distribution curves found with different drug concentrations against a microbial species. The disk "strength" was selected in part by correlation with treatment response and with drug concentrations achievable in blood. However, drug concentrations in urine, cerebrospinal fluid, bile, or mucous membranes might be very different from those in blood. Consequently, the results of single-disk tests were sometimes misleading to clinicians.

3   With single disks, resistant mutants present in low frequency could be missed, whereas similar mutants would be readily detected in liquid test media.

4   In any disk test it is relatively difficult (and rarely attempted) to determine whether a drug is primarily bacteriostatic or significantly bactericidal for the clinical isolate. Such determinations are far easier with tests in liquid media subjected to subculture on solid media.

5   The results of disk tests are often irrelevant or misleading in the selection of possibly synergistic drug combinations (see below).

6   Agar diffusion susceptibility tests, particularly of pseudomonads and of Enterobacteriaceae, appear to be subject to far more complex influences of the test media than in liquid media. The latter may therefore be preferable, and reference strains may be included in the test (5).

7   In some cases a single disk may represent the behavior of a clinical isolate toward an entire class of drugs. However, with the proliferation of cephalosporins and aminoglycosides, differences between individual members of a class of drugs may be great enough to warrant testing more than one member of a class. The selection of appropriate drugs presents a major logistics problem to clinical laboratories whether disk tests or tests in liquid media are employed.

For these and other reasons, in 1980 there was a trend away from the universal use of standardized single-disk (Kirby-Bauer) tests and toward microdilution tests in liquid media. Commercially or locally prepared microdilution kits are kept frozen until used and appear to have a reasonable shelf-life. They permit a fairly accurate description of the amount of drug in a liquid medium necessary to inhibit a uniform, standardized bacterial inoculum (MIC). Such kits also make possible convenient subculture into drug-free media and thus a semiquantitative estimate of bactericidal effects (MBC).

The laboratory report on MICs must be accompanied by guidelines for their interpretation (6). This will be essential for the many physicians who have become too accustomed to the sensitive-resistant pattern in drug susceptibility reports based on disk zone size.

The quantitative microdilution test is gaining popularity particularly in tertiary care centers with their high proportion of compromised hosts infected with opportunistic organisms of unpredictable drug resistance. In this setting the quantitative estimates of susceptibility of an isolate and the bactericidal capability of different drugs may be of substantial help in selecting drug and dose. Another setting for quantitative broth dilution tests might be the evaluation of drugs in combination, discussed below.

TESTS FOR DRUG COMBINATIONS

Before proceeding to this complex and frustrating portion of my assignment, I must briefly review some basic features of combined antibiotic action. They have been repeatedly voiced in the past (7–10), and only a few points will be mentioned here.

1   Although it is evident that drugs in combination can sometimes accomplish what single drugs fail to do, there is no generally accepted definition of antimicrobial synergism (7–10). Any definition depends on the criteria used in laboratory evaluation of the effect of combinations (see below). For the sake of clinical therapy, it may not be essential to separate different types of positive summation of drug effects as long as a combination achieves a result which cannot be achieved by a single drug in a readily tolerated dose. I shall therefore use the noncommittal term *beneficial action*.

2   Beneficial summation of drug effects can manifest itself in several ways. Each of these requires a different method of measurement in the laboratory: bacteriostatic action, early rate of bactericidal action, total bactericidal effect, or therapeutic effect in experimental models. Varying emphasis has been placed on the relative importance of these parameters to predict beneficial summation applicable to the treatment of human infections (7, 11–19). The nature of the infection may determine the required effect.

3   The criteria for quantifying beneficial combined effects vary with laboratory methods:

   a   Bacteriostatic action, measured by checkerboard titration, often uses the formula $\frac{1}{4}$ MIC of drug A + $\frac{1}{4}$ MIC of drug B > 1 MIC of either A or B alone.

   b   Rate of bactericidal action, estimated by time-kill curves (exposure of organism to drug in broth followed by subculture on drug-free solid media, with colony counts), often uses the criterion of a hundredfold (2 log) reduction in count by the combination below that of the single more active drug during 8 to 18 h.

   c   Total bactericidal effect, estimated as in b but for a longer time, to determine whether few or no organisms survive (>99.99 percent killing). The results of the tests outlined in a to c may correlate well (20), but often they do not (7–10, 18). For the time being, the choice of a laboratory test must depend on the views of an individual clinician or laboratory investigator.

4   Certain generalized predictions, based on experience, are possible regarding probable beneficial combinations for certain microbial genera or species, but the variation of behavior from strain to strain is great. Therefore, a beneficial drug combination can be stated only for a specific microbial isolate submitted to laboratory test or to experimental therapy. Universally beneficial drug combinations do not exist.

5   Each laboratory method mentioned above is subject to many variables. Results are greatly influenced by inoculum size, composition of microbiologic media, pH, and temperature and time of incubation and sampling. None of these are currently standardized, creating great difficulties in interpreting the results.

It is evident that much future effort will be required to develop uniformity for the different methods which propose to assess whether a combination is likely to be beneficial against a given microorganism. More importantly, however, there is no consensus regarding the principal aims of combined antimicrobial therapy. In some infections, e.g., tuberculosis, the principal aim is to prevent or delay the emergence of variants resistant to a single member of the combination. This might apply occasionally to other infections with very large microbial populations (14, 17, 21, 22). In other types of infectious diseases, e.g., endocarditis or sepsis in the immunosuppressed host, a main goal is to achieve greater bactericidal effects than is possible with a single drug (8, 10, 13, 15, 16, 23–27).

One or both of these goals and perhaps others may be important in certain clinical situations. It therefore seems unlikely that a single, universally applicable method of testing for beneficial drug combinations can be devised. The checkerboard titration method provides information mainly on enhanced bacteriostasis and the suppression of possible variants which are resistant to either drug alone (11, 14); however, it tells nothing about either the rate or the completeness of bactericidal action (9, 10).

Because of our interest in endocarditis and sepsis in the immunodeficient host, we have focused on combined antimicrobial action which results in enhanced bactericidal effects. The dynamics of such combined effects often involve enhancement by one drug of penetration of a second drug (9, 10). The second drug unable to reach its site of action alone (e.g., aminoglycosides unable to reach ribosomes) may lack any manifest inhibitory effect on the test organism in a concentration which can be achieved in vivo. Consequently, no useful information is provided by testing for inhibition by disk test or MIC estimation in liquid media (5, 18, 28, 29). Nevertheless, beneficial bactericidal action may result from the addition of this drug to another drug which permits it to penetrate to its site of action (e.g., the addition of a cell-wall-active drug). To be detected this type of beneficial bactericidal effect requires time-kill curve methods.

We proposed a method based on experience available in 1955 for testing the activity of drug combinations (29). Its main features were a two-stage test for inhibitory and cidal activity and the use of only a few concentrations of each drug, chosen on the basis of levels achievable in vivo with minimal toxicity. Only a very few drug combinations were applied to a given microorganism, based on current patterns of drug response. The efficacy of a drug combination chosen in such a way could be monitored by serum bactericidal assays (see below). Variations of such tests, involving time-kill curves in two-stage tests, have been employed in many settings (10, 12, 13, 15, 18, 19, 23, 25). Usually these tests have employed an aminoglycoside plus a cell-wall-active drug.

Such tests are easy to conceive but difficult to standardize and interpret:

1   It may be impossible to devise "routine" drug combinations and concentrations that are applicable to many different microorganisms, at different times, in different settings. Often such tests have to be tailored to a specific patient.

2   The results are greatly influenced by inoculum size, time of incubation and subculture, and other laboratory variables.[1] An example is shown in Figure 1. At time I the apparent rate of bactericidal action is greater for drug A than for A + B. At time II A + B permits fewer survivors than A alone. Which finding is more relevant in clinical therapy?

3   As a quantitative criterion it has been suggested that the viable bacterial count with a beneficial combination should be 2 log lower than with a single drug. But at which time? In which part of the time-kill curve? Tests for drug combinations are requested more often in clinical infections in which bactericidal drug effects appear necessary for cure, in which bactericidal serum assays are appropriate (see below), or in which there is failure to respond to initial antimicrobial therapy and microbial tolerance is suspected (12, 15, 16, 23, 25, 30). Microbial isolates which may qualify for tests against drug combinations are listed in Table 1, but in some circumstances (or with the passage of time) others might be considered. Serratia isolates, for example, might be tested with mixtures of polymyxin with rifampin or with trimethoprim-sulfamethoxazole.

---

[1] A particularly knotty technical problem concerns the determination of bactericidal drug activity against fastidious organisms, especially fastidious anaerobes. Growth of such organisms is easily inhibited under any suboptimal circumstances. Consequently, truly lethal effects, comparable to those required in vivo, may be difficult or even impossible to prove in vitro.

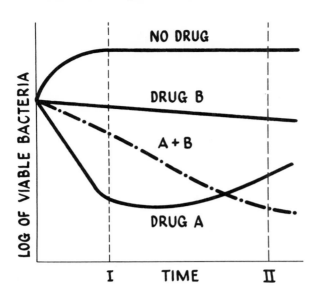

Figure 1 Schematic representation of count of viable bacteria against time, indicating the effect of drug A, drug B, or the two drugs, A + B.

Table 1   Clinical isolates which may be submitted to testing with antibiotic combinations for possible guidance in therapy

Organism	Drug combination for initial trial
Streptococcus, group D, group B, viridans (?); *Listeria* sp.	Penicillin G (or ampicillin) + aminoglycoside
Staphylococcus aureus, *Staph. epidermidis*	Nafcillin (or vancomycin) + aminoglycoside (or rifampin)
Diphtheroids	Vancomycin +(?) aminoglycoside (or rifampin)
Klebsiella sp., *Pseudomonas* sp.	Cephalosporin (or ticarcillin) + aminoglycoside
Enterobacter sp., *Serratia* sp., Proteus sp.	Ticarcillin (or cephalosporin) + aminoglycoside

Initial drug concentration, µg/ml of broth medium*					
Penicillin G†	20	Nafcillin	15	Amikacin	15
Ampicillin	20	Cefazolin	30	Vancomycin	10
Ticarcillin	50	Gentamicin	5	Rifampin	5

* These drug concentrations are tested as single drugs and in combinations. If rapid and complete bactericidal action occurs, the amounts in combination are progressively reduced in subsequent tests.

† For viridans streptococci, 3 µg/ml.

The listing in Table 1 is intended as a proposal for experimentation, *not* as a feasible outline for routine tests. It is suggested that the drug concentrations listed be tested both as single drugs and in combination. Half the amounts are also placed in a combination. If either combination appears to exert beneficial effects, the components of the mixture are used in therapy and bactericidal serum assays are performed against the patient's isolate. If the serum assay indicates probable effective therapeutic levels of drugs, downward adjustment of dosage or withdrawal of one drug may be contemplated. This is certainly not a rigorously defined system for the control of combined antibiotic therapy, but it may be an aid in the selection of drug treatment in difficult infections. Although the past quarter century has provided remarkably little progress in the rational design and laboratory control of treatment with drug combinations, one must hope that the future will bring progress.

MICROBIAL DRUG ACTIVITY IN SERUM

Estimation of drug concentration in serum may serve two distinct—but at times related—purposes. One is to adjust the dose regimen so that levels fall within an accepted range while avoiding excessive, possibly toxic levels on the one hand and unacceptably low levels on the other. Such measurements may be carried out by microbiologic, chemical, or immunologic assay. Perhaps the commonest application is the use of radioimmunoassay to determine aminoglycoside levels in persons with impaired renal function (31). The results permit adjustment of dose regimen, although simple serum creatinine levels may provide almost equally useful information.

The second purpose is a direct assessment of the antibacterial activity in the serum of treated patients to tell the physician whether he has chosen a proper drug and an adequate dose regimen. The serum of a patient under treatment is taken at various times and set up in dilutions which are inoculated with the microorganism isolated from that same patient. If the serum is able to kill the inoculated bacteria rapidly, it may be assumed that optimal antimicrobial therapy is at work. The practical problems of such tests and the limits of their interpretations are discussed below.

The *serum bactericidal assay* originated in the treatment of experimental infections with penicillin (21, 32). These studies attempted to establish whether treatment results could be predicted by the measurement of drug concentration in the blood of infected experimental animals treated with penicillin. The studies also tried to determine whether bactericidal drug levels were required during the entire treatment period, and this question was answered in the negative. While effective antibacterial concentrations in blood were clearly related to the eradication of infections, such concentrations had to be present only during part of the treatment period. At least with penicillin, the suppression of microbial replication in animal tissues lasted much longer than demonstrable levels of drug in the blood (32).

At about the same time Schlichter proposed a serum assay to predict cure in penicillin-susceptible infective endocarditis (33, 34). He pointed to the need of bactericidal drug activity in blood to cure endocarditis due to viridans streptococci, although the level of bactericidal activity or its duration in the treatment period were not clearly defined. Our group in San Francisco proposed that serum bactericidal activity was an important correlate of cure in endocarditis caused by enterococci or staphylococci treated with drug combinations (15, 35, 36). It was also suggested that viridans streptococci could be killed at a faster rate by combinations of penicillin with an aminoglycoside than with penicillin alone. This feature has attracted attention intermittently for over a quarter of a century since (24, 26, 36), but its practical application has not been resolved.

Between 1950 and 1960 it became widely accepted that serum bactericidal levels in excess of 1:5 dilution were desirable and probably necessary for cure of endocarditis. Such levels were generally anticipated at the time of peak drug concentrations in the blood, about 1 h after an intramuscular or intravenous bolus dose. However, it remained unclear for how much of the total treatment time such levels had to persist. In an excellent study (performed in 1964 but not published until 1979) cure of experimentally induced gonococcal urethritis in volunteers was best predicted by the aggregate time penicillin concentrations remained higher than three to four times the MIC for the infecting strain (22). It is not yet evident whether such a requirement can be defined for chronic infections requiring prolonged bactericidal therapy.

METHOD OF ASSAY

Results of serum bactericidal tests varied considerably from one laboratory to another, and there was little agreement of standardized techniques for the test. It was evident that results depended greatly on the degree of protein binding of the drug, the composition of the test medium, and the size of the microbial inoculum. Since the early 1970s significant progress in the standardization of serum bactericidal assays has been achieved, principally through the work of Reller and Stratton (37, 38) and of Vosti and his associates (39, 40). A micro method was found to give results comparable to the standard tube dilution assay (40, 41).

An optimal diluent for serum assays was found to be Mueller-Hinton broth, supplemented with Mg^{2+} and Ca^{2+} and mixed in equal proportions with pooled human serum (37, 38). An optimal inoculum size consisted of a final concentration of organisms between 5×10^4 and 5×10^5 per milliliter. Such an inoculum permits estimation of 99 to 99.9 percent killing efficacy, which is believed to be a satisfactory index of bactericidal activity with an incubation of 1 to 2 days. It is not established, however, whether such an inoculum size is optimal for all types of microorganisms. While it gives meaningful results with streptococci and staphylococci, perhaps a tenfold lower inoculum may be appropriate for some gram-negative enteric bacteria (25, 35, 42).

INTERPRETATION OF THE SERUM BACTERICIDAL ASSAY AND ITS SUGGESTED CLINICAL IMPLICATIONS

There is no consensus—and few data on which to base one—regarding either the levels of bactericidal activity or the aggregate time necessary to maintain it in order to achieve optimal treatment and cure in different infections. In endocarditis, sepsis with bacteremia, and perhaps hematogenous osteomyelitis, peak levels (obtained within 1 h of a bolus injection) of 1:8 or 1:16 serum bactericidal activity are believed to be desirable. Evidence for this is based mainly on penicillins given at intervals of not more than 4 h. These general rules apply probably to endocarditis with viridans streptococci treated with these penicillins plus an aminoglycoside (at 8- to 12-h intervals). In such settings trough levels (obtained just before the next intravenous bolus) are usually measurable in serum levels of 1:2 or 1:4. There are anecdotal reports which relate such serum bactericidal levels to cure, but the tests were not performed in a standardized fashion (8, 10, 24). In rabbit models of endocarditis caused by a penicillin-sensitive streptococcus, cure was associated with peak bactericidal levels of 1:8 to 1:16 serum dilutions and trough levels, at 6 h, of 1:2 (26, 43).

In staphylococcal endocarditis treated in premethicillin days with selected drug combinations (15) peak bactericidal serum levels of 1:8 or greater resulted in a cure rate of 70 percent. It is not known how long during the treatment period such levels were present. The desire to maintain almost continuous bactericidal serum levels in staphylococcal endocarditis has led to the recommendation that nafcillin (or an equivalent drug) be administered as a bolus every 2 h in sufficient dose to maintain peak bactericidal levels of 1:16 or greater. Individual cases treated with methicillin have been cured with peak serum bactericidal levels of not more than 1:5 serum dilution. Optimal peak and trough concentrations are not defined and may well differ for different drugs (19). This has also applied to staphylococcal infections which failed to respond to initial therapy and were suspected of tolerance (12, 23, 30).

One of the important applications of serum bactericidal levels has been their application to the control of antimicrobial levels during a switch from intravenous to oral drug administration. This is, of course, of considerable concern particularly in infections where the need for long-term treatment carries the risk of introducing superinfection as a consequence of indwelling venous lines. At least two studies have addressed themselves to the problem in hematogenous osteomyelitis of children. Tetzlaff et al. suggested that serum bactericidal levels of antistaphylococcal drugs be maintained at 1:8 dilution during oral treatment of skeletal infections of children (44). Such peak levels may not be easily achieved with highly protein-bound lactamase-resistant penicillins, and there is no proof that they are required for cure. Prober and Yeager found that nafcillin (40 mg/kg intravenously every 4 h) given to children with staphylococcal hematogenous osteomyelitis uniformly resulted in peak serum bactericidal levels of 1:16 or greater (45). Nine of thirteen children were switched from intravenous treatment to oral dicloxacillin (25 mg/kg with probenecid every 6 h) and achieved similar peak bactericidal levels. Apparently all children in their series had a complete remission of clinical signs of osteomyelitis at the end of 6 weeks of treatment. Again the needed aggregate time of a given level of bactericidal activity required for "cure" is not known.

In severely neutropenic patients receiving chemotherapy for cancer, the impression exists that bactericidal concentrations of antimicrobials in serum are preferable to bacteriostatic ones. Klastersky (16, 42), Murillo et al. (25), and others have selected drug combinations to be used empirically in the treatment of suspected sepsis by using the criteria of bactericidal action of drug combinations active against the commonest opportunistic pathogens in their patients.

From these limited clinical reports it is evident that many more correlative studies will be needed to establish a firm foundation for the use of serum bactericidal titers as a quantitative guide to antimicrobial therapy. For the time being it is clear that no fixed time of serum assay or level of bactericidal activity can be given which would be universally applicable. Particularly when two drugs with different dosage schedules or pharmacokinetic patterns are administered, it would seem appropriate to obtain bactericidal serum assays at several points during 24-h cycles.

SUMMARY OF POSSIBLE MAJOR APPLICATIONS OF SERUM BACTERICIDAL ASSAYS

1 In diseases where serum bactericidal activity is definitely needed for cure, e.g., infective endocarditis

2 In immunodeficient or granulopenic hosts where serum bactericidal activity is probably important, e.g., in patients developing infections during cancer chemotherapy

3 For the assessment of synergistic action of drug combinations in vivo, where the endpoint must be bactericidal effect

4 To control efficacy of a change in therapeutic regimen, e.g., when oral therapy is substituted for parenteral or when a given drug regimen is no longer tolerated and must be changed to another

5 In infections where serum bactericidal activity probably aids in the eradication of infection, e.g., acute osteomyelitis or bacterial meningitis

CODA

It has been 50 years since Fleming published his initial observations and gave a name to penicillin. For 40 years antimicrobial drugs have been used on an enormous scale and have revolutionized the practice of medicine. More than 30 years ago it was recognized that in certain infectious processes combinations of drugs could effect a cure whereas single drugs failed. While some of the principles of combined drug effects have been known for over a quarter of a century, there is a remarkable lack of precise definitions and of rigorous laboratory tests to guide the therapeutic use of antibiotics in combinations. The field remains more an art than a science.

Sir George Pickering (46) pointed out that "Medicine, like theology, cannot tolerate ignorance. If it does not know the answer, it must invent it." In this review I have attempted to invent as little as possible. Nevertheless, my bias, or ignorance, will be apparent.

REFERENCES

1 Ericsson HM, Sherris JC: Antibiotic sensitivity testing. *Acta Pathol Microbiol Scand B Suppl* 217:1, 1971.

2 Bauer AW et al: Antibiotic susceptibility testing by a standardized single disc method. *Am J Clin Pathol* 45:493, 1966.

3 Matsen JM, Barry AL: Susceptibility testing: Diffusion test procedures, in Lennette EH et al (eds): *Manual of Clinical Microbiology*, ed 2. Washington, American Society of Microbiology, 1974, p 418.

4 Thornsberry C et al: New developments in antimicrobial agents susceptibility testing. *Cumitech 6*, 1977.

5 Washington JA: Infectious diseases 1979— Antimicrobial susceptibility tests. *J Infect Dis* 140:261, 1979.

6 Witebsky FG et al: Broth dilution minimum inhibitory concentrations: Rationale for use of selected antimicrobial concentrations. *J Clin Microbiol* 9:589, 1979.

7 Jawetz E: Combined antibiotic action: Some definitions and correlations between laboratory and clinical results. *Antimicrobial Agents and Chemotherapy.* Washington, American Society of Microbiology, 1967, p 203.

8 Jawetz E: The use of combinations of antimicrobial drugs. *Ann Rev Pharm* 8:151, 1968.

9 Moellering RC Jr: Antimicrobial synergism—An elusive concept. *J Infect Dis* 140:639, 1979.

10 Rahal JJ Jr: Antibiotic combinations: The clinical relevance of synergy and antagonism. *Medicine* 57:179, 1978.

11 Bererbaum MC: A method for testing for synergy with any number of agents. *J Infect Dis* 137:122, 1978.

12 Faville RJ et al: *Staphylococcus aureus* endocarditis. Combined therapy with vancomycin and rifampin. *JAMA* 240:1963, 1978.

13 Glew RH, Moellering RC Jr: Effect of protein binding on the activity of penicillins in combination with gentamicin against enterococci. *Antimicrob Agents Chemother* 15:87, 1979.

14 Greenwood D: Interactions between antibacterial drugs below the minimal inhibitory concentration. *Rev Infect Dis* 1:807, 1979.

15 Jawetz E, Brainerd HD: Staphylococcal endocarditis: Results of combined antibiotic therapy in 14 consecutive cases. *Am J Med* 32:17, 1962.

16 Klastersky J et al: Significance of antimicrobial synergism for the outcome of gram negative sepsis. *Am J Med Sci* 273:157, 1977.

17 Klein M, Kimmelman LJ: The correlation between the inhibition of drug resistance and synergism in penicillin and streptomycin. *J Bacteriol* 54:363, 1947.

18 Norden CW et al: Comparison of techniques for measurement of in vitro antibiotic synergism. *J Infect Dis* 140:629, 1979.

19 Sande MA, Johnson ML: Antimicrobial therapy of experimental endocarditis caused by staphylococcus aureus. *J Infect Dis* 131:367, 1975.

20 Weinstein RJ et al: Comparison of methods for assessing *in vitro* antibiotic synergism against *Pseudomonas* and *Serratia*. *J Lab Clin Med* 86:853, 1975.

21 Eagle H: Speculations as to the therapeutic significance of the penicillin blood level. *Ann Intern Med* 28:260, 1948.

22 Jaffe HW et al: Pharmacokinetic determinants of penicillin cure of gonococcal urethritis. *Antimicrob Agents Chemother* 15:587, 1979.

23 Denny AE et al: Serious staphylococcal infections with strains tolerant to bactericidal antibiotics. *Arch Intern Med* 139:1026, 1939.

24 Malacoff RF et al: Streptococcal endocarditis (nonenterococcal, non-group A). *JAMA* 241:1807, 1979.

25 Murillo J et al: Comparison of serum bactericidal activity among three antimicrobial combinations. *Antimicrob Agents Chemother* 13:992, 1978.

26 Sande MA, Irvin RG: Penicillin-aminoglycoside synergy in experimental *Streptococcus* viridans endocarditis. *J Infect Dis* 129:573, 1974.

27 Scheld WM et al: Response to therapy in an experimental rabbit model of meningitis due to listeria monocytogenes. *J Infect Dis* 140:287, 1979.

28 Gunnison JB, Jawetz E: Sensitivity tests with combinations of antibiotics: Unsuitability of disc method. *J Lab Clin Med* 42:163, 1953.

29 Jawetz E et al: A laboratory test for bacterial sensitivity to combinations of antibiotics. *Am J Clin Pathol* 25:1016, 1955.

30 Sabath LD et al: A new type of penicillin resistance of *Staphylococcus aureus*. *Lancet* 1:443, 1977.

31 **Reymann MT et al:** Correlation of aminoglycoside dosages with serum concentrations during therapy of serious gramnegative bacillary disease. *Antimicrob Agents Chemother* 16:353, 1979.

32 **Jawetz E:** Dynamics of the action of penicillin in experimental animals. *Arch Int Med* 77:1, 1946.

33 **Schlichter JG, McLean H:** A method of determining the effective therapeutic level in the treatment of subacute bacterial endocarditis with penicillin. *Am Heart J* 34:209, 1947.

34 **Schlichter JG et al:** Effective penicillin therapy in subacute bacterial endocarditis and other chronic infections. *Am J Med Sci* 217:600, 1949.

35 **Jawetz E:** Assay of antibacterial activity in serum. *Am J Dis Child* 103:81, 1962.

36 **Jawetz E, Gunnison JB:** The determination of sensitivity to penicillin and streptomycin of enterococci and streptococci of the viridans group. *J Lab Clin Med* 35:488, 1950.

37 **Reller LB, Stratton CW:** Serum dilution test for bactericidal activity: 11. Standardization and correlation with antimicrobial assays and susceptibility tests. *J Infect Dis* 136:196, 1977.

38 **Stratton CW, Reller LB:** Serum dilution test for bactericidal activity: 1. Selection of a physiologic diluent. *J Infect Dis* 136:187, 1977.

39 **Pien FD, Vosti KL:** Variation in performance of the serum bactericidal test. *Antimicrob Agents Chemother* 6:330, 1974.

40 **Prober CG et al:** Comparison of a micromethod for performance of the serum bactericidal test with the standard tube dilution method. *Antimicrob Agents Chemother* 16:46, 1979.

41 **Provonchee RB, Zinner SH:** Rapid method for determining serum bactericidal activity. *Appl Microbiol* 27:185, 1974.

42 **Klastersky J et al:** Antibacterial activity in serum and urine as a therapeutic guide in bacterial infections. *J Infect Dis* 129:187, 1974.

43 **Carizosa J, Kaye D:** Antibiotic concentration in serum, serum bactericidal activity, and results of therapy of streptococcal endocarditis in rabbits. *Antimicrob Agents Chemother* 12:479, 1977.

44 **Tetzlaff TR et al:** Oral antibiotic therapy for skeletal infections of children: II. Therapy of osteomyelitis and suppurative arthritis. *J Pediatr* 92:485, 1978.

45 **Prober CG, Yeager AS:** Use of the serum bactericidal titer to assess the adequacy of oral antibiotic therapy in the treatment of acute hematogenous osteomyelitis. *J Pediatr* 95:131, 1979.

46 **Pickering G:** Therapeutics—Art or science? *JAMA* 242:649, 1979.

Shock in gram-negative bacteremia: Predisposing factors, pathophysiology, and treatment

WILLIAM R. McCABE
RICHARD N. OLANS

Shock may occur during the course of a number of bacterial, fungal, viral, and rickettsial infections. A variety of causes and pathogenetic mechanisms (Table 1) may lead to the development of shock. Despite the large number of infections in which shock may develop, it is infrequent, except as a terminal or agonal event. Gram-negative organisms are unique among infectious agents, however, because of their capacity to produce shock and its often characteristic pattern of development. Shock occurs in approximately 40 percent of patients with gram-negative bacteremia (1, 2) and typically appears within the first 4 to 10 h after the onset of bacteremia. In contrast, shock is infrequent in other types of infection and tends to appear later, only after the infection is well established. In addition, shock associated with other types of infections is often accompanied by clinical findings, e.g., valvular insufficiency, diarrhea, and peritonitis, which provide ready explanation for vascular collapse while the mechanisms leading to shock in gram-negative bacterial infections are rarely clinically apparent.

The progressively increasing prevalence of gram-negative bacteremia, coupled with the relatively constant (±40 percent) rate of complicating shock, make it one of the most frequent overall causes of shock seen in medical practice. Studies in larger tertiary care medical centers have revealed that the prevalence of gram-negative bacteremia has increased by fifteenfold or more since the early 1950s (3). Reports from several major medical centers have demonstrated rates of gram-negative bacteremia in excess of 1 per 100 hospital admissions (2-5). Although substantially lower rates have been observed in small community hospitals (6), these differences in prevalence appear to reflect a greater concentration of patients with more severe underlying disease and greater utilization of measures which predispose to bacteremia in large referral centers than in smaller hospitals. Accurate estimation of the overall frequency

These studies were supported in part by United States Public Health Service Research Grants 5 R01 AI14789 and 7 R01 AI14789.

Table 1 Shock associated with infections

1 Failure of myocardial pump function: myocarditis
  a Bacterial (diphtheria, bacterial endocarditis, leptospirosis, etc.)
  b Viral (enteroviruses, Coxsackie, etc.)
  c Rickettsial (Rocky Mountain spotted fever, etc.)
  d Parasitic (Trichinella, Toxoplasma)

2 Valvular insufficiency
  a Bacterial endocarditis (acute and subacute)

3 Inadequate cardiac filling
  a Purulent pericarditis
  b Constrictive pericarditis

4 Diminution of fluid volume
  a Fluid loss or sequestration
    (1) Diarrhea (cholera, shigellosis, salmonellosis, enterotoxic *E. coli*, etc.)
    (2) Peritonitis
    (3) Pancreatitis
  b Increased vascular permeability
    (1) Rickettsial diseases (typhus, Rocky Mountain spotted fever, etc.)
    (2) Hemorrhagic fevers (viral)

5 Decreased venous return
  a Gram-negative bacteremia
  b Candidemia (?)

6 Hypoxia
  a Pneumonia
    (1) Bacterial
    (2) Viral
  b Intravascular hemolysis (clostridial sepsis)

of gram-negative bacteremia and septic shock among the 33 million annual acute hospital admissions in this country is precluded by these limitations. Clinical observations suggest that only cardiac disease exceeds gram-negative bacteremia as a cause of shock among hospitalized patients. Recent studies have demonstrated fatality rates of 47 percent among patients with gram-negative bacteremia complicated by the development of shock in contrast to fatality rates of 7 percent among patients with bacteremia not complicated by shock (1). Thus, not only is gram-negative bacteremia one of the most frequent causes of shock, but the occurrence of shock also markedly increases the lethality of gram-negative bacteremia.

CLINICAL FEATURES OF BACTEREMIA AND SHOCK

Although shock is a dramatic and highly lethal complication of bacteremia, its frequency and occurrence early in the course of bacteremia make it prudent to consider shock as an integral part of the syndrome of gram-negative bacteremia. For clinical purposes, development of shock should be anticipated and prepared for whenever the diagnosis of gram-negative bacteremia is seriously considered. The recent demonstration that early effective antibiotic treatment of bacteremia significantly reduces the frequency with which shock develops clearly establishes the importance of prompt diagnosis and therapy (1). Diagnosis of gram-negative bacteremia can be established only by isolation of infection microorganism(s) from blood cultures, but the relatively high fatality rate and rapid course of bacteremia often require the diagnosis to be made on the basis of clinical findings to allow prompt initiation of therapy. For this reason, a thorough understanding of factors which predispose to the development and outcome of bacteremia and its modes of presentation are essential.

Bacteremia

Predisposing factors   Available evidence indicates that bacteremia caused by gram-negative bacilli is an "opportunistic" type of infection which occurs primarily in hosts with altered defense mechanisms or when the organism is provided access to sites normally protected by host defenses. Both host factors and therapeutic measures predispose to the development of gram-negative bacteremia and determine its outcome (7). Distinction between the relative importance of host factors which predispose to bacteremia and the infectious hazards of various therapeutic modalities is often difficult because of the greater use of therapeutic agents and devices which predispose to, or produce infection in, the most critically ill patients, who are most susceptible to opportunistic infections (3).

Among host factors predisposing to the development and outcome of gram-negative bacteremia (Table 2), the severity of the host's underlying disease at the onset of bacteremia has been shown to be of paramount importance. Recognition of the importance of underlying host disease as a determinant in gram-negative bacteremia resulted in the development of a system which classified patients as having rapidly fatal, ultimately fatal, or nonfatal underlying diseases (8, 9). This classification has served as a necessary standard for comparative evaluation of therapy and factors affecting the development and outcome of bacteremia. Although attack rates of bacteremia increase with increasing age, it is unclear whether this is solely a reflection of age or the result of more severe underlying disease and greater use of therapeutic measures which predispose to the development of infection in the elderly (3). Granulocytopenia, irrespective of its cause, markedly predisposes to the development and fatal outcome of gram-negative bacteremia (3, 10). Both the frequency and severity of bacteremia are markedly increased in patients with total granulocyte counts of 1000 to 1500 per cubic millimeter or less (10). Considerable emphasis has been placed on the greater risk of acquisition of infections and their greater severity in immunocompromised patients and those with neoplastic disease (11–13). Despite the attention paid to infections in such patients, there is no evidence that this is due to malignancy per se rather than a reflection of disease- or therapy-

**Table 2 Factors predisposing to acquisition
and outcome of gram-negative bacteremia**

Host factors		Treatment factors	
Acquisition	*Severity*	*Acquisition*	*Severity*
Severity of underlying host disease	Severity of underlying host disease	Urinary catheters and manipulation	Corticosteroid therapy
Age	Granulocytopenia	Intravenous catheters	Drug- or irradiation-induced granulocytopenia
Loss of skin integrity by burns, etc.	Age	Respiratory tract manipulation	
	Azotemia	Corticosteroid therapy	
	Diabetes mellitus	Cytotoxic or antimetabolite therapy	
	Congestive heart failure	Gastrointestinal procedures	
		Surgical procedures	
		Irradiation	
		Drug- or irradiation-induced granulocytopenia	

associated granulocytopenia, more frequent use of procedures capable of inducing infection (intravenous catheters, etc.), and more frequent and protracted hospitalization with its attendant hazards. In contrast to other types of infection, no specific defect in host defense mechanisms, other than granulocytopenia, has been clearly established to predispose to gram-negative bacteremia. Azotemia, congestive heart failure, diabetes, and nosocomially acquired bacteremia are associated with a less favorable prognosis independent of the classification of severity of underlying host disease (1, 14). Failure to mount a significant febrile response during the first 24 h of bacteremia is also associated with a less favorable outcome (1, 14).

Much of the increasing frequency of gram-negative infections is attributable to the increasing use of certain therapeutic agents which adversely affect host defenses or medical devices which serve as a source of entry for gram-negative bacilli into normally protected body sites. Three types of widely used medical devices, indwelling urethral catheters (15), indwelling venous catheters (16, 17) (intravenous catheters, central venous pressure lines, and hyperalimentation lines), and ventilatory equipment (18) are perhaps the most frequent sources of gram-negative bacteremia. Granulocytopenia, induced by chemotherapy or irradiation, increases both the frequency of development and the severity of bacteremia (10). Similarly, corticosteroid therapy appears to be associated with an increased frequency and severity of bacteremia (1). Although prior therapy with antimetabolites or cytotoxic agents such as cyclophosphamide, etc., is associated with a less favorable outcome (1), it is unclear whether these adverse effects occur in the absence of the granulocytopenia which they may induce. A number of gastrointestinal procedures, proctosigmoidoscopy, etc., have also been shown to be associated with bacteremia (19), but these bacteremias tend to be transient and of little clinical significance. Increasing frequency of bacteremia has also been shown to parallel increasing frequency of prior therapy with antibiotics and cytotoxic agents and hospitalization on general and thoracic surgical services (1).

Clinical presentations of bacteremia The manifestations of gram-negative bacteremia may be extremely protean, varying from a fulminant, rapidly lethal presentation to one in which the bacteremia may be unrecognized for several days (1–5, 7–10). Some of the modes of presentation are listed in Table 3 and illustrate the variety of initial symptoms that may be observed. In its most readily identifiable form, bacteremia presents with rigors, high fever, prostration, and occasionally nausea, vomiting and/or diarrhea 1 to 2 h after manipulation of a urinary catheter or infected wound. Shock usually occurs during the first few hours after appearance of the initial signs of bacteremia. This dramatic sequence is usually recognizable, but only about one-third of patients present with this typical pattern. The onset of bacteremia is less apparent in the majority of the patients; almost all patients are febrile, but the degree of fever may be minimal in the elderly and in patients with uremia or receiving corticosteroids (1). Fever, in the absence of other findings, may be the sole indicator of bacteremia in patients with leukemia or other hematologic diseases, neoplasias, indwelling venous or urethral catheters, or gastrointestinal or genitourinary disorders. In some patients, an unexplained increase in the rate and depth of respiration, usually associated with respiratory alkalosis, may herald the onset of

Table 3   Clinical findings suggestive of gram-negative bacteremia

Chills, fever, and hypotension
Fever only (particularly in patients with granulocytopenia, neoplastic
  and hematologic diseases, and with intravascular or urinary catheters)
Hyperpnea, tachypnea, and respiratory alkalosis*
Hypotension*
Oliguria or anuria*
Acidosis*
Hypothermia*
Change in mentation (confusion, stupor, agitation, etc.)*
Thrombocytopenia*
Disseminated intravascular coagulation*
Adult respiratory disease syndrome
Evidence of urinary tract infection
Evidence of pulmonary infection
Ecthyma gangrenosum

* Without recognized cause.

bacteremia (20, 21). Bacteremia also may present only as unexplained hypotension, oliguria or anuria, or metabolic acidosis. In the elderly, change in mental status, manifested by confusion, stupor, agitation, etc., may be indicative of bacteremia. Hypothermia may also be an initial manifestation, but it rarely persists for more than a few hours (1). Thrombocytopenia is present at the onset in 60 percent of patients with bacteremia (1), and bacteremia may rarely present as frank disseminated intravascular coagulation (DIC). In other patients, manifestations of local infections, such as urinary or respiratory tract infections, may be so flagrant that they tend to mask features of bacteremia. Thus, while many of the presenting features of gram-negative bacteremia may be relatively nonspecific, they should alert the physician to this diagnostic possibility. Unfortunately, those patients at greatest risk for development of lethal bacteremia are the very patients in whom clinical presentations are often the least typical. Fever may be minimal in patients with uremia, in those receiving corticosteroids, and in the elderly; and the clinical signs of infection may be less apparent in granulocytopenic patients than in the more immunocompetent patient (22). The etiologic agent of bacteremia does not influence the mode of presentation, and the specific etiologic agent cannot be predicted on the basis of clinical findings. However, ecythyma gangrenosum (tender, indurated skin lesions with black necrotic centers, or bullous or vesicular lesions surrounded by an erythematous margin) is almost specific for bacteremia caused by *P. aeruginosa* or *Aeromonas* spp. (23).

Bacteremic shock

Predisposing factors   Factors predisposing to shock are less clearly defined than those predisposing to bacteremia. Although shock is more frequent in patients with rapidly fatal and ultimately fatal diseases than in those with nonfatal underlying diseases, this relation is not as striking as that of the lethality to the severity of underlying host disease (24). Shock is more frequent in patients over 50 years of age than in younger patients (24). At the onset of bacteremia hypothermia is not associated with a greater incidence of shock, but failure to mount a fever in excess of 99.6°F during the first 24 h is associated with an increased frequency of shock (24). Also associated with an increased frequency of shock are previous therapy with antibiotics, corticosteroids, antimetabolites, or cytotoxic agents; and diabetes, congestive heart failure, and azotemia (24). More surprising, perhaps, are factors demonstrated to be unrelated to shock. No difference has been detected in the frequency of shock in bacteremia caused by various species of bacilli (24). Similarly, no correlation was demonstrated between the magnitude of bacteremia, as determined by colony counts of blood cultures, and development of shock in two studies (2, 24); and four investigations have failed to show any relation between circulating "free" endotoxin and shock (25–28). Therefore, it is difficult to identify prospectively patients at greater risk of development of shock or to identify potential initiators of the hemodynamic alterations in shock solely on the basis of predisposing factors.

Evaluation of factors influencing the outcome of shock have demonstrated that inappropriate antibiotic therapy (1), delayed admission to an intensive care unit, significant lactate accumulation (20, 29), and decreased cardiac output which fails to increase after therapy (20) are associated with increased fatality rates.

Clinical presentation of bacteremic shock   The initial signs and symptoms of bacteremia should alert the physician to possible subsequent development of shock. The transition from manifestations of bacteremia to those of shock may be abrupt and dramatic or insidious. In some instances, bacteremia may be unrecognized until shock occurs, or shock may even be unrecognized until oliguria, respiratory changes, or coagulation abnormalities appear. Early, subtle findings of shock include an unexplained increased rate and depth of respiration, often associated with respiratory alkalosis (21), and unexplained alterations in mental status in the elderly. Awareness of these early clues may allow initiation of earlier and more effective therapy.

Two distinct clinical patterns may be observed in bacteremic shock. The first, *warm shock*, is characterized by evidence of circulatory hyperdynamicity. Patients are often alert with somewhat plethoric facies and extremities. Hyperventilation is usual, their skin is warm and dry, and their pulses strong and bounding (21). The physician is often surprised at the discovery of marked hypotension in such patients. The second type is more consistent with the classical presentation of shock. In this form, *cold shock*, the patient is obtunded, ashen, or cyanotic in appearance, has cold, clammy skin, and a rapid but weak and thready pulse (21). Both types of shock are associated with distinct and different patterns of hemodynamic alterations (see below). Although it was originally felt that these represented different syndromes, more recent evidence suggests instead that both represent two different phases in the spectrum of shock.

Epi- or paraphenomena   DISSEMINATED INTRAVASCULAR COAGULATION (DIC) This syndrome, with concomitant activation of the fibrinolytic and coagulation systems, may occur in a variety of conditions. Overall, infections with gram-negative bacteria appear to be the most frequent of the numerous causes of DIC (30, 31), but DIC is not a frequent event in gram-negative bacteremia. DIC associated with bacteremia is almost always associated with shock. Recent studies have demonstrated thrombocytopenia in approximately 60 percent and laboratory evidence of DIC in approximately 12 percent of patients with gram-negative bacteremia. DIC of a degree sufficient to produce bleeding occurred in less than 3 percent of these patients (1). Clinically, DIC presents as oozing from venipuncture sites, skin or subcutaneous bleeding, or bleeding from the mucous membranes of the mouth, nose, or gastrointestinal tract. It is assumed that activation of Hageman factor by gram-negative bacilli is the initial step with subsequent activation of the fibrinolytic and intrinsic clotting systems producing concomitant intravascular coagulation and fibrinolysis. Laboratory findings consist of thrombocytopenia, demonstration of circulating fibrin split products, and decreased levels of coagulation factors II, V, and VII (30, 31).

"SHOCK" LUNG: ADULT RESPIRATORY DISTRESS SYNDROME (ARDS)   Pulmonary abnormalities often occur after recovery from bacteremic shock. The usual pattern is that of a patient who appears stable after recovery from shock but abruptly develops tachypnea, dyspnea, and rales diffusely throughout the lungs after a latent period of 12 to 24 h. Chest roentgenograms demonstrate diffuse homogeneous pulmonary infiltrates, and blood gases reveal marked reductions in arterial P_{O_2} (40 to 60 mmHg), low arterial P_{CO_2} levels, and often respiratory alkalosis. The hypoxemia is not correctable by administration of 100 percent oxygen alone, and mechanical ventilation using high pressures is required for improvement. Considerable decrease in lung compliance and impaired ventilation-perfusion relations also occur. Histologic changes consist of alveolar thickening, intraalveolar fluid accumulation, and round cell infiltration (32, 33). Although ARDS may result from a variety of insults, bacteremic shock appears to be the most common cause. ARDS increases the fatality rate of gram-negative bacteremia, and ARDS caused by bacteremia has a higher fatality rate than that resulting from other causes (34). The exact mechanisms responsible for ARDS have yet to be delineated.

PATHOPHYSIOLOGY OF BACTEREMIC SHOCK

Initial stimulus

Despite extensive investigation, precise definition of the initial events and identification of the substance(s) that triggers the hemodynamic changes of bacteremic shock remain unclear. It is often assumed that the endotoxins (lipopolysaccharides, LPS) of gram-negative bacteria cause many of the manifestations and initiate the events resulting in the development of shock. The similar clinical findings and comparable frequency of shock in gram-negative bacteremia, irrespective of the etiologic agent suggest that these may result from a component common to all gram-negative bacteria (35). In addition, many of the findings in gram-negative bacteremia—fever, shock, leukocytosis, intravascular coagulation, complement activation, and kinin generation—can be induced by injection of dead bacteria or purified LPS extracted from gram-negative bacteria and has led to the belief that LPS is responsible for inducing the hemodynamic changes of septic shock (35).

Endotoxin has been shown to be present in two distinct physical states in vitro and in infections. *Bound endotoxin* constitutes an integral portion of the bacterial cell wall, but it can elicit the same activities as isolated, purified LPS. *Free endotoxin* is LPS which has been released and is no longer associated with the intact bacterial cell. Definition of the role of endotoxin in the pathogenesis of shock and other manifestations of bacteremia is complicated by difficulties in distinguishing between effects induced by intact bacteria and free endotoxin. Although this distinction may appear primarily semantic, it has important clinical implications: Effects produced by intact bacteria can be prevented or modified by antibiotic therapy, but the effects of free endotoxin, or toxemia, are not affected by antibiotics. Support for the importance of LPS is primarily derived from the similarities of manifestations of bacteremia irrespective of the etiologic agent, production of many of the clinical findings of bacteremia by purified LPS, and the demonstration of circulating free endotoxin in some infections (36). Although impressive, these represent only an association between clinical features and free endotoxin and not a cause-and-effect relation.

In contrast, several studies have suggested that LPS may not play a crucial role in the development of shock and lethality in gram-negative infections. Studies by Senterfitt and Shands evaluated the course of systemic *Salmonella* infections in control mice and in mice whose susceptibility to endotoxin had been increased a thousandfold by administration of BCG vaccine. If endotoxin present in, or released by, proliferating *Salmonella* were responsible for lethality, much smaller numbers of bacteria would be expected to produce death in mice, with a thousandfold increase in susceptibility to LPS than in controls; but similar numbers of *Salmonella* were found at the time of demise in control and sensitized mice (37). Extensions of these studies have evaluated *K. pneumoniae* and *E. coli* infections in C3H/HeJ mice, which are genetically resistant to endotoxin and in control, C3H/FeJ mice with and without BCG sensitization. Susceptibility to LPS varied approximately 5000-fold among the various groups, but despite these marked differences in sensitivity to LPS, animals in each experimental group died at similar times following bacterial challenge. In addition, similar total body counts of bacteria were found in animals in each group at the time of demise (38). Since similar numbers of bacteria were used for infection and animals died at a similar time postinfection with similar total body counts of the infecting bacteria, similar exposure to endotoxin from the infecting strains must have occurred. The demonstration that similar numbers of endotoxin-containing bacteria were required to produce lethality in groups of mice whose sensitivity to endotoxin varied 5000-fold suggests that endotoxin was not the cause of death in these infections (38). Quarles et al. (39) evaluated the effects of perfusion of hemodialysis chambers containing cultures of S. *marcescens* implanted between the carotid artery and jugular vein of goats. Perfusion of these cultures with plasma ultrafiltrates produced chills, fever, alterations in white blood cell count, and oliguria. Initially, these manifestations were considered to result from LPS released into the perfusing fluid, but follow-up studies using graded-porosity membrane filtration of the effluent indicated that the toxic moiety had a molecular weight between 300 and 10,000, which is considerably smaller than the molecular weights of several hundred thousand to 1 million found for biologically active endotoxin. These studies suggest that substances other than endotoxin may be responsible for clinical manifestations usually attributed to endotoxin.

Several clinical studies also cast doubt on the importance of free endotoxin in the pathogenesis of bacteremic shock. Although endotoxinlike material has been demonstrated in the circulation, many of these studies have used assays of equivocal specificity or failed to correlate assay results with manifestations attributed to LPS. Five such investigations have attempted to correlate clinical findings with circulating free endotoxin (25–28, 36). The epinephrine-induced skin necrosis bioassay for circulating free endotoxin was used by Porter et al. in patients with severe gram-negative bacteremia (25), and McGill et al. modified this assay to obtain greater sensitivity for studies of an even larger group of patients (26). Patients with severe gram-negative bacterial infections with and without bacteremia, with circulating free endotoxin, did not have fever, shock, or fatal outcome more frequently than similar patients with negative assays (25, 26). Using the *Limulus* gelation assay, which he helped develop, Levin found a greater incidence of shock and death among patients with bacteremic and nonbacteremic gram-negative bacterial infections who had positive assays for LPS than in patients without circulating LPS (36), but Stumacher et al. were unable to confirm these findings using the same assay to study an even larger group of patients. Patients with bacteremic and nonbacteremic gram-negative bacterial infections with positive *Limulus* assays did not have a greater frequency of shock and death than patients with similar infections with negative assays (27). Elin et al. were also unable to correlate circulating free endotoxin, detected by the *Limulus* assay, with shock and death among patients with gram-negative bacterial infections (28).

Thus, both experimental and clinical studies provide conflicting evidence about the role of free endotoxin in the pathogenesis of shock and other manifestations of gram-negative bacteremia. The popular and simplistic concept that the release of free endotoxin from gram-negative bacteria during the course of infection is responsible for producing shock and other clinical manifestations does not appear to be supported by critical experimental or clinical findings. Although LPS, either free or associated with intact bacteria, may play a role in producing some of the manifestations of infection, this must involve more complex mechanisms than simple direct quantitative effects of circulating LPS. Also, it is unlikely that the pathogenetic mechanisms involved in the production of manifestations of bacteremia will be delineated until it is recognized that more complex mechanisms than simple toxemia are involved.

Endogenous mediators of effects of bacteremia

Attempts to elucidate mechanisms involved in the pathogenesis of shock have served as potent stimuli for investigators. Such studies have identified a large number of substances postulated to serve as mediators in producing changes observed in shock. Histamine, epinephrine, norepinephrine, serotonin, glucocorticoids, acetylcholine, slow reacting substance, anaphylotoxins, prostaglandins, endorphins, lysosomal enzymes, lymphocytes, and components of the coagulation, fibrinolytic, complement, and kinin systems have all been suggested as causes of some of the pathophysiologic changes in shock. Delineation of the importance of these mediators in bacteremic shock is complicated in that many of the studies relating to them have evaluated changes occurring after LPS challenge rather than during infection and/or in relatively artificial animal models. An even greater problem in the evaluation of these mediators is determining whether changes represent primary pathogenetic effects or merely reflect compensatory host responses.

In contrast to uncertainty about many of the proposed mediators, activation of components of the coagulation, complement, and kinin systems has been demonstrated in gram-negative bacteremia in human beings (40, 41). Gram-negative bacilli are capable of activating Hageman factor (Factor XII), which then results in sequential and interrelated activation of the intrinsic coagulation, fibrinolytic, complement, and kinin systems. Activated Hageman factor can initiate conversion of plasminogen to plasmin and activate the intrinsic coagulation system (43), thus providing the early changes of DIC. Both gram-negative bacilli and plasmin can activate the complement cascade. Complement activation by bacteria can proceed either by classical or alternate (properdin) pathways, but studies early in the course of bacteremia have demonstrated only activation of the alternate pathway (42). Complement activation may lead to release of two vasoactive anaphylotoxins that may contribute to hemodynamic alterations. Hageman factor, plasmin, and plasmin-degraded Hageman factor fragments may lead to bradykinin generation. In human beings bradykinin produces hemodynamic effects, i.e., increased vascular permeability and vasodilation without significant alterations in cardiac output, similar to those observed early in bacteremic shock (44). Studies of patients with gram-negative bacteremia have demonstrated that significant decreases in Hageman factor, C3, and bradykinin precursors preceded the development of shock and were more marked in patients with bacteremia complicated by the development of shock (40, 41). Mason et al. found significant decreases in Hageman factor and bradykinin precursors in serum obtained shortly after the onset of bacteremia in patients who subsequently developed shock but only slight decreases in bacteremia without shock (40). McCabe found significant decreases of C3 levels in acute serum specimens in bacteremic patients who subsequently developed shock or died but normal levels in those with uncomplicated bacteremia. It was subsequently demonstrated that these changes involved only the alternate pathway without significant changes in classical pathway components (42). Although these findings do not prove that activation of the coagulation, complement, and kinin systems are responsible for the development of shock, they do offer strong indications of their importance. The similarity of the hemodynamic changes produced by bradykinin to those observed in bacteremic shock, the demonstration of activation of C3, Hageman factor, and bradykinin prior to the development of shock, and correlation between the magnitude of these changes and the development of shock strongly suggest that these mediators do play a role in bacteremic shock.

Animal models

Interest in the effects of endotoxin and attempts to elucidate mechanisms involved in bacteremic shock have resulted in a veritable deluge of studies of the response to LPS in almost every species of animal. Mice, rats, hamsters, and guinea pigs have been most popular for microcirculatory studies, while dogs and, more recently, nonhuman primates have been used most often for measurement of overall hemodynamic responses.

Injection or application of LPS results in alternating cycles of hyper- and hyporeactivity of the microcirculation (45), with more pronounced and protracted vasodilatation after larger doses. In the dog, injection of endotoxin results in a rapid, striking decrease in arterial pressure. The fall in arterial pressure primarily results from decreased venous return secondary to hepatic and splanchnic pooling caused by hepatic venous constriction. Concentrations of agents resembling histamine and catecholamine increase shortly after LPS administration. The decreased systemic arterial pressure improves after approximately 15 min and may be the result of catecholamine release. Thus, it is unclear whether catecholamine release represents a primary event or response to hypotension. This improvement in arterial pressure is only temporary, and even more severe hypotension that proves fatal during the next 3 to 24 h reappears (46).

Hemodynamic changes following administration of lethal doses of LPS to nonhuman primates differ from those observed in canines. Changes in arterial pressure are less precipitous, with a gradual decrease to shock levels, often with periods of recovery. Hepatosplanchnic pooling and portal hypertension are not observed although decreases in peripheral resistance, venous return, and cardiac output are major components of shock in primates (46). Catecholamine release does not occur until late. Hyperventilation, metabolic acidosis, and pulmonary changes consistent with early shock lung have also been reported (46).

Despite attempts to extrapolate findings from these experimental models, it is uncertain how closely they relate to bacteremic shock in human beings. The assumption that LPS administration produces effects identical to those occurring during clinical infections has tenuous validity. In addition, despite its ready availability and relatively low cost, the dog has been a particularly unfortunate choice as a model of human bacteremic shock because of its unusual enterohepatic circulation, resulting in hepatosplanchnic pooling of large quantities of blood unique to this species. The primate model more closely approximates changes observed in human patients, but even these studies have primarily evaluated lethal challenge with LPS rather than infection. Although challenge with viable bacteria has been undertaken, it has used inocula of bacteria similar to the lethal dose of killed bacteria and has not evaluated infections produced by small numbers of bacteria which induce a progressive, lethal infection.

Hemodynamic and other changes in bacteremic shock

The development of techniques for evaluation of the hemodynamic alterations in human beings has provided important breakthroughs in clarifying the pathophysiologic changes in bacteremic shock. Recognition of the need to study hemodynamic changes and evaluate therapeutic measures in human bacteremic shock rather than relying on animal models has materially enhanced our understanding of this syndrome (47). Initial physiologic studies of bacteremic shock yielded apparently conflicting results (48, 49) until it was recognized that these variable results reflected observations made during different stages of shock (20). Despite marked heterogeneity of underlying diseases and clinical status of patients investigated, two relatively consistent patterns of hemodynamic alterations were demonstrated. The first type usually presents as warm shock and is characterized by evidences of a hyperdynamic circulation. Typical findings include (1) increased or, less often, normal or decreased cardiac output, (2) marked decrease in peripheral resistance, (3) high or normal central venous pressure, (4) hyperventilation, and (5) lactate accumulation. Respiratory alkalosis is usually present, but metabolic acidosis may be found (20, 49). The second type presents with a clinical picture more typical of the classical pattern of shock with ashen or cyanotic color and cold clammy extremities. Pathophysiologic alterations include (1) decreased cardiac output, (2) increased peripheral resistance, (3) decreased central venous pressure, (4) hyperventilation, and (5) lactate accumulation (48). Respiratory alkalosis is found occasionally, but metabolic acidosis is usual. The first type was originally felt to represent shock in patients with normal blood volumes while the second pattern was believed to represent the response to bacteremia in hypovolemic patients (20).

Subsequently, more patients have been evaluated shortly after the onset of bacteremic shock, and hemodynamic and other measurements obtained sequentially throughout their course indicate that these two patterns of hemodynamic changes merely represent two phases in the evolution of bacteremic shock (50). It is now felt that the earliest hemodynamic alterations are those of a hyperdynamic state with a fall in vascular resistance and an increase in cardiac output. The decrease in peripheral resistance or vascular tone, which reflects the pressure-flow relationship in the body, is disproportionate to the increase in cardiac output (47) and results in inadequate tissue and organ perfusion. Hyperventilation with subsequent respiratory alkalosis is a relatively consistent early finding and is often a valuable early clue to the development of septic shock (21). Modest increases in serum lactate levels may be found early and, if shock proceeds uncorrected, lactate levels continue to increase and frank metabolic acidosis develops (48). The duration of this hyperdynamic phase is variable, and it may not be detected clinically until the patient has progressed into the later, more flagrant phase of shock. The substance(s) initiating or mediating these changes have not been identified, but evidence of generation of bradykinin, which produces similar hemodynamic changes, has been demonstrated early in the course of bacteremic shock in human beings.

The factors responsible for the transition from shock associated with a hyperdynamic circulation to a state of decreased cardiac output and increased peripheral resistance have yet to be defined. Recent studies have suggested that a fall in tissue oxygen consumption (51) and/or myocardial depression (52) may lead to these changes. In most patients with bacteremic shock, oxygen consumption is increased; but in the most seriously ill patients with hyperdynamic circulation, who often progress to the latter phase, there is a decrease in oxygen consumption, which results from failure of extraction rather than failure of oxygen delivery and which does not appear to be due to arteriovenous shunting. Although the cause of the decreased oxygen extraction has not been identified, this change may be implicated in the progression of shock (47, 51). There is also evidence that circulating substances which depress myocardial function may be found in the later phase of bacteremic shock (52) and that there is a blunted cardiac output in response to a volume load also in the later phases of bacteremic shock (53). In addition, factors which produce depression of myocardial function in vitro have been demonstrated in the serum of patients with bacteremic shock. Endotoxin has been excluded as the depressant factor(s). One cardiodepressant substance has been shown to be composed partially of ʟ-leucine, but complete characterization has not yet been accomplished (54).

MANAGEMENT OF BACTEREMIC SHOCK

Optimal care of the patient with shock involves a series of sequential steps, among which differential diagnosis is most crucial. The assumption of similar pathogenetic mechanisms and treatment for all types of shock proved fallacious and hazardous in the past. Unfortunately, this tendency to oversimplify the approach to treatment or to focus on only one aspect of bacteremic shock has not been completely reversed. Many recent studies of bacteremic shock have dealt almost exclusively with the management of hemodynamic alterations, and only a few have provided detailed consideration of the treatment of the cause of the shock—bacteremia (20, 49, 51). A surprising number of reports dismiss the subject of antibiotic therapy with terse statements like "massive doses of antibiotic therapy were administered" or "are recommended," apparently without recognizing that the effectiveness of the antibiotic is more crucial than the massiveness of its dose. This and other problems clearly emphasize the necessity for a logical, sequential, but multifaceted approach to the diagnosis and treatment of bacteremic shock, as outlined in Tables 4 and 5.

Diagnosis

Prompt recognition and diagnosis of gram-negative bacteremia are crucial for optimal therapy. The typical and the less obvious presentations of bacteremia must be recognized. Since bacteremia can be established only by blood cultures, treatment often must be initiated on the basis of clinical findings. Nonspecific tests for the bacterial nature of febrile episodes, such as the nitroblue tetrazolium (55, 56) and *Limulus* assays (27, 28), have failed to fulfill their early promise for diagnosis or identification of the type of bacterial disease. Except for the usefulness of the *Limulus* assay in gram-negative meningitis (57), these tests lack the specificity necessary to assist in the selection of antibiotic therapy. More specific immunologic assays, such as counterimmunoelectrophoresis, enzyme-linked immunosorbent assay (ELISA), etc., are of value for diagnosis of some infections, but it is unlikely that they can be modified to provide sufficient breadth to recognize the large number of species and serologic types of gram-negative bacilli that produce bacteremia. Inability to develop a rapid, specific diagnostic test for bacteremia means that meticulous patient evaluation and sound clinical judgment remain the major bases of diagnosis and treatment. Although quite nonspecific, total and differential leukocyte counts may reveal a marked "shift to the left" and toxic granulation, which strongly suggest serious bacterial infection. Examination of stained preparations of urine and sputum can help identify or exclude sites of origin of sus-

Table 4 Management of bacteremic shock

1 Establishment of diagnosis
    a Diagnosis of bacteremia
        (1) Epidemiologic, clinical, and physical findings
        (2) Collection of blood, urine, and other appropriate specimens for Gram stain and/or culture
    b Diagnosis of etiology of shock when preceding bacteremia not recognized
        (1) Hypovolemia
        (2) Hemorrhage
        (3) Cardiac
        (4) Hypersensitivity, anaphylaxis
        (5) Endocrine (adrenal insufficiency)
        (6) Other (pulmonary embolism)
        (7) Bacteremia
2 Appropriate antibiotic therapy
    a Check available culture and sensitivity data
    b Consider diagnosis, possible site of origin, nosocomiality, and possibility of anaerobes
    c Ensure collection of appropriate cultures before administration of antibiotics
3 Volume expansion: 1000 ml of crystalloid solution over 15–20 min if congestive failure absent
4 Monitoring volume expansion: insertion of Swan-Ganz or central venous pressure (CVP) catheter
    a Increase in wedged PA pressure of >8 mmHg or to levels >22 mmHg suggests possible cardiac decompensation
    b Increase in CVP of >50 mmH$_2$O or to level >120–140 mmH$_2$O with volume expansion suggests potential hazard of fluid overload
5 Continue volume expansion (15–20 ml/min) until recovery or wedged pulmonary artery pressure ≥22 mmHg or CV pressure ≥120 mmH$_2$O
6 Vasoactive agents (see Table 5)
7 Continued evaluation of mental status and urinary output (indwelling urethral catheter, "closed" sterile drainage system essential)
8 Ventilation: supplemental O$_2$ with or without intubation and assisted ventilation
9 Digitalis if congestive heart failure develops
10 Drainage of purulent accumulations; removal of foreign bodies
11 Modification of antibiotics as indicated by cultures, susceptibility tests, and renal function

pected bacteremia. Such preparations provide evidence of an inflammatory reaction, without which symptomatic infection is rare, and provide clues concerning possible etiologic agents. Gram stains made from the intravascular portion of intravenous catheters also may be of value. Finally, when there are large numbers of circulating bacteria, stains of the buffy coat may reveal the infecting organism.

The necessity for prompt recognition and therapy of bacteremia does not negate the requirement for bacteriologic confirmation and determination of the antimicrobial susceptibility of the infecting organism. Prompt collection of

Table 5   Drugs used in management of bacteremic shock

Agent	Dose	Effects	Response
Dopamine	2–50 μg/kg/min	Alpha, beta$_1$, and "dopaminergic" effects; positive inotropic > chronotropic effects; renal and splanchnic vasodilation with doses <8 μg/kg per minute without increase in blood pressure or heart rate; vasoconstriction, reversal of renal vasodilation and ↑ in blood pressure with doses per minute of ⩾10 μg/kg	↑ in blood pressure; ↑ in urine flow; improved sensorium
Isoprotenerol	1–2 μg/min	Beta$_1$ and beta$_2$, positive inotropic > chronotropic effects; vasodilation, ↑ strength and rate cardiac contractions with ↑ cardiac output and venous return	↓ CVP, ↑ cardiac output, ↑ urine output, improved sensorium; risk of tachycardia and arrhythmias
Dobutamine	2–15 μg/kg/min	Alpha and beta$_1$; positive inotropic effects > chronotropic effects	↑ cardiac output, ↑ urine output, improved sensorium
Norephinephrine	40–200 μg/min	Alpha and beta$_1$; positive inotropic effects > chronotropic effects	↑ blood pressure, ↑ cardiac output, ↑ coronary perfusion, marked peripheral vasoconstriction
Corticosteroids as single dose: Dexamethasone	6 mg/kg/min	?	Value debatable
Methylprednisolone	30 mg/kg/min	?	Value debatable

appropriate specimens for Gram's stain and culture before administration of antibiotics cannot be neglected. Cultures and microscopic examination of blood, urine, sputum, intravenous catheters, and wound drainage can be obtained rapidly even in the most urgent situations. Since bacteremia usually develops from localized infections, identification of the site of original infection is a crucial aspect of initial evaluation.

Occasionally, the onset of bacteremia may not be recognized because of the subtlety of initial manifestations until the patient presents with shock of uncertain etiology. Although the etiology of shock is usually apparent, it may be cryptic in a few patients. In the authors' experience, the greatest difficulty in differential diagnosis has occurred with elderly, dehydrated patients referred from chronic care facilities. These patients are frequently hypovolemic, often have low-grade fevers, and may have local infections, such as decubiti and urinary tract infections, caused by gram-negative bacilli. In contrast, distinction between bacteremic and hemorrhagic or cardiogenic shock usually does not present a problem, but exceptions do occur. Occasionally, fever may be associated with gastrointestinal bleeding, and a few hours may elapse before hematemesis or melena appear. The frequent use of intravenous and bladder catheters in patients with severe cardiac disease may serve as a source for bacteremia or lead to confusion regarding the etiology of shock. In addition, T wave and ST segment abnormalities and elevations of serum glutamic oxaloacetic transaminase and lactic dehydrogenase may develop in bacteremic shock and be misconstrued to reflect evidence of myocardial infarction. Adrenal insufficiency often presents with fever and hypotension, and bacterial infection may be suspected until the typical electrolyte changes and eosinophilia are observed. Hyperglycemia also occurs in gram-negative bacteremia and may lead to a suspicion of diabetes. Confusion also may arise in patients with pulmonary embolism where tachypnea and hyperpnea may be attributed to bacteremia and pulmonary infiltrates considered to represent gram-negative bacterial pneumonia. Thus, other types of shock may occasionally be confused with bacteremia, but careful clinical assessment usually will identify the cause of shock in these confusing cases. If bacteremia cannot be excluded, however, antibiotics should be administered until results of blood and other cultures are available.

Antibiotic therapy

Early administration of an effective antibiotic is the most crucial of all measures used for the treatment of gram-negative bacteremia and shock. The importance of appropriate antibiotic therapy has been unequivocally established in a series of investigations. Although the influence of the patients' underlying disease in determining outcome and insufficient numbers of patients to compensate for these modifying effects precluded demonstration of the importance of appropriate therapy in early studies (9), subsequent investigations documented enhanced survival in bacteremia treated with appropriate antibiotics (1, 2, 4, 14). Extension of these studies has also established the importance of appropriate antibiotics in the prevention and treatment of bacteremic shock. Recent investigations have demonstrated that appropriate antibiotic therapy, even when initiated after the onset of shock, significantly improved survival rates over those of patients who received inappropriate agents (1). The occurrence of 40 and 60 percent of fatalities within 24 and 48 h, respectively, after the onset of bacteremia emphasizes the importance of early, appropriate therapy (1). Even more convincing was the demonstration that early appropriate treatment afforded a twofold reduction in the frequency of shock among patients in all categories of severity of underlying disease (1).

Identification of the "most appropriate antibiotic(s)" is complicated by claims based on information generated in support of recently introduced antibiotics and from studies in a single type of disease. Recent studies of 612 patients with gram-negative bacteremia failed to demonstrate any differences in efficacy between a variety of individual antibiotics or various antibiotic combinations provided the infecting organism was susceptible and adequate antibiotic levels were maintained (1). This appears to conflict with the increasingly popular recommendations, particularly in neutropenic patients with underlying malignancy, for the treatment of bacteremia with combinations of antibiotics (13, 58–60). In actuality, however, there is very little real difference between results in these studies. When in vitro synergy can be demonstrated with specific combinations, increased efficacy of the combination usually occurs in experimental and clinical infections caused by the same organism (13, 58–60). The problem lies in the fact that synergy cannot be accurately predicted clinically and must be demonstrated retrospectively after the infecting organism has been isolated. Thus, although treatment with synergistic combinations was associated with enhanced effectiveness, the combinations actually used were no more efficacious than a single antibiotic. Of the four studies comparing the efficacy of single antibiotics with combinations in the treatment of gram-negative bacteremia, no significant differences in survival rates could be demonstrated (13, 58–60). Enhanced survival rates could be shown only for the subgroup (±50 percent) of patients treated with combinations subsequently shown to be synergistic, but not for the entire group receiving antibiotic combinations (58, 59). The lack of improved survival rates in the entire group receiving antibiotic combinations apparently reflects the inability prospectively to select a synergistic combination often enough to exert a significant impact on overall survival rates. In view of the increased toxicity of certain combinations (61) and the demonstration of the appearance and spread of strains resistant to both components of combinations after their extensive use (62), it is probably wise to temper enthusiasm for blanket use of combinations in gram-negative bacteremia.

There are clinical situations, however, where treatment with more than one antibiotic is indicated. They include infections in which both aerobic and anaerobic bacilli may be involved and, perhaps, infections caused by P. aeruginosa. Similarly, sepsis which may be caused by cocci or gram-negative bacilli also requires therapy adequate to include both potential etiologic agents until culture reports are available.

Selection of an effective antibiotic is not a problem in patients for whom previous culture and susceptibility results are available. In other patients, however, initial antibiotic therapy is selected on the basis of (1) identification of the site of origin of bacteremia, (2) knowledge of those bacteria which produce infections most often at these sites, (3) susceptibility patterns of the most likely pathogens, and (4) awareness of the usual nosocomial pathogens in specific areas of the hospital and their antimicrobial susceptibilities. The most frequent etiologic agents of bacteremia originating from various sites and the antibiotic to which these organisms are most often susceptible are listed in Table 6.

The urinary tract is the most frequent source of gram-negative bacteremia, E. coli predominating as the etiology of bacteremia originating from this site. Members of the *Klebsiella-Enterobacter-Serratia* and *Proteus* families and P.

Table 6 Choice of antibiotics for suspected gram-negative bacteremia by site of infection

Site	Likely etiologic agent	Antibiotic of choice	Alternative
Urinary tract	E. coli, K. pneumoniae, Proteus sp., P. aeruginosa	Aminoglycoside:* Amikacin (5 mg/kg IV every 8 h) or gentamicin (1.5 mg/kg IV every 8 h) or tobramycin (1.5 mg/kg IV every 8 h)	Cephalosporin
Gastrointestinal tract:			
Bowel†	E. coli, Bacteroides sp., K. pneumoniae, Proteus sp., P. aeruginosa	Aminoglycoside* + clindamycin (450–600 mg every 6 h IV)	Cefoxitin (2 g IV every 4–6 h) or chloramphenicol (50 mg/kg IV daily) A cephalosporin
Biliary tract†	E. coli, K. pneumoniae, Proteus sp.	Aminoglycoside*	
Reproductive tract†	E. coli, K. pneumoniae, Bacteroides sp.	Aminoglycoside* + clindamycin	Cefoxitin or chloramphenicol or (?) doxycycline (200 mg/day IV)
Respiratory tract:			
Tracheostomy, assisted ventilation	P. aeruginosa, Acinetobacter sp., Serratia sp., K. pneumoniae	Aminoglycoside* or aminoglycoside* + carbenicillin (4–6 g IV every 4–6 h)	
Aspiration†	E. coli, Bacteroides sp., Fusobacterium sp., K. pneumoniae, Proteus sp.	Aminoglycoside* + penicillin (6 million units IV daily)	Cefoxitin or chloramphenicol
Skin:			
Decubiti†	E. coli, Bacteroides sp., K. pneumoniae, Proteus sp.	Aminoglycoside* + clindamycin	Cefoxitin or chloramphenicol
Burns	P. aeruginosa, Enterobacter cloacae	Aminoglycoside* or aminoglycoside* + carbenicillin	
Intravascular devices, agranulocytosis, leukemia†	P. aeruginosa, Acinetobacter sp., Serratia sp.	Aminoglycoside* or aminoglycoside* + carbenicillin	

* Modify dosage interval with renal insufficiency. Change to least toxic antibiotic after receipt of culture reports and sensitivities.
† Gram-positive cocci often involved.

aeruginosa are much less frequent causes of urinary tract infections and usually appear only after treatment in chronic, recurrent infections or in patients with structural genitourinary abnormalities, indwelling catheters, or repetitive manipulations. *E. coli* is also the most frequent etiologic agent of bacteremias originating from the gastrointestinal and female genital tracts; but anaerobic bacilli, especially *B. fragilis*, are relatively more frequent in bacteremias originating from these sites. This influences antibiotic selection since most agents used in the treatment of gram-negative bacteremia have little activity against *B. fragilis*. Although the aminoglycosides (amikacin, tobramycin, and gentamicin) are usually selected for empiric therapy of suspected bacteremia from these sites, clindamycin and other antibiotics effective against *B. fragilis* should also be added. The biliary tract is a relatively frequent site of origin of bacteremia in the elderly. Anaerobes may be isolated in cultures from diseased gallbladders, but since they rarely are a cause of bacteremia, treatment of bacteremia originating from the biliary tract usually does not include coverage for *B. fragilis*.

Bacteremias originating from the skin and respiratory tract are often secondary to nosocomial infections of these sites with antibiotic-resistant organisms. In addition, infections of the skin, those resulting from intravenous catheters, and pulmonary infections associated with tracheostomies and mechanical ventilatory equipment are more often produced by bacteria, such as *P. aeruginosa*, *S. marcescens*, and *Acinetobacter*, that are skin inhabitants or are found in the environment. Gram-negative pneumonias secondary to aspiration are more often caused by constituents of the gastrointestinal flora, such as *E. coli*, *K. pneumoniae*, and *Bacteroides*. Decubitus ulcers may also be a source of bacteremia, anaerobes and *E. coli* being the most frequent etiologic agents. Since these types of infections are often nosocomial, results of preceding cultures and susceptibility tests frequently are available to assist in selection of therapy. It should also be recognized that some infections believed to be community-associated may actually be caused by strains acquired during previous hospital admissions. Similarly, antibiotic-resistant bacilli may be prevalent in some chronic care facilities and result in infections which necessitate transfer to the hospital. The frequency of antibiotic resistance in nosocomial gram-negative infections usually leads to the selection of the aminoglycoside with the broadest spectrum of activity for treatment. Resistance of gram-negative bacilli to individual aminoglycosides varies from hospital to hospital, the highest rates occurring in large referral centers, and this greatly influences whether gentamicin, tobramycin, or amikacin is selected for initial empiric therapy. The high proportion of strains in which synergy can be demonstrated often leads to the use of carbenicillin or ticarcillin and an aminoglycoside (63) when *P. aeruginosa* is strongly suspected as the etiologic agent of bacteremia.

Antibiotic resistance and the need for an agent with the broadest spectrum against potential etiologic agents has led to extensive use of aminoglycosides for empiric therapy of suspected bacteremia, but these agents do have distinct disadvantages. Gentamicin, tobramycin, and amikacin have all been shown to be nephrotoxic and ototoxic. These side effects appear to be less frequent with tobramycin than with gentamicin, but the relative toxicity of amikacin has not yet been firmly established. Of equal or greater concern, however, is the lack of predictability and the relatively low serum levels (in relation to the inhibitory concentrations for many gram-negative bacilli) achievable with tobramycin and gentamicin (64). This may explain the relatively lesser effectiveness of gentamicin in a recent review by Kreger et al. (1). The greater ratio of serum levels to organism susceptibility and the increasing frequency of resistance to gentamicin and tobramycin may lead to their replacement by amikacin as the agent of choice for empiric therapy of suspected bacteremia. Irrespective of the aminoglycoside used, however, there is indisputable evidence that monitoring of serum levels is essential to give optimal therapy and to minimize drug toxicity (64, 65). In addition, dosage of aminoglycosides must be modified markedly in patients with renal insufficiency.

The newly introduced cephalosporins, cefamandole and cefoxitin, do not appear likely to replace aminoglycosides as agents of choice for initial therapy of bacteremia because of significant gaps in their spectrum against gram-negative bacilli (66, 67). Newer cephalosporins, currently under investigation, have an even wider spectrum of activity against aerobic bacilli and B. *fragilis* than the aminoglycosides and may become the agents of choice for empiric therapy in the near future (68, 69).

Equally important is substitution of the least toxic antibiotic (that achieves adequate serum levels) to which the infecting organism is susceptible once results of cultures and sensitivities have been obtained. The demonstration of equal efficacy of most antibiotics (that achieve adequate serum levels) to which the infecting organism is susceptible supports this approach (1). Automated instrumentation has been developed to detect bacteremia and allow determination of antibiotic susceptibility more rapidly than by routine methods, but these expensive instruments may not be routinely available. Other methods developed for rapid identification and susceptibility testing for use in smaller laboratories allow more rapid identification of inappropriate therapy and earlier change to a less toxic effective agent (70, 71).

The duration of antibiotic therapy is determined primarily by the nature of the original local infection. Antibiotics should be continued for a minimum of 5 afebrile days or even longer if local infection persists. The diagnosis of focal infection, removal of foreign bodies, and drainage of purulent accumulations is crucial to the management of bacteremia and shock (see below).

Volume expansion and cardiovascular monitoring

Inadequate perfusing volume resulting from decreased peripheral resistance not accompanied by an equivalent increase in cardiac output is the major functional defect in bacteremic shock (47). Treatment is directed toward correction of this defect by volume expansion and improvement of cardiac output. Fluid administration, 1000 ml of crystalloid solution over a 15- to 30-min period, should be started once bacteremic shock is suspected if congestive failure is not present. Appropriate cultures, specimens for creatinine, electrolytes, and arterial pH, P_{CO_2}, and P_{O_2} determinations should be obtained, and a central venous pressure

(CVP) or, preferably, a flow-directed pulmonary artery catheter placed during this time. Pulmonary artery catheters allow measurements of wedged pulmonary artery pressure (WPAP) or pulmonary diastolic pressures and provide a more reliable index than CVP determinations of left atrial and ventricular filling pressures and of the hazard of cardiac decompensation. Facilities for more sophisticated measurements, e.g., cardiac output determinations, may be of assistance but are not essential for management of bacteremic shock. Volume expansion, even in the absence of a decrease in blood volume, usually improves cardiac output provided fluid overload does not occur. Absolute CVP and WPAP values are less crucial than changes in pressure in response to fluid infusions. If the CVP or WPAP do not exceed 140 mmH$_2$O or 22 mmHg, respectively, volume expansion with both crystalloid and colloid (albumin or low-molecular-weight dextran) solutions is continued at a rate of 15 to 20 ml/min. A sudden or continuous progressive increase in CVP of >50 mmH$_2$O or to levels greater than 120 to 140 mmH$_2$O or an increase in WPAP > 8 mmHg or to levels greater than 22 mmHg suggest possible fluid overload and impending cardiac decompensation (20, 29, 48, 49). Frequent auscultation of the chest and examination of the jugular pulse should accompany pressure monitoring. Volume expansion is continued until recovery or evidence of impending fluid overload. It is not necessary to raise the blood pressure to levels present before the development of shock; systolic levels of 20 mmHg less than normal values are usually adequate. Monitoring to ensure a urinary output of 40 to 50 ml/h usually requires placement of an indwelling catheter, but scrupulous attention must be directed toward use of a closed-drainage system and prevention of infection. Since peripheral blood pressure measurements may not adequately reflect central aortic pressure, continuous assessment of mental status and urinary output provides important clues to the adequacy of perfusion of these organs.

Vasoactive agents

If volume expansion does not produce prompt improvement, vasoactive agents should be added to increase cardiac output further. Almost uniformly glowing reports of efficacy of each new vasoactive drug for the treatment of bacteremic shock have accompanied their introduction, but there is little proof of the superiority of any individual agent in enhancing survival. There is general agreement, however, that the vasopressors metaraminol and norepinephrine increase peripheral vasoconstriction and further compromise blood flow and should not be used except in limited, specific circumstances.

Dopamine   Dopamine has become the most widely used vasoactive agent in the treatment of bacteremic shock. It is of particular interest because of the variety of dose-dependent pharmacologic activities produced. At low doses, 2 to 5 μg/kg per minute, it is a beta-adrenergic agonist that increases myocardial contractility more than it increases heart rate. Dopamine also produces non-beta-adrenergic dilatation of the renal and splanchnic vasculature. At doses greater than 8 to 10 μg/kg per minute, alpha-adrenergic effects of generalized vasoconstriction appear, and at doses of 30 μg/kg per minute vasoconstriction is comparable to that of norepinephrine (72). Therapy is begun by continuous intravenous infusion of dopamine at a rate of 2 to 5 μg/kg per minute, and the infusion rate is varied to produce the desired effect, e.g., restoration of blood pressure and urine output. It is preferable to use doses less than those producing marked vasoconstriction.

Isoproterenol Isoproterenol exerts both beta$_1$ and beta$_2$ effects; its activity in increasing cardiac output is accompanied by equivalent vasodilatation. Its positive inotropic effects are beneficial, but its vasodilatory activity is undesirable in the treatment of early bacteremic shock. In addition, its pronounced effects in increasing tissue oxygen consumption and in increasing heart rate may be arrhythmogenic and have led to a marked decrease in its use in bacteremic shock. The dose of isoproterenol is 1 to 2 μg/min (73).

Dobutamine Dobutamine is a recently introduced beta agonist that acts directly on beta$_1$-adrenergic receptors and has primarily a positive inotropic effect with little chronotropic activity. It has been shown to increase myocardial contractility and reduce left ventricular filling pressure in patients with heart failure (74). Although of potential promise, dobutamine has had limited use in the treatment of bacteremic shock.

Norepinephrine As discussed earlier, the marked vasoconstriction induced by norepinephrine is contraindicated and has prevented its use in bacteremic shock. It has been suggested that there may be indication for temporary increases in perfusion pressure with its accompanying increase in coronary flow in patients with severe coronary insufficiency and bacteremic shock. Except for this possible indication, vasoconstrictors are contraindicated.

Corticosteroids The effectiveness and hazards of corticosteroids in the therapy of septic shock has been a controversial issue. Some studies suggest improved survival (75, 76) while others indicate no benefit from the use of steroids (77, 78) in the treatment of bacteremia and shock. Many of the errors in design or performance in these studies have been delineated (79). Recently, Schumer indicated in his study an increased survival among patients with bacteremic shock randomly treated with one or two doses of 3 mg/kg of dexamethasone or 30 mg/kg of methylprednisolone (80). Other recent studies of patients with comparable underlying diseases and bacteremic shock of equivalent severity found that "pharmacologic" doses of corticosteroids not only failed to improve survival but were associated with a significant increase in fatality rates (1). These disparate results in various studies of steroid therapy in septic shock, ranging from significantly increased fatality rates to significantly improved survival rates, are not readily explicable. The effects of steroids in bacteremic shock thus remain incompletely delineated and await further well-designed and controlled studies for clarification.

Other vasoactive agents A number of other vasoactive agents, such as phentolamine, phenobenzamine, propranolol, chlorpromazine, and vasoconstrictors, have also been used in the treatment of bacteremic shock in the past. The brief popularity of these agents has often been based on a limited number of reports of apparently beneficial effects which are not substantiated by more extensive experience. It may well be that the seemingly beneficial effects of many vasoactive agents result from factors other than the pharmacologic effects of the agents themselves (see below). More recently, the potent vasodilator, nitroprusside, has been used to improve left ventricular performance by decreasing left ventricular afterload and preload in the presence of marked vasoconstriction, but its merit in shock has yet to be established.

Other measures

Ventilation   One of the initial steps in the management of the patient with bacteremic shock is to ensure an adequate airway and to administer oxygen. A number of studies have indicated that inadequate respiratory gas exchange is an important contributing factor to an adverse outcome. Patients with labored or feeble respiratory excursions, respiratory acidosis, or hypoxia ($P_{O_2} < 70$ mmHg) should be carefully examined to exclude airway obstruction and be started on mechanical ventilatory assistance.

Digitalis and management of congestive failure   Digitalis has not been shown to be of benefit in the treatment of bacteremic shock in the absence of congestive heart failure. If vigorous volume expansion results in fluid overload, digitalis remains the cornerstone of treatment. Extreme caution is required in the use of diuretics to ensure that excessive diuresis is not produced and the beneficial effects of volume expansion dissipated. In the authors' experience, occasional patients have been "ping-ponged" from shock to congestive failure by over-vigorous volume expansion, become hypotensive again after zealous diuresis, and then resubjected to fluid overload. For this reason, it is preferable to ensure adequate digitalization before resorting to diuretics.

Drainage of purulent collections; removal of foreign bodies   Recognition and adequate management of local sites of infection is as crucial to the treatment of bacteremia as antibiotic administration. Foreign bodies should be removed, obstructing lesions corrected, and purulent accumulations drained as rapidly as possible. Intravenous catheters and other intravascular lines should be removed immediately and replaced when they are essential to patient management. Since bacteria will settle out on such lines, it is preferable to replace them again after 48 h of antibiotic treatment. Indwelling Foley catheters should also be changed.

Bacteremia always originates from a local infection although the site may not be apparent. Careful examination by radiologic techniques, ultrasound, gallium scanning, and computerized axial tomography should be undertaken as soon as feasible. Since bacteremia may persist despite effective antibiotic therapy in patients with abscesses, etc., surgical debridement, removal of retained products of conception, and drainage of purulent accumulations should be accomplished as soon as possible. Despite reluctance to subject patients with shock and large abscesses to surgery, failure to respond within 1 to 2 h to resuscitative measures should prompt emergent surgical drainage. Similarly, surgical ligation and removal of the infected thrombus is often required in suppurative thrombophlebitis. There are also instances, e.g., the postpartum female with retained products of conception, profound shock, and DIC, in which immediate hysterectomy is crucial for the prevention of fatal outcome.

Management of pyrexia   A great deal of attention is often devoted toward reducing fever in septic patients. Except for increased metabolic activity, fevers have relatively limited adverse effects in adults, except at 106°F and above. The increased metabolic activity resulting from rigors induced by antipyretics and shivering produced by cooling mattresses often negate any effects that might be achieved by reducing fever.

Special care facilities and expert consultation   The large number of reports suggesting use of a variety of therapeutic measures, e.g., hypothermia, hyperbaric oxygen, various pharmacologic agents, etc., whose merit could not be confirmed subsequently suggests that a well-trained team for the management of shock may be more crucial than the specific therapeutic modalities used. This is supported by indications that early transfer to an intensive care setting is associated with enhanced survival (29). There is concern, however, for the routine management of bacteremic shock in units where attention may be focused primarily on the management of hemodynamic alterations rather than treatment of the cause. Those primarily involved in management of circulatory and cardiovascular problems often do not have a comprehensive understanding of the intricacies of antimicrobial therapy. As has been shown, management of the cause of this type of shock, i.e., bacteremia, is as important as management of hemodynamic complications; it is essential to ensure optimal treatment of both bacteremia and shock. The demonstration that adherence to recommendations by expert consultants for antibiotic therapy improved survival rates in bacteremia provides further support for the necessity of optimal antibiotic treatment (12).

Granulocyte replacement   Development of techniques for collection of granulocytes has led to their use as adjuncts in the treatment of patients with chemotherapy-induced granulocytopenia. Despite variables which make comparisons difficult, granulocyte transfusions appear to exert some beneficial effects (81). Such therapy should be limited to patients with absolute granulocyte counts under 1000 per cubic millimeter. Attempts to use granulocyte transfusions for prophylaxis have been encouraging but inconclusive (82).

Treatment of complications

DIC   The syndrome of DIC has provoked considerable attention and has been postulated to be an important cause of multiple organ failure. The initial enthusiasm for heparin treatment of DIC has been tempered, however, by evidence of the inability of such treatment to reduce fatalities in either experimental models or human patients despite improvement in coagulation factors. If heparin therapy is undertaken, it is essential that the patient be carefully monitored for increased hemorrhage and that appropriate blood products be administered concomitantly (83, 84).

ARDS Once the need for mechanical ventilation has been established, the patient is intubated and begun on volume-cycled ventilation. It is usually noted that a large respiratory minute ventilation is required and that little improvement or, often, a decrease in P_{O_2} is noted despite increasing oxygen concentration. Positive end-expiratory pressure (PEEP) is usually initiated at this point at a pressure of 5 cmH$_2$O and continued for ± 30 min to observe response. PEEP is increased at increments of 5 cmH$_2$O until adequate Pa$_{O_2}$ values are achieved. Inspired oxygen concentrations are decreased when Pa$_{O_2}$ reaches 70 mmHg, and attempts are made to maintain values of 60 to 70 mmHg. After the patient's condition has been stabilized for 24 h, the level of PEEP is decreased by small increments at 12- to 24-h intervals until treatment can be discontinued. It may be possible to wean some patients rapidly while others may require weeks of therapy with PEEP.

Oliguria Oliguric renal failure may complicate bacteremic shock and may be difficult to distinguish from prerenal azotemia. The response in urinary output to volume expansion usually serves to identify a prerenal cause. Early tubular necrosis should be treated with intravenous infusion of 12.5 g of mannitol over 5 min and repeated after 2 h if a urine flow of 30 to 40 ml/h is not achieved. Furosemide, 240 mg, is given intravenously at the time of the second infusion of mannitol. If there is no response to the mannitol and furosemide, a second dose of 480 mg of furosemide is given intravenously, but no further efforts at diuresis are made if this proves unsuccessful. If these measures are ineffective, standard methods, including dialysis, for management of renal failure are instituted.

PREVENTION

The optimal management of gram-negative bacteremia, as with many other infections, is its prevention. Although attempts at developing vaccines against gram-negative bacilli are in progress, they are far from clinically useful. The best hope for reducing the frequency of such infections is the prevention of hospital-acquired gram-negative bacillary infections. Major efforts in controlling nosocomial infections should be directed toward the three most frequent sources of infection, indwelling intravenous and bladder catheters and ventilatory therapy equipment. Their use should be limited to settings in which they are absolutely necessary, and they should be discontinued as soon as possible. Bladder catheters should be inserted under sterile conditions and only closed-drainage systems used (85). Continuous bladder irrigation with dilute (0.25%) acetic acid or antibiotic solutions does not obviate the need for these precautions. The use of antibiotic irrigants only postpones the development of bladder infections, is associated with selection of more resistant bacteria, and when used concomitantly, does not improve the effectiveness of closed-drainage systems (86). Intravenous catheters should be inspected regularly and should be changed every 48 to 72 h. The use of special intravenous teams to decrease the rate of intravenous-related sepsis has been recommended (87), but other research indicates that meticulous attention to aseptic technique during insertion and maintenance adequately improves infection rates (88). All ventilatory equipment should be disposable or sterilized before use. All fluid reservoirs should be regularly changed and cleaned. Prevention of decubiti, replacement of quaternary ammonium compounds with organic iodine antiseptics (89), and strict adherence to aseptic techniques in the care of tracheostomies, wounds, tube drainage, and catheters are other important control measures. Limitation of excessive use of antibiotics can help diminish the proliferation of multiply resistant organisms in the hospital environment. Antibiotic prophylaxis has generally proved ineffective in the prevention of gram-negative bacteremia, but there are limited instances, e.g., necessity for emergency urologic procedures in patients with urinary infections and silver sulfonamide topical therapy in burn patients, where this may be of value. Extensive attempts have been made to prevent infections in patients made granulocytopenic by cancer chemotherapy. Most of these measures are extremely expensive and of limited effectiveness. The slight decrease in infections in neutropenic patients managed in laminar flow units and with oral antimicrobials to reduce the fecal flora appears to be primarily the result of the oral agents (90). Reduction of infections in patients with neoplastic disease has also been reported with oral trimethoprim-sulfamethoxazole (91). It has yet to be determined, however, whether extensive prolonged use of oral antibiotics within a limited area will result in the appearance of a resistant flora. As McGowan et al. have pointed out, much more study is needed to determine those measures which are most effective in the control of hospital-acquired bacteremia (92). Regular surveillance of infections and commitment of all hospital personnel are necessary to diminish the incidence of nosocomial gram-negative infections.

REFERENCES

1 Kreger BE et al: Gram-negative bacteremia: IV. Re-evaluation of clinical features and treatment in 612 patients. *Am J Med.* 68:344, 1980.

2 DuPont HL, Spink WW: Infections due to gram-negative organisms: An analysis of 860 patients with bacteremia at the University of Minnesota Medical Center 1958–1966. *Medicine* 48:307, 1969.

3 Kreger BE et al: Gram-negative bacteremia: III. Re-assessment of etiology, epidemiology and ecology in 612 patients. *Am J Med.* 68:332, 1980.

4 Myerowitz RL et al: Recent experience with bacillemia due to gram-negative organisms. *J Infect Dis* 124:239, 1971.

5 Finland M: Changing ecology of bacterial infections as related to antibacterial therapy. *J Infect Dis* 122:419, 1970.

6 Scheckler WE: Nosocomial infections in a community hospital. *Arch Intern Med* 138:1792, 1978.

7 McCabe WR: Gram-negative bacteremia. DM Disease-a-Month. December 1973. Chicago, Year Book 1973.

8 McCabe WR, Jackson GG: Gram-negative bacteremia: I. Etiology and ecology. *Arch Intern Med* 110:845, 1962.

9 McCabe WR, Jackson GG: Gram-negative bacteremia: II. Clinical, laboratory and therapeutic observations. *Arch Intern Med* 121:856, 1962.

10 Bodey GP et al: Quantitative relationships between circulating leukocytes and infection in patients with acute leukemia. *Ann Intern Med* 64:328, 1966.

11 Levine AS et al: Management of infections in patients with leukemia and lymphoma. Current concepts and experimental approaches. *Semin Hematol* 9:141, 1972.

12 **Singer C et al:** Bacteremia and fungemia complicating neoplastic disease. *Am J Med* 62:731, 1977.

13 **Schimpff S et al:** Empiric therapy with carbenicillin and gentamicin for febrile patients with cancer and granulocytopenia. *N Engl J Med* 284:1061, 1971.

14 **Bryant RE et al:** Factors affecting gram-negative rod bacteremia. *Arch Intern Med* 127:120, 1971.

15 **Martin CM et al:** Prevention of gram-negative rod bacteremia associated with indwelling urinary tract catheterization, in *Antimicrobial Agents and Chemotherapy*. Washington, American Society of Microbiology, 1964, p 617.

16 **Collins RN et al:** Risk of local and systemic infection with polyethylene catheters. *N Engl J Med* 279:340, 1968.

17 **Goldman DA, Maki DG:** Infection control in total parenteral nutrition. *JAMA* 223:1360, 1973.

18 **Pierce AK et al:** Long-term evaluation of decontamination of inhalation-therapy equipment and the occurrence of necrotizing pneumonia. *N Engl J Med* 282:528, 1970.

19 **LeFrock JL et al:** Transient bacteremia associated with sigmoidoscopy. *N Engl J Med* 289:467, 1973.

20 **MacLean LD et al:** Patterns of septic shock in man—A detailed study of 56 patients. *Ann Surg* 166:543, 1967.

21 **Simmons DH et al:** Hyperventilation and respiratory alkalosis as signs of gram-negative bacteremia. *JAMA* 174:2196, 1960.

22 **Sickles EA et al:** Clinical presentation of infection in granulocytopenic patients. *Arch Intern Med* 135:715, 1975.

23 **Dorff GJ et al:** Pseudomonas septicemia. Illustrated evolution of its skin lesion. *Surg Gynecol Obstet* 128:37, 1969.

24 **Kreger BE et al:** Shock in Gram-negative bacteremia. In preparation.

25 **Porter PJ et al:** Endotoxin-like activity of serum from patients with severe localized infections. *N Engl J Med* 271:445, 1964.

26 **McGill M et al:** The use of a bioassay for endotoxin in clinical infections. *J. Infect Dis* 121:103, 1970.

27 **Stumacher RJ et al:** Limitations of the usefulness of the limulus assay for endotoxin. *N Engl J Med* 288:1261, 1973.

28 **Elin RJ, Robinson RA:** Lack of clinical usefulness of the limulus test in the diagnosis of endotoxemia. *N Engl J Med* 293:521, 1975.

29 **Nishijima H et al:** Hemodynamic and metabolic studies on shock associated with gram negative bacteremia. *Medicine* 52:287, 1973.

30 **Corrigan JJ et al:** Changes in blood coagulation system associated with bacteremia. *N Engl J Med* 279:851, 1968.

31 **Yoshikawa T et al:** Infection and disseminated intravascular coagulation. *Medicine* 50:237, 1971.

32 **Pontoppidan H et al:** Acute respiratory failure in the adult. *N Engl J Med* 287:690, 743, 749, 1972.

33 **Clowes GHA Jr:** Pulmonary abnormalities in sepsis. *Surg Clin North Am* 54:993, 1974.

34 **Kaplan RH et al:** Incidence and outcome of the respiratory distress syndrome in gram-negative sepsis. *Arch Intern Med* 139:867, 1979.

35 **McCabe WR:** Antibiotics and endotoxic shock. *Bull NY Acad Med* 51:1084, 1975.

36 **Levin J et al:** Gram-negative sepsis: Detection of endotoxemia with the limulus test. *Ann Intern Med* 76:1, 1972.

37 **Senterfitt VC, Shands J:** Salmonellosis in mice infected with *Mycobacterium tuberculosis* BCG:I. The role of endotoxin in infection. *J Bacteriol* 96:287, 1968.

38 **Craven DE, McCabe WR:** Unpublished studies.

39 **Quarles JM et al:** Hemodialysis culture of *Serratia marcescens* in a goat–artificial kidney–fermentor system. *Infect Immun* 9:550, 1974.

40 **Mason JW et al:** Plasma kallikrein and Hageman factor in gram-negative bacteremia. *Ann Intern Med* 73:545, 1970.

41 **McCabe WR:** Serum complement levels in bacteremia due to gram-negative organisms. *N Engl J Med* 287:261, 1972.

42 **Fearon DT et al:** Activation of the properdin pathway in patients with gram-negative bacteremia. *N Engl J Med* 292:937, 1975.

43 **Morrison DC, Cochrane CG:** Direct evidence for Hageman factor (factor XII) activation by bacterial lipopolysaccharides (endotoxins). *J Exp Med* 140:797, 1974.

44 **Miller RL et al:** Biochemical mechanisms of generation of bradykinin by endotoxin. *J Infect Dis* 128S:136S, 1973.

45 **Zweifach BW:** Vascular effects of bacterial endotoxin, in Landy M, Braun W (eds): *Bacterial Endotoxins*. Rahway, NJ, Institute of Microbiology, Rutgers, The State University, 1964.

46 **Hinshaw LB:** Release of vasoactive agents and vascular effects of endotoxin, in Kadis S et al (eds): *Microbial Toxins, Vol 5, Bacterial Endotoxins*. New York, Academic, 1971.

47 **Siegel JH et al:** Physiological and metabolic correlations in human sepsis. *Surgery* 86:163, 1979.

48 **Udhoji VN, Weil MH:** Hemodynamic and metabolic studies on shock associated with bacteremia: Observations on sixteen patients. *Ann Intern Med* 62:966, 1965.

49 **Motsay GJ et al:** Hemodynamic alterations and results of treatment in patients with gram-negative septic shock. *Surgery* 67:577, 1970.

50 **Gunnar RM et al:** Hemodynamic measurements in bacteremia and septic shock in man. *J Infect Dis* 128S:295S, 1973.

51 **Siegel JH, Greenspan M:** Abnormal vascular tone, defective oxygen transport and myocardial failure in human septic shock. *Ann Surg* 165:504, 1967.

52 **Lefer AM:** Mechanisms of cardiodepression in endotoxin shock. *Circ Shock Suppl* 1:1, 1979.

53 **Weisel RD et al:** Myocardial depression during sepsis. *Am J Surg* 133:512, 1977.

54 **Goldfarb RD:** Characteristics of shock-induced circulating cardiodepressant substances: A brief review. *Circ Shock Suppl* 1:23, 1979.

55 **Silva J Jr et al:** Quantitative nitro blue tetrazolium test in febrile patients. *Arch Intern Med* 135:1569, 1975.

56 **Steigbigel RT et al:** The nitroblue tetrazolium reduction test versus conventional hematology in the diagnosis of bacterial infection. *N Engl J Med* 290:235, 1974.

57 **Nachum R et al:** Rapid detection of gram-negative bacterial meningitis by the limulus lysate test. *N Engl J Med* 289:931, 1973.

58 **Anderson ET et al:** Antimicrobial synergism in the therapy of gram-negative rod bacteremia. *Chemotherapy* 24:45, 1978.

59 **Klastersky J et al:** Significance of antimicrobial synergism in the outcome of gram-negative sepsis. *Am J Med Sci* 273:157, 1977.

60 **Bodey GP et al:** β-Lactam antibiotics alone or in combination with gentamicin for therapy of gram-negative bacillary infections in neutropenic patients. *Amer J Med Sci* 271:179, 1976.

61 **EORTC Antimicrobial Therapy Project Group:** Three antibiotic regimens for the treatment of infection in febrile granulocytopenic patients with cancer. *J Infect Dis* 137:14, 1978.

62 **Greene WH et al:** *Pseudomonas aeruginosa* resistant to carbenicillin and gentamicin. Epidemiologic and clinical aspects in a cancer center. *Ann Intern Med* 79:684, 1973.

63 **Klastersky J et al:** Antimicrobial activity of the carbenicillin/gentamicin combination against gram-negative bacilli. *Am J Med Sci* 260:373, 1970.

64 **Reymann MT et al:** Correlation of aminoglycoside dosages with serum concentrations during therapy of serious gram-negative bacillary disease. *Antimicrob Agents Chemother* 16:353, 1979.

65 **Kaye D et al:** The unpredictability of serum concentrations of gentamicin. *J Infect Dis* 130:150, 1974.

66 **Eickhoff TC, Ehret JM:** "In vitro" comparison of cefoxitin, cefamandole, cephalexin and cephalothin. *Antimicrob Agents Chemother* 9:994, 1976.

67 **Wallick H, Hendlin D:** Cefoxitin, a semisynthetic cephamycin antibiotic: Suscepti-

bility studies. *Antimicrob Agents Chemother* 5:25, 1974.

68 **Neu HC et al:** HR 756, a new cephalosporin active against gram-positive and gram-negative aerobic and anaerobic bacteria. *Antimicrob Agents Chemother* 15:273, 1979.

69 **Neu HC et al:** Antibacterial activity of a new 1-oxa cephalosporin compared with that of other β-lactam antibiotics. *Antimicrob Agents Chemother* 16:141, 1979.

70 **Wasilauskis BL, Ellner PD:** Presumptive identification of bacteria from blood cultures in four hours. *J Infect Dis* 124:499, 1971.

71 **Barry AL et al:** Rapid determination of antimicrobial susceptibility for urgent clinical situations. *Am J Clin Pathol* 59:693, 1973.

72 **Goldberg I:** Dopamine—clinical uses of an endogenous catecholamine. *N Engl J Med* 291:707, 1974.

73 **Kardos GG:** Isoproterenol in the treatment of shock due to bacteremia with gram-negative pathogens. *N Engl J Med* 274:868, 1966.

74 **Sonnenblick EH et al:** Drug therapy: Dobutamine: A new synthetic cardioactive sympathetic amine. *N Engl J Med* 300:17, 1979.

75 **Weil MH et al:** Shock caused by gram-negative microorganisms: Analysis of 169 cases. *Ann Intern Med* 60:384, 1964.

76 **Christy JH:** Treatment of gram-negative shock. *Am J Med* 50:77, 1971.

77 **Bennett IL et al:** A double-blind study of the effectiveness of cortisol in the management of severe infections. *Trans Assoc Am Physicians* 75:198, 1962.

78 **Klastersky J et al:** Effectiveness of betamethasone in the management of severe infections. *N Engl J Med* 284:1248, 1971.

79 **Weitzman S, Berger S:** Clinical trial design in studies of corticosteroids for bacterial infections. *Ann Intern Med* 81:36, 1974.

80 **Schumer W:** Steroids in the treatment of clinical septic shock. *Ann Surg* 184:333, 1976.

81 **Alavi JB et al:** A randomized clinical trial of granulocyte transfusions for infection in acute leukemia. *N Engl J Med* 296:706, 1977.

82 **Buckner CD et al:** The role of a protective environment and prophylactic granulocyte transfusions in marrow transplantation. *Transplant Proc* 10:255, 1978.

83 **Corrigan JT, Kiernat JF:** Effect of heparin in experimental gram-negative septicemia. *J Infect Dis* 131:138, 1975.

84 **Mant MJ, King EG:** Severe acute disseminated intravascular coagulation. A reappraisal of its pathophysiology, clinical significance and therapy based on 47 patients. *Am J Med* 67:557, 1979.

85 **Kunin CM, McCormack RC:** Prevention of catheter-induced urinary-tract infections

by sterile closed drainage. *N Engl J Med* 274:1156, 1966.

86 **Warren JW et al:** Antibiotic irrigation and catheter-associated urinary-tract infections. *N Engl J Med* 299:570, 1978.

87 **Bentley DW, Lepper MH:** Septicemia related to indwelling venous catheter. *JAMA* 206:1749, 1968.

88 **Corso JA et al:** Maintenance of venous polyethylene catheters to reduce risk of infection. *JAMA* 210:2075, 1969.

89 **Malizia WF et al:** Benzalkonium chloride as a source of infection. *N Engl J Med* 263:800, 1960.

90 **Schimpff SC et al:** Infection prevention in acute nonlymphocytic leukemia. Laminar air flow room reverse isolation with oral, nonabsorbable antibiotic prophylaxis. *Ann Intern Med* 82:351, 1975.

91 **Gurwith MJ et al:** A prospective controlled investigation of prophylactic trimethoprim/sulfamethoxazole in hospitalized granulocytopenic patients. *Am J Med* 66:248, 1979.

92 **McGowan JE et al:** Nosocomial bacteremia: Potential for prevention of procedure-related cases. *JAMA* 237:2727, 1977.

The management of patients with mycotic aneurysm

WALTER R. WILSON
J. T. LIE
O. WAYNE HOUSER
DAVID G. PIEPGRAS
JOSEPH E. GERACI

Mycotic aneurysms occur rarely. During the 16 years from 1963 to 1979 we were able to identify only 32 patients at Mayo Clinic with this disorder. Our criteria for the diagnosis of mycotic aneurysm were the presence of at least two of the following: (1) isolation of bacteria on culture of an aneurysm obtained at surgery or postmortem examination, (2) the presence of organisms on Gram's stain of tissue, and (3) evidence of erosive arteritis on histopathologic examination. The purpose of this chapter is to present what we believe is a rational and prudent approach, based on our experience with these 32 patients, to the diagnosis and medical and surgical management of patients with mycotic aneurysms.

HISTORICAL ASPECTS AND DEFINITIONS

Broadly defined, *mycotic aneurysm* is an infective, erosive arteritis or an infection of a preexisting aneurysm caused by almost any organism, not just fungal organisms, as the literal meaning of the word *mycotic* implies. In 1877 Goodhart postulated that an infective process may play a role in bacterial aneurysm formation (1). In 1885 Sir William Osler in his "Gulstonian Lecture on Malignant Endocarditis" introduced the term *mycotic aneurysm* to describe those aneurysms resulting from septic embolization of microorganisms originating from bacterial endocarditis. At the time of Osler's presentation, *mycotic* referred to any infectious process, and Osler used the term to describe the case of endocarditis, commenting that the debris in the patient's aortic arch aneurysm resembled the vegetations found on infected heart valves. The word *aneurysm* may also be a misnomer because many of these lesions do not necessarily result in the formation of a true aneurysm, which is defined as a permanent abnormal localized dilatation of an artery due to congenital or acquired weakness of the vessel wall. For historical reasons and because it is an established part of our vocabulary in clinical medicine, the term *mycotic aneurysm* will be retained in the present discussion.

PATHOGENESIS AND PATHOLOGY

An understanding of the pathogenesis and pathology of mycotic aneurysms is important in the formulation of an appropriate treatment plan for patients with this disorder. Most mycotic aneurysms develop in patients with infective endocarditis (IE), but other conditions may result in the formation of mycotic aneurysms. The successful management of patients depends upon identification, treatment, and, if possible, elimination of the portal of entry.

Mycotic aneurysms may develop in a variety of ways. The most common mechanism (approximately 80 percent of cases) involves septic embolization from bacterial endocarditis to the vasa vasorum or intraluminal space of arteries. In 1887 Eppinger (3) found the same microorganism in the wall of a mycotic aneurysm as in an infected heart valve. In 1940 Lippincott (4) identified gram-positive cocci in the vasa vasorum of a case of dissecting mycotic aneurysm of the abdominal aorta. Most authors favor the theory of bacterial entry via the vasa vasorum rather than the intraluminal route of infection (5–8), but the two are not mutually exclusive. The experimental studies of Molinari et al. (9) suggest that either route may result in the formation of mycotic aneurysms. In bacteremic patients a second mechanism involves infection of a preformed, usually atherosclerotic aneurysm through the vasa vasorum or through the intima. A third mechanism involves contiguous spread, either directly or via lymphatics, from a localized abscess or area of cellulitis. A fourth mechanism involves injury and bacterial contamination of an artery as a result of vascular surgery, catheter-induced vascular trauma, penetrating trauma, or arterial injection of narcotics in drug abusers (10, 11). Finally, mycotic aneurysms may occur in the apparent absence of an identifiable focus of infection even at autopsy. This type of mycotic aneurysm has been termed *primary* or *cryptogenic* (12, 13), but it is likely in these cases that some occult source of extravascular infection served as the portal of entry (14, 15).

Mycotic aneurysms may occur in any artery. Vessel branching points favor the impaction of emboli and are preferred sites. In descending order of frequency the vessels involved are aorta, cerebral arteries, visceral arteries, and arteries of the lower and upper extremities (16, 17) (Figures 1 to 3). Multiple vessel involvement is characteristic of mycotic aneurysm. In the collective series of 217 cases reviewed by Stengel and Wolferth multiple aneurysms were found in 49 patients (23 percent) (16).

Histologically, an exuberant inflammatory reaction and destruction of the normal architecture of the vessel wall are the hallmarks of a mycotic aneurysm (Figure 4). In the more acute lesions, the cellular infiltrate is predominately polymorphonuclear, and microabscesses are not uncommon. In some cases, especially in the large, elastic arteries, the inflammatory process may be conspicuously centered around the vasa vasorum, and the elastic lamella is almost totally erased. In the less acute lesions and when rupture has not occurred, the inflammatory infiltrate is typically a mixture of polymorphonuclear leukocytes, lymphocytes, and plasma cells. Vascular and fibroblastic granulation tissue in the adventitia and subsequent fibrosis may offer a last line of resistance and avert rupture. A healed mycotic aneurysm, if such exists, is a false aneurysm

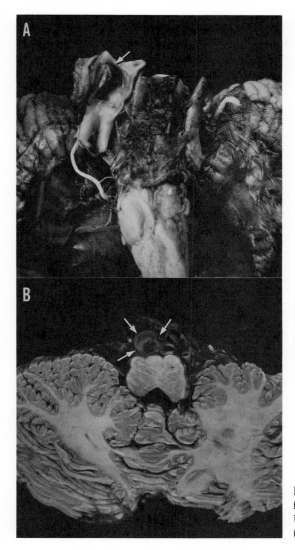

Figure 1 Cerebral mycotic (infected) aneurysms. (a) Right vertebral artery (arrow). (b) Basilar artery (arrows).

since its wall is devoid of a tunica media. The transition from the uninvolved segment of the vessel wall to the area of aneurysmal destruction may be abrupt or gradual; it is not uncommon to discover microscopically that the weakened vessel wall is more extensive than the gross appearance of the artery would indicate.

GENERAL PRINCIPLES OF DIAGNOSIS

A number of general principles of diagnosis apply to all patients with mycotic aneurysm.

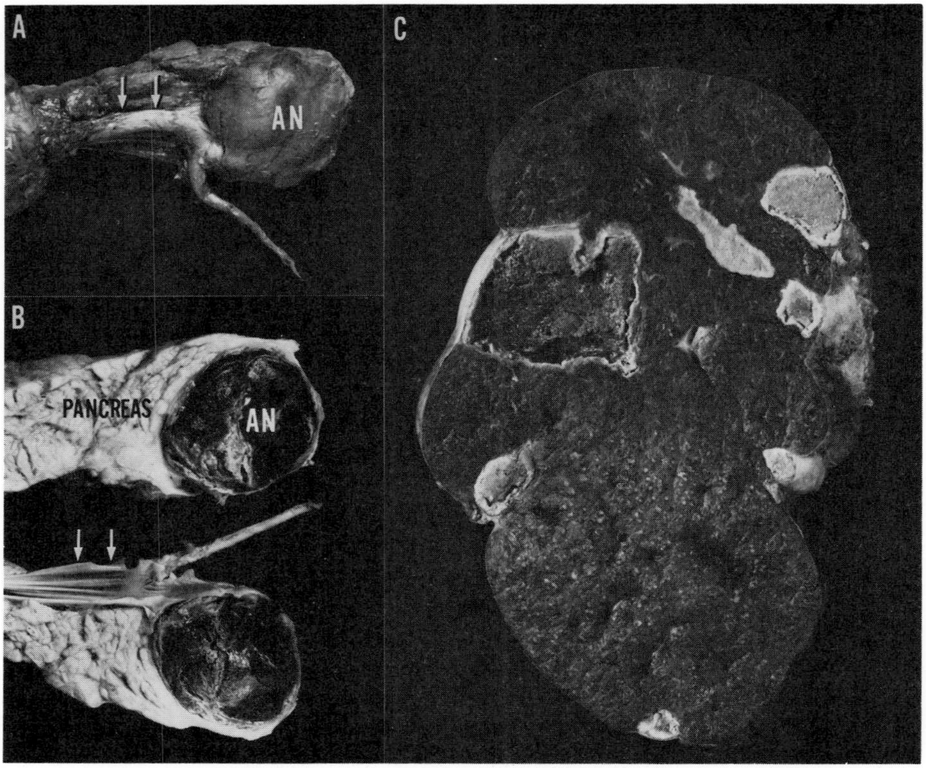

Figure 2 (*a*) Unopened mycotic aneurysm (AN) of the splenic artery (arrows). (*b*) Bisected mycotic aneurysm (AN) filled with thrombus of the splenic artery (arrows). (*c*) Cut surface of spleen showing multiple infarcts.

Clinical diagnosis

The appearance of a tender, pulsatile mass located near a major artery strongly suggests the presence of a mycotic aneurysm. Aside from this physical finding, there are few clinical features which suggest the diagnosis.

Laboratory diagnosis

Routine laboratory tests are of minimal value in the diagnosis of mycotic aneurysm. Anemia, leukocytosis, and an elevated erythrocyte sedimentation rate may be present, but results of these and other routine tests usually reflect the underlying condition predisposing to mycotic aneurysm. Angiography may be helpful in the diagnosis of mycotic aneurysms and is discussed below. Mycotic aneurysms often occur multiply. Once the diagnosis of mycotic aneurysm has been made, it is important to suspect that other aneurysms may be present and to obtain appropriate diagnostic studies.

Infective endocarditis is the underlying condition most often associated with mycotic aneurysm. It is vitally important to establish or exclude this diagnosis and to identify the causative microorganism by isolation from blood culture. The selection of appropriate antimicrobial therapy is guided by identification of the isolate and the results of in vitro susceptibility tests. Streptococci and staphylococci are the most common causative organisms isolated from patients with staphylococcal infectious endocarditis (IE), and, not surprisingly, these organisms are the most frequent bacteria associated with mycotic aneurysm formation. Among patients with IE who have not received prior antimicrobial therapy, streptococci were isolated from the first blood culture in 96 percent of cases and from one of the first two cultures in 98 percent (18). In this same study staphylococci were isolated from the first culture in approximately 90 percent of instances and from one of the first two cultures in all cases of IE caused by this microorganism. These and other data (19) suggest that in patients with IE who have not received prior antimicrobial therapy it is rarely necessary to obtain more than three sets of blood cultures drawn within 24 h, or more than a total of six sets of blood cultures drawn within 48 h. Wound, urinary tract, and other infections may serve as a portal of entry in cases of mycotic aneurysm, and it is important to obtain appropriate cultures from these sites before antimicrobial therapy is begun.

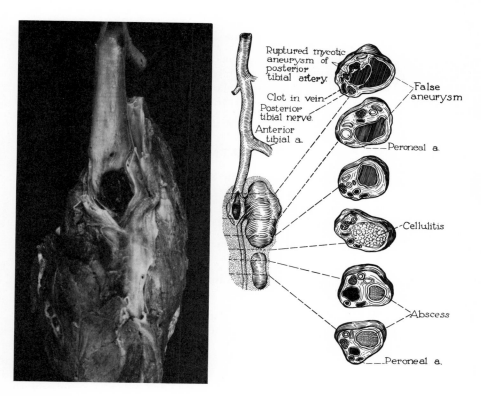

Figure 3   Mycotic (infected) aneurysm of the posterior tibial artery. (*Left*) Photograph of the actual specimen. (*Right*) Companion diagram.

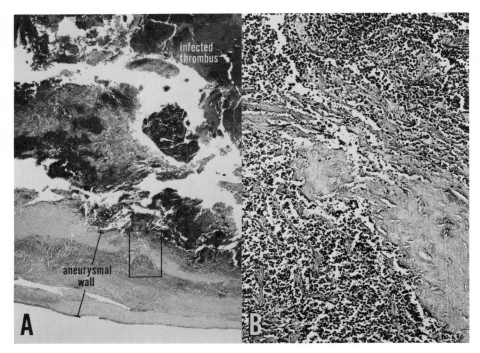

Figure 4   Photomicrographs of mycotic aneurysm of the aorta. (*a*) Low-magnification view of the aneurysmal wall and the content (infected thrombus) of the aneurysm. H&E, ×16. (*b*) High-magnification view of the boxed area in (*a*), showing extensive destruction of the vessel wall with intense polymorphonuclear infiltrate. H&E, ×160.

GENERAL PRINCIPLES OF TREATMENT

The management of patients with mycotic aneurysm presents several special problems:

1   The diagnosis of mycotic aneurysm is often not suspected antemortem.

2   The anatomic location of most mycotic aneurysms complicates the surgical approach.

3   Following excision of a mycotic aneurysm, vascular reconstruction may be necessary and the risk of recurrent infection is high.

4   When limb viability is questionable, surgeons are often faced with a difficult decision of whether to amputate or attempt vascular reconstruction.

Medical treatment

Few data exist concerning the optimal antimicrobial therapy of patients with mycotic aneurysm. In general, the same guidelines used for patients with IE should be followed for the treatment of patients with mycotic aneurysm. Numerous excellent references are available outlining standard antimicrobial therapy regimens for patients with IE (20). Once antimicrobial therapy has been initiated, it is important to obtain additional in vitro susceptibility tests to assure that bactericidal therapy is being administered. Minimum bactericidal concentration, serum bactericidal test, serum antibiotic assay, and, if necessary, in vitro synergy testing using combinations of antibiotics should be performed; adjustments in therapy should be made accordingly.[1]

The optimal length of preoperatively administered antimicrobial therapy for patients with mycotic aneurysm differs from person to person. The risk of postoperative recurrence of infection may be less in patients who have completed a full course of antimicrobial agents preoperatively, but physicians must consider the risk of rupture of the mycotic aneurysm if surgery is delayed by prolonging this therapy. We believe that to minimize the risk of rupture it is generally preferable to subject patients to surgery early in the course of antimicrobial therapy rather than late. Postoperatively, antimicrobial therapy should be continued for a minimum of 2 weeks and probably 4 to 6 weeks (11). Infections caused by penicillin-sensitive streptococci could probably be treated adequately for 2 weeks postoperatively; *Staphylococcus aureus* and enterococcal infections should be treated for 4 to 6 weeks postoperatively.

Close attention to the control of any coexisting arterial hypertension with the use of antihypertensive agents including beta-blocking drugs is important in the management of patients with mycotic aneurysm. If possible, anticoagulant therapy should be avoided.

Surgical treatment

The surgical treatment of choice for patients with mycotic aneurysm is proximal and distal ligation and excision. Depending upon the anatomic location and artery involved, ligation and excision may not be feasible, and vascular reconstruction may be imperative. The risk of recurrent infection in the suture lines of reconstructed areas is high, with subsequent rupture and fatal hemorrhage. The risk of recurrence of infection is less with the use of autogenous venous grafts than with the use of synthetic material (10, 11, 21–24), and saphenous or other vein interposition is preferable to synthetic material when vascular reconstruction is required. If bypass grafts are constructed with synthetic material, grafts should be positioned whenever possible in an extraanatomic location which traverses uninfected tissue planes.

The diagnosis, management, and outcome of patients with mycotic aneurysm depend upon the anatomic location of the aneurysm. Intracranial, intrathoracic, intraabdominal, and peripheral mycotic aneurysms will be discussed separately below.

MYCOTIC ANEURYSMS OF THE HEAD AND NECK

The following case illustrates some of the clinical aspects of intracranial mycotic aneurysms and emphasizes the difficulties of management.

---

[1] See the article by Ernest Jawetz, p. 109.

Case 1

In December 1978, a 33-year-old unemployed right-handed male was admitted to his local hospital with a 3-week history of fever, malaise, and generalized headaches. Abnormal physical findings present at admission were a temperature of 38.4°C, Osler's nodes on two fingers, and a grade 2/6 murmur of mitral incompetence. Several blood cultures yielded *Streptococcus fecalis*. Cardiac echocardiography demonstrated vegetations and incompetence of the mitral valve. A diagnosis of mitral valve infective endocarditis was made, and the patient was treated by his local physician for 4 weeks with intravenous penicillin and intramuscular streptomycin. The patient responded well to antimicrobial therapy with rapid disappearance of fever. His headaches persisted, however, and now became localized to the right parietooccipital area. The patient was dismissed from his local hospital on January 10, 1979. Blood cultures obtained at 1 week and 1 month following dismissal from hospital were reportedly negative. Following discharge he had no evidence of recurrence of infective endocarditis, but he continued to complain of right-sided, moderately severe headaches which were partially relieved by aspirin.

On April 29, 1979, he awoke to answer the telephone, felt light-headed, had severe bitemporal headache, and noted the loss of left lateral visual field vision. He was referred to Mayo Clinic for evaluation and admitted to hospital on April 30, 1979.

Abnormal admission physical findings were a left homonymous hemianopsia and a grade 3/6 holosystolic murmur of mitral incompetence. No neck stiffness was present. A computerized tomographic scan of the head on May 2 revealed blood in the right lateral and third and fourth ventricles and an intracerebral hematoma in the posterior medial temporal lobe adjacent to the atrium of the right lateral ventricle. On May 3 a transfemoral four-vessel angiogram demonstrated a fusiform dilatation of a calcarine branch of the right posterior cerebral artery (Figure 5) associated with a vascular right temporal mass compatible with a hematoma. An EEG revealed diffuse nonspecific abnormalities. Because of increased intracranial pressure, lumbar puncture was not performed. Multiple blood cultures were obtained and were subsequently negative.

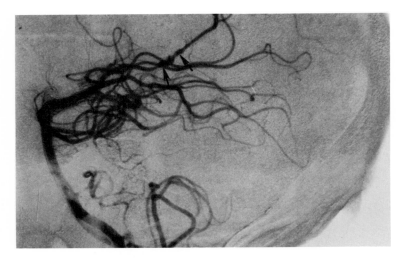

Figure 5 Cerebral angiogram demonstrating fusiform dilatation of a calcarine branch of the right posterior cerebral artery (May 3).

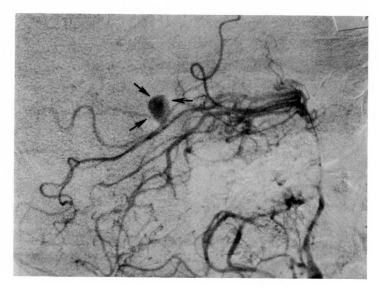

Figure 6 Cerebral angiogram demonstrating marked increase in size of posterior cerebral artery aneurysm (May 18).

The patient was treated with phenobarbital, intravenous penicillin, intramuscular streptomycin, and supportive care. Neurosurgery was considered but was deferred. His severe bitemporal headache persisted, and on the second hospital day he developed moderately severe, progressive neck stiffness and a fluctuating mental status. These symptoms persisted until May 12, when he had a 30-min period of unresponsiveness. A repeat CT scan of the head showed a considerable increase in the amount of intraventricular blood and an enlargement of the intracerebral hematoma compared with the CT scan of May 2.

On May 18 a transfemoral four-vessel angiogram was repeated. The aneurysm had increased markedly in size compared with May 3 (Figure 6).

On May 22 the patient underwent right parietooccipital craniotomy and evacuation of an intracerebral hematoma. In the bed of the hematoma lay a mycotic aneurysm. The artery was ligated proximally and distally, and the aneurysm was resected. The histopathology of the posterior cerebral artery specimen was consistent with a mycotic aneurysm. Gram-positive cocci were seen on Gram's stains, but culture of the specimen was negative. The patient's immediate postoperative course was complicated by a subgaleal hematoma, which was drained.

Antimicrobial therapy with penicillin and streptomycin was instituted on May 9 and continued for 12 days postoperatively. The patient improved gradually and was discharged from hospital on June 29. At the time of dismissal, his mental status was normal, and he had normal muscle strength on the left. The left homonymous hemianopsia persisted.

Comment Several features of this case merit emphasis. The patient complained of persistent localized headaches during treatment for IE. In a patient with IE and localized severe headaches, the possibility of mycotic aneurysm should have been considered earlier and angiography performed. The patient's headache persisted after dismissal from hospital, but the onset of significant bleeding from the aneurysm was delayed—more than 3 months after completion of antibiotic therapy—emphasizing the importance of close follow-up of patients treated for IE. The diagnosis of mycotic aneurysm was first made by angiography on May 3, but aneurysmectomy was not performed until May 22, almost 3 weeks later. In the interim, the patient experienced at least one additional intracerebral bleed. In retrospect, a more aggressive neurosurgical approach probably should have been pursued following initial diagnosis. Neurosurgery was deferred because of the high surgical risk, and it was hoped that the bleeding had stopped. However, the initial surgical risk was outweighed by the risk of imminent rupture of the mycotic aneurysm, which usually results in massive, fatal, intracerebral bleeding.

Frequency, anatomic location, microbiologic etiology, and underlying conditions

Intracerebral mycotic aneurysms are recognized uncommonly. The frequency has decreased since the advent of antimicrobial therapy. Mycotic aneurysms are said to constitute 2.5 to 6.2 percent of all intracranial aneurysms (25–27). Bohmfalk et al. (28) could locate only 85 cases of intracranial aneurysm reported from 1954 to 1977 and added four cases of their own. During the 17 years from 1952 to 1968, 385 patients were treated at Mayo Clinic for infective endocarditis; three of these (0.8 percent) developed intracranial mycotic aneurysms (29). This percentage is similar to our more recent experience. From 1963 through 1979 we encountered eight cases of intracranial mycotic aneurysms among 628 patients (1.2 percent) with IE treated at Mayo Clinic. Intracranial mycotic aneurysm associated with intravenous heroin abuse and IE has also been reported (30, 31). The true incidence of intracranial mycotic aneurysm probably exceeds the number of cases diagnosed. It is likely that some patients with IE develop an intracranial mycotic aneurysm which is asymptomatic and undergoes spontaneous healing with antimicrobial therapy and which would therefore go undetected (32). The majority of intracranial mycotic aneurysms occur distal to the first bifurcation of the middle or posterior cerebral artery (28). Six of our patients had mycotic aneurysm involving the middle cerebral artery; three had aneurysm of the posterior cerebral artery. In all eight patients, the aneurysm was located distal to the first bifurcation. In approximately 85 percent of patients, intracranial mycotic aneurysm occurs singly, and in the 15 percent of patients with multiple intracranial mycotic aneurysms the second aneurysm may appear after completion of therapy for the first aneurysm (28).

Intracranial mycotic aneurysm may involve the cavernous sinus (28, 33, 34). This type of mycotic aneurysm is uncommonly associated with IE and is usually the result of cavernous sinus thrombophlebitis from a variety of causes. Rarely, intracranial mycotic aneurysm of extravascular origin may occur in diverse anatomic sites secondary to penetrating head trauma, otitis media, or purulent or tuberculous meningitis (35–38).

The microbiologic spectrum of intracranial mycotic aneurysm usually reflects that of IE. Among patients with positive blood cultures, streptococci or staphylococci were isolated from 89 percent of patients described by Bohmfalk et al. (28). *Staph. aureus* is the most common cause of intracranial mycotic aneurysm associated with cavernous sinus thrombosis. A variety of microorganisms have been isolated from patients with purulent meningitis and mycotic aneurysm. Very rarely, intracerebral mycotic aneurysm may be caused by fungi (39–40).

Diagnosis

Clinical signs The most important factor in the successful management of patients with intracranial mycotic aneurysm is early diagnosis prior to rupture. Most reports suggest that a "warning leak" indicating the presence of an intracranial mycotic aneurysm is rare and that the diagnosis of mycotic aneurysm is made usually after a sudden massive, often fatal, subarachnoid or intracerebral hemorrhage.

On the contrary, our experience suggests that if one maintains a high index of suspicion, the diagnosis of intracranial mycotic aneurysm may be made early before massive hemorrhage occurs. In six of our eight patients, the diagnosis of intracranial mycotic aneurysm was made antemortem. In the remaining two patients, the diagnosis was made at postmortem examination, but both these latter patients had the sudden onset of severe headache with rapid development of neurologic signs progressing to coma before angiography could be accomplished.

The presence of severe, localized headache in a patient with IE strongly suggests the possibility of an intracranial mycotic aneurysm (Table 1). Mild nonspecific, intermittent, generalized headaches occur frequently in patients with IE. Among 100 consecutive patients with IE seen at Mayo Clinic in the previous 3 years, 43 complained of nonspecific mild headache. Severe, localized headache occurs much less frequently. Jones et al. reported that only 3.6 percent of patients (14 out of 385) complained of severe headache and 3 of these 14 had intracranial mycotic aneurysm (29). Among 213 patients with IE seen at Mayo Clinic from 1975 to 1979, seven (3.2 percent) complained of severe, localized, unremitting headache, and four of these had mycotic aneurysm. Of the remaining three patients, two had subarachnoid hemorrhage and one had intracerebral bleeding from suspected mycotic aneurysm but none was demonstrated by angiography (two patients) or at postmortem examination (two patients).

Homonymous hemianopsia occurred in four of our eight patients (Table 1), and in three of these four patients, headache and visual field defects were the predominant complaints. One patient developed homonymous hemianopsia just before a massive fatal hemorrhage which occurred while the patient was being transferred to the operating room for neurosurgery.

Five patients had stiff neck; cerebrospinal fluid examination was performed in four of these; three had erythrocytes in the cerebrospinal fluid. Among our

Table 1 Clinical presentation of eight patients with intracranial mycotic aneurysm

Finding	No. of patients
Severe localized headache	8
Fever	7
Stiff neck	5
Homonymous hemianopsia	4
Papilledema	4
Dilated pupil(s)	2
Hemiplegia	1
Seizure	1
Coma	1

patients, the appearance of severe, localized headache, homonymous hemianopsia, the presence of erythrocytes in the cerebrospinal fluid, and other neurologic signs suggests that warning leaks of intracranial mycotic aneurysm may occur. These warning leaks should initiate immediate action to confirm or exclude the presence of intracranial mycotic aneurysm.

An important feature of intracranial mycotic aneurysm is that some patients will develop fresh mycotic aneurysms after appropriate antimicrobial therapy has been instituted (26, 28, 32, 41–43). Moreover, other patients may not develop signs of mycotic aneurysmal bleeding until well after such therapy has been completed. In two of our eight patients, symptoms of mycotic aneurysm bleeding occurred 11 days and 3 months, respectively, after completion of antimicrobial therapy for IE. One should suspect mycotic aneurysm in patients with a previous history of IE who develop suggestive signs even if previous angiographic studies failed to demonstrate an intracranial mycotic aneurysm.

Laboratory diagnosis Skull roentgenograms were obtained in all eight of our patients and were nondiagnostic. Electroencephalograms were obtained in six of the eight patients and showed nonspecific changes.

Computerized tomography (CT) of the head was performed on multiple occasions in two of our eight patients with intracranial mycotic aneurysm. The scans demonstrated blood in the ventricles or areas of intracerebral hemorrhage. The CT findings were not specific for intracranial mycotic aneurysm. While the CT scan is not yet able to detect mycotic aneurysm, this technique is of considerable value in assessing the extent of bleeding from leaking or ruptured mycotic aneurysm. As CT technology improves, the use of this technique in patients with IE and the usefulness of CT scanning in the diagnosis of intracranial mycotic aneurysm may improve. Conceivably, CT scanning could detect areas of inflammation or leakage around intact aneurysms or small hematomas, infarcts, or other changes present in patients with IE suggestive of aneurysm formation; these changes could then be evaluated further with angiography.

Cerebral angiography is the only reliable means of establishing the diagnosis of intracranial aneurysm. In six of our eight patients, the diagnosis of intracranial mycotic aneurysm was confirmed antemortem by cerebral angiography. Neither of the two patients diagnosed at postmortem had undergone cerebral angiography before death.

Some authorities suggest that all patients with IE (including those with no neurologic symptoms) undergo cerebral angiography at least once, and preferably three times, during their treatment and follow-up (28–32, 44). These authors believe that repeated cerebral angiography would provide a more accurate estimate of the true incidence of intracranial mycotic aneurysm in patients with IE; the natural history could be defined better, including the effect of appropriate antimicrobial therapy; and, finally, some neurologic disasters caused by sudden, unexpected massive hemorrhage might be avoided.

We do not believe that cerebral angiography should be performed in all patients with IE. In our experience, symptomatic intracranial mycotic aneurysm occurs rarely in patients with IE, and in the majority of our patients the diagnosis was suspected and confirmed antemortem. While the risk of neurologic complications resulting from cerebral angiography is small, occasional severe complications occur. One prudent course might be as outlined in Figure 7; i.e., all patients with IE who have neurologic complaints or abnormal neurologic physical findings should undergo prompt CT scan, with and without contrast, and cerebral angiography. If these studies are negative, follow-up CT scan and angiography should be performed at the completion of antimicrobial treatment or earlier if indicated. If these studies demonstrate the presence of an aneurysm, patients should be managed according to Figure 7. Patients with no central nervous system complaints should undergo CT scan, with and without contrast, as soon as their condition permits. Patients with abnormal CT scan suggesting bleeding or inflammation should undergo prompt cerebral angiography. Follow-up CT scan and angiography in asymptomatic patients who have a normal initial CT scan should be obtained only if central nervous system complaints or abnormal neurologic physical findings develop subsequently.

Treatment and prognosis

Antimicrobial therapy   Guidelines for the antimicrobial therapy of patients with intracranial mycotic aneurysms are discussed above.

Surgical therapy   While the true natural history of intracranial mycotic aneurysm is not known, it is believed that the majority of these lesions rupture if not resected. Bingham (32) suggests, however, that the outcome in patients with intracranial mycotic aneurysm is similar in those treated with adequate

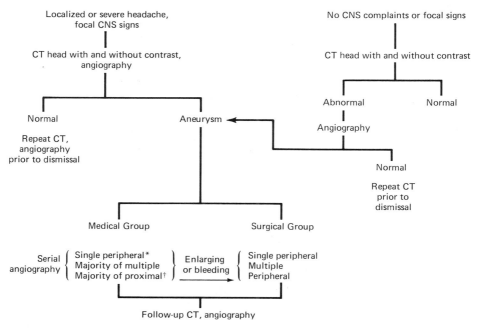

Figure 7   Evaluation and management of patients with infective endocarditis. * Distal to first bifurcation; † Proximal to first bifurcation.

antimicrobial therapy alone to those treated with antibiotics plus surgical excision of the aneurysm. Bingham described instances of thrombosis, decrease in size, and presumed fibrosis without rupture of intracranial aneurysm in patients treated with adequate antimicrobial therapy and postulates that some cases of failure with medical therapy alone may have resulted from the use of ineffective or inadequate antimicrobial agents. Our schema for the surgical management of patients with IE and intracranial aneurysm is outlined in Figure 7. A single peripheral aneurysm should be followed with frequent serial angiograms and excised promptly if the aneurysm enlarges or bleeds. Intracranial mycotic aneurysms may evolve rapidly, and surgeons must be prepared to intervene promptly. Multiple peripheral aneurysms present a complex problem surgically. They should be monitored closely with frequent serial angiography and CT scans. If one or more of the aneurysms enlarge, prompt surgical excision should be attempted.

Aneurysms which occur proximal to the first bifurcation are less amenable to surgical excision. Attempts at clipping the aneurysmal dilatation may lead to fragmentation and rupture because of the infected friable arterial wall (26, 28, 45). Proximal aneurysms frequently arise from major vessels, and ligation may result in severe neurologic insult. Proximal aneurysms should be followed closely with serial angiograms and CT scans, and if signs of enlargement or leakage develop, surgical therapy should be attempted. Occasionally, proximal aneurysms stabilize and thrombose with antimicrobial therapy, and medical cures have been reported (28, 32, 42, 43). Aneurysms of the cavernous sinus may decrease in size with appropriate antimicrobial therapy alone (28, 34, 46).

Bohmfalk reported in his review of 85 cases that the overall mortality for intracranial mycotic aneurysms was 60 percent (28). In this same review, rupture occurred in 65 percent and the mortality among these patients was 80 percent. Patients with multiple or a single peripheral aneurysm had similar mortality rates, 38.5 and 42 percent, respectively. The mortality for patients with proximal aneurysm was 58 percent. The mortality among our patients was 75 percent (six of eight patients). The only two survivors had early diagnosis of mycotic aneurysm and underwent elective surgical excision. One other patient underwent urgent surgery for ruptured mycotic aneurysm and died immediately postoperatively. The other five cases did not undergo surgery. All died from massive intracerebral hemorrhage.

THORACIC MYCOTIC ANEURYSM

Intrathoracic mycotic aneurysms frequently involve vital contiguous structures and differ from other mycotic aneurysms in that simple excision without reconstructive or bypass surgery is virtually impossible. Consequently, intrathoracic mycotic aneurysms are among the most technically difficult and frustrating surgical problems encountered. The following case illustrates some of the special problems.

Case 2

A 72-year-old male was admitted to Mayo Clinic hospitals on June 29, 1979, complaining of a 1-month history of fever and suprasternal chest pain. In December 1977 he developed Raynaud's phenomenon, myalgias, and arthralgias and showed an 18-kg weight loss. A diagnosis of vasculitis was made elsewhere, and the patient was treated with prednisone with marked improvement. The prednisone was tapered and discontinued in April 1979.

Abnormal physical findings on admission included a temperature of 38.9°C, petechiae on the extremities, a bluish discolored lesion on the right thumb, and a tender pulsatile mass above the right clavicle. Chest radiographs showed calcification and torsion of the thoracic aorta with possible aneurysmal dilatation behind the heart.

The initial clinical impression was relapse of systemic vasculitis. Treatment was initiated with prednisone (60 mg per day), and the patient improved somewhat. Five days later, blood cultures obtained on admission yielded *Staph. aureus*. Subsequently, all 16 blood cultures drawn during the 5-day period prior to the report of the first positive blood culture yielded *Staph. aureus*. The prednisone was tapered rapidly to 15 mg per day and oxacillin (2 g every 4 h) was administered intravenously.

The in vitro susceptibility studies demonstrated tolerance of the *Staph. aureus* to oxacillin (MIC 0.78 μg/ml; MBC >100 μg/ml; MBC/MIC = >128). Therapy was changed to vancomycin and subsequently to cephalothin, 2 g intravenously every 4 h. The MIC to cephalothin was 0.8 μg/ml; MBC 1.56 μg/ml; MBC/MIC = 2.

On July 6 the pulsatile supraclavicular mass increased in size abruptly, and the patient complained of considerable localized pain. Chest radiographs showed a soft tissue density in the right apex and a slight shift of the trachea to the left. Using a retrograde approach through the femoral artery, an aortic arch angiogram was performed which revealed a 4-cm-diameter false aneurysm of the right innominate artery near the origin of the subclavian artery (Figure 8). A 4.5- by 5-cm aneurysm was also noted in the abdominal aorta opposite the second and third lumbar vertebrae.

On July 8 the patient underwent resection of the innominate artery aneurysm. Surgical exposure was possible through an incision at the base of the neck, and the chest was entered through a midline incision. Before resecting the mycotic aneurysm, a saphenous vein bypass graft was constructed between the innominate artery proximal to the aneurysm and the right common carotid artery. A second saphenous vein bypass graft was constructed from the proximal innominate artery to the right subclavian artery. The innominate artery was then ligated proximally and distally to the mycotic aneurysm, and the infected arterial segment was excised. Histopathologic examination of the arterial specimen showed infective arteritis typical of mycotic aneurysm. Cultures of the specimen yielded *Staph. aureus*.

Postoperatively, the patient was treated with intravenous cephalothin for 28 days. Postoperative recovery was uneventful. The patient experienced no neurologic or other vascular complications related to the operative procedures.

In February 1980 the patient underwent resection of a 6-cm atherosclerotic abdominal aortic aneurysm with interposition of Dacron graft. Preoperative blood cultures were negative. Histopathologic examination of the abdominal aneurysm showed atherosclerotic disease with no evidence of mycotic aneurysm, and cultures and Gram's stain of the aneurysm were negative. The patient had no complaints referable to the previous resection of the innominate artery mycotic aneurysm.

Comment   In this patient, simple excision of the mycotic aneurysm without the establishment of bypass conduits was not feasible. Because of the lower risk of infection, the use of an autogenous venous bypass is preferable to the use of synthetic material. Whenever possible, bypass grafts should be constructed in an extraanatomic position so that the bypass graft does not traverse the infected area. The anatomic location of the mycotic aneurysm in this patient precluded an extraanatomic site.

Frequency, anatomic location, microbiologic etiology, and underlying conditions

Of the 32 patients with mycotic aneurysms in our study, 13 (42 percent) had intrathoracic mycotic aneurysms, distributed as shown in Table 2. The majority of patients with intrathoracic mycotic aneurysm had IE or infectious complications following recent cardiac surgery. Seven of thirteen patients had IE; two had recent cardiac surgery (aortic valve replacement and repair of multiple ventriculoseptal defects, respectively); and one had resection of the colon for carcinoma; in three patients the portal of entry was unknown.

Diagnosis

Clinical signs   Few clinical signs or physical findings suggest the diagnosis of intrathoracic mycotic aneurysm. Constant localized chest pain or a tender pulsatile mass in a patient with IE is suggestive, but because of their anatomic location most intrathoracic mycotic aneurysms do not produce visible pulsa-

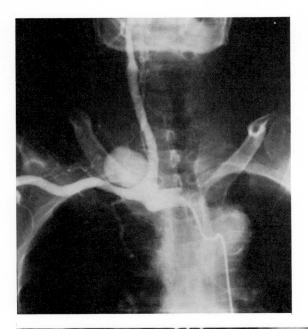

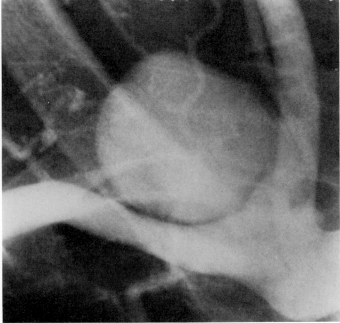

Figure 8   Aortic arch angiogram demonstrating a 4-cm "false" aneurysm of the right innominate artery.

Table 2   Distribution of intrathoracic mycotic aneurysms by site and agent

	No. of patients
Site:	
Sinus of Valsalva	5
Right coronary cusp	2
Left coronary cusp (Figure 9)	2
Right noncoronary cusp	1
Aortic arch	3
Aortic root	2
Innominate artery	1
Subclavian artery	1
Right coronary artery	1
Agent:	
Viridans streptococci	5
Staph. aureus	4
Neisseria gonorrhoeae	1
Staph. epidermis	1
Pseudomonas aeruginosa	1
Clostridium septicum	1

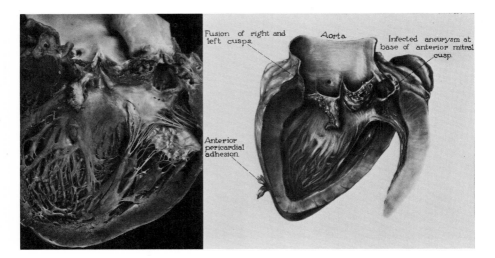

Figure 9   Mycotic (infected) aneurysm of the sinus of Valsalva. (*Left*) Photograph of the actual specimen. (*Right*) Companion diagram. Note involvement of all three aortic valve cusps by infective endocarditis and erosion of anterior leaflet of mitral valve by mycotic aneurysm of the left sinus of Valsalva.

tions. Sinus of Valsalve aneurysms involve the right coronary cusp more often than the left and rupture into the right ventricle or right atrium. Occasionally, a left coronary cusp aneurysm may rupture into the left ventricle. Among our patients with sinus of Valsalva aneurysm, two had ruptured into the right atrium and one into the left ventricle. The appearance of sudden-onset aortic insufficiency in a patient with IE usually is related to acute destruction of the aortic valve, but one should also consider the possibility of ruptured sinus of Valsalva aneurysm.

Laboratory diagnosis Routine chest radiography or tomography may reveal a soft tissue mass or mediastinal vascular widening. In 4 of our 13 cases the diagnosis of aneurysm was suspected because of abnormal appearance of chest radiograms or tomograms. [^{67}Ga]Gallium citrate imaging has been reported to be helpful in the diagnosis of intrathoracic mycotic aneurysm (47). Performed in one of our patients with intrathoracic aneurysm, it demonstrated the presence of a myocardial abscess and a mycotic aneurysm of the aortic root. Both were confirmed at surgery. Although experience with the use of ultrasound techniques including B- and M-mode echocardiography is limited in these patients at Mayo Clinic, these modalities have thus far not been helpful in the diagnosis of intrathoracic aneurysm. Technical improvements and increased experience may enhance the usefulness of these noninvasive diagnostic tools. Angiography is the only reliable means of demonstrating intrathoracic aneurysm. Angiography demonstrated aneurysm in four of our 13 patients (31 percent). One of these had a sinus of Valsalva aneurysm. In the majority of patients intrathoracic mycotic aneurysm is diagnosed at surgery or postmortem examination. Among our 13 patients, six (46 percent) were diagnosed during thoracic surgery and three (23 percent) were discovered at postmortem findings.

Treatment and Prognosis

Antimicrobial therapy The antimicrobial therapy of patients with intrathoracic mycotic aneurysm depends upon isolation of the microorganism and results of in vitro susceptibility tests. The same general principles outlined above apply.

Surgical therapy The mainstay of treatment for intrathoracic mycotic aneurysm is surgical excision. The natural history of sinus of Valsalva aneurysm associated with IE is not known. Since presumably the majority of these aneurysms, like other intrathoracic mycotic aneurysms, rupture if untreated, attempts should be made to repair these lesions surgically. Shumacker (48) and Gonzales-Lavin et al. (49) described their surgical approach to patients with sinus of Valsalva aneurysm. After evacuation of clots contained within the aneurysm and debridement, unruptured aneurysms may be sutured closed, approximating snugly the reunited margins of the aneurysm to the cuff of the rigid aortic valve prosthesis. This technique was used successfully in two of our five patients with sinus of Valsalva aneurysm. In the remaining three patients rupture occurred and surgical closure was not possible. All three patients died during operation or immediately postoperatively.

In cases of sinus of Valsalva rupture or in patients with aortic root mycotic aneurysm with extensive infection, necrosis, and abscess, there may not be enough viable tissue capable of holding sutures to permit surgical repair or aortic valve replacement. In these patients, radical surgical techniques may offer the only possibility of stabilizing, at least temporarily, cardiac hemodynamics, which may allow additional time for antimicrobial therapy and healing of cardiac and aortic tissue.

One surgical approach in these patients was reported in detail (50). Briefly, the infected material or prosthetic valve is excised, debridement of the area is meticulously carried out, and aneurysmal tissue is sutured closed. A new aortic prosthesis is then implanted in the ascending aorta, the coronary ostia are sutured closed, and coronary artery perfusion is reestablished by a segment of autogenous saphenous vein anastamosed end-to-side to the right coronary and end-to-side to the aorta distal to the prosthesis. Another segment of vein is used to construct a Y extension from the right coronary artery graft to the left anterior descending coronary artery. This technique has been used in three patients seen at Mayo Clinic with myocardial and aortic root abscess. Two of the three are alive with minimal cardiac symptoms 17 and 25 months, respectively, postoperatively. Another radical surgical technique which has been used at our institution is ligation and resection of the aortic root mycotic aneurysm, saphenous vein bypass circulation to the coronary arteries as described above, and establishment of a bypass synthetic-material conduit extending from the left ventricle to the descending thoracic aorta. An aortic valve prosthesis is implanted in the conduit. Many other surgical reconstructive techniques have been described for management of aortic root and arch aneurysms (49, 51–53).

Mycotic aneurysm may occur rarely in association with coarctation of the aorta, and the aneurysm is usually located distal to the area of coarctation (54, 55). These mycotic aneurysms develop rapidly and rupture if not treated surgically. The aneurysm should be excised, and preferably the aorta should be rejoined by primary anastomosis. Other cases have been treated successfully by resection and homograft, Dacron, or Teflon graft prosthesis interposition (54, 56, 57).

Very rarely, mycotic aneurysms involve the coronary arteries (58, 59). These aneurysms usually thrombose and may result in myocardial infarction. The single patient in our series had an aneurysm of the right coronary artery which had thrombosed. The patient died of purulent pericarditis, and the diagnosis of mycotic aneurysm was made at postmortem examination. There was no evidence of myocardial infarction. Kawasaki's disease, endemic in Japan, is an acute febrile illness of unknown etiology which occurs predominantly in children under 5 years old and is being recognized increasingly in the United States (60). Studies in Japan using contrast angiography have demonstrated that as many as 30 percent of patients may develop coronary artery aneurysm and that 1 to 2 percent of patients die of complications of these aneurysms, including myocardial infarction, dysrhythmia, and aneurysmal rupture (61, 62). Of the fatal cases, 95 percent die within 6 months from the onset of the acute illness.

Treatment is supportive. One study suggests that the use of aspirin 30 mg/kg daily may be effective in reducing the frequency of coronary artery aneurysm formation (63).

Despite improved techniques which have facilitated earlier diagnosis and more aggressive surgical treatment, the mortality of intrathoracic mycotic aneurysm is high (48, 49). The mortality among our 13 patients was 69 percent (9 patients). The high mortality is the result of early rupture or recurrence of infection at the suture lines with subsequent rupture. The close proximity of major arteries makes vascular reconstruction technically difficult, and it is frequently impossible to resect the infected tissue and establish extraanatomic arterial bypass grafts. Despite the obvious technical problems imposed on the thoracic surgeon, early diagnosis, excision, and vascular reconstruction offer the only possibility of survival for most patients with intrathoracic mycotic aneurysm.

INTRAABDOMINAL MYCOTIC ANEURYSM

Intraabdominal mycotic aneurysms are more accessible surgically than intracerebral or intrathoracic mycotic aneurysms, but because of their anatomic location and the rich intraabdominal collateral circulation, these aneurysms may be occult and the first indication of their presence may be a sudden rupture and fatal hemorrhage. Case 3 illustrates some of the features pertinent to the diagnosis and management of intraabdominal mycotic aneurysms.

Case 3

In November 1976 a 63-year-old male banker from the Philippines was admitted to a Mayo Clinic hospital with a 7-month history of lumbosacral back pain, a 14-kg weight loss, and intermittent fever. In 1973 he had undergone an aortoiliac bilateral Dacron bypass procedure at another hospital for severe arteriosclerotic occlusive disease and bilateral leg claudication. Before coming to Mayo Clinic he received a 2-week course of chloramphenicol administered orally with defervescence. After discontinuation of chloramphenicol the fever returned. Cotrimoxazole therapy was then administered for 2 weeks; the fever subsided but reappeared following discontinuation of the drug. The patient had had several urinary tract infections in the 3 to 4 years before coming to Mayo Clinic.

Physical findings on admission included an oral temperature of 38.3°C, a diffusely tender abdomen, and femoral and carotid bruits. Peripheral pulses in the lower extremities were normal.

Pertinent laboratory values on admission included hemoglobin 9.6 g/dl, WBC 8400 per cubic millimeter, erythrocyte sedimentation rate 120 mm/h, and urinalysis showing 60 WBC per high-powered field and proteinuria. Roentgenograms of the lumbosacral spine showed a destructive process eroding the anterior margins of the body of the twelfth thoracic and first lumbar vertebrae. An excretory urogram showed a left suprarenal mass displacing the kidney laterally and inferiorly. Twenty-four hours after admission a urine culture yielded *Escherichia coli* (greater than 10^5 colonies per milliliter), and *E. coli* was isolated from five blood cultures obtained during the first 2 days of hospitalization. The in vitro antimicrobial susceptibilities of the isolates from the urine and blood were identical. Ampicillin MIC was 1.56 μg/ml, MBC 3.12 μg/ml, and SBT 1:32. Peak serum ampicillin concentration was 32 μg/ml.

A CT scan of the abdomen revealed a large mass in the paraaortic area which began in the lower chest and extended to the lower pole of the left kidney with displacement of the kidney laterally (Figure 10).

An aortogram was performed which delineated a large sacular false aneurysm measuring 6 cm in anteroposterior diameter and 10 cm long arising from the posterior wall of the aorta (Figure 11). The aorta was narrowed and pushed anteriorly by the false aneurysm. The orifice between the aorta and the aneurysm was 3 cm long (Figure 12). The origins of the celiac, superior mesenteric, and left renal artery were narrowed. The aneurysm extended to approximately 4 cm above the previously implanted aortoiliac graft.

Antimicrobial therapy was initiated with gentamicin (1.5 mg/kg) administered intravenously every 8 h and chloramphenicol (1 g intravenously every 6 h) and was changed to ampicillin (1 g intravenously every 3 h) when the in vitro susceptibility test results were reported. The patient's intermittent fever persisted despite antimicrobial therapy. After 15 days of antimicrobial therapy the patient underwent abdominal exploration with resection of the aneurysm.

Surgical exploration confirmed the anatomic location and size of the aneurysm noted on the CT scan and aortogram. There was no evidence of hemorrhage from the aneurysm. The thoracic origin of the aneurysm was ligated, and a 19-cm Dacron graft was anastomosed to the healthy appearing thoracic aorta above the area of excised aneurysm. The distal end of the graft was sutured to the abdominal aorta just above the orifice of the left renal artery. The superior mesenteric artery was anastomosed to the graft. The celiac artery was atheromatous and could not be anastomosed to the graft. A 6-mm-diameter Dacron graft was sutured into the celiac artery and anastomosed with the aortic graft. The right renal artery could not be preserved and was oversewn. The previously placed aortoiliac graft was not involved by the aneurysm, appeared to be functioning normally, and was preserved.

Histopathologic examination of the excised arterial specimen showed an infected atherosclerotic aneurysm. Gram-negative bacilli were noted in the vessel wall on

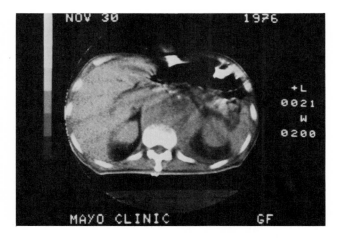

Figure 10 Abdominal CT scan showing large mass in periaortic area displacing the left kidney laterally.

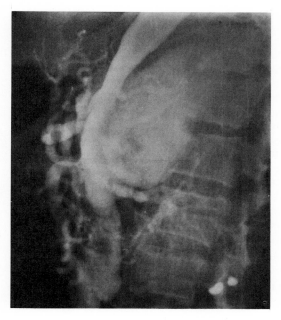

Figure 11   Abdominal aortogram showing 6-cm (AP diameter) by 10-cm (length) aneurysm arising from posterior wall of abdominal aorta.

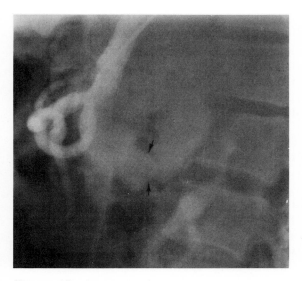

Figure 12   Aortogram demonstrating 3-cm (length) orifice between aorta and aneurysm.

Gram's stain. Cultures of the specimen yielded *E. coli* with identical in vitro susceptibilities to the *E. coli* isolated previously from blood and urine specimens.

The patient's postoperative course was complicated by oliguric renal failure secondary to acute tubular necrosis. Serum creatinine gradually returned to near normal
levels of 1.5 mg/dl at the time of dismissal from the hospital. Treatment with ampicillin administered intravenously was continued for 18 days postoperatively.

Because the aortic Dacron graft was interposed in an infected area, it was felt that
the graft was probably infected with *E. coli*. Accordingly, the patient was begun on
oral amoxicillin therapy 1 g administered orally three times daily to be taken indefi-
nitely in an attempt to suppress residual infection. The patient maintained close
contact with Mayo Clinic physicians by correspondence. In January 1980 the patient
wrote and stated that he felt well, had no fever or back pain, was back at work, and
had gained 9 kg. He continued to take amoxicillin. Followup urine and blood cultures
were reportedly negative on multiple occasions.

Comment Although it would have been preferable to excise the abdominal
mycotic aneurysm and establish extraanatomic bypass circulation, the extensive involvement of vital intraabdominal arteries by the aneurysm made this
approach impossible. The portal of entry for the *E. coli* infection was thought
to be the urinary tract. The patient had mild prostatic hypertrophy which was
not severe enough to require corrective surgery.

Frequency, anatomic location, microbiologic etiology, and underlying conditions

Intraabdominal mycotic aneurysm occurs infrequently. Parkhurst and Decker
(64) reported an incidence of 12 mycotic aneurysms in 12,792 autopsies. Most
cases of intraabdominal mycotic aneurysm involve the aorta. Five (16 percent)
of our 32 patients with mycotic aneurysm had intraabdominal aneurysm. The
abdominal aorta was involved in three cases and the inferior mesenteric artery in
one, and one patient had involvement of the abdominal aorta and right iliac
artery. Mycotic aneurysm is one of the most common causes of mesenteric
artery aneurysm (65, 66). Other sites of involvement include the splenic, renal,
iliac, inferior mesenteric, and hepatic arteries (16, 67–71). The mean age of our
patients was 70 years (range 57–84), and all patients had extensive atherosclerotic disease; *E. coli* (two patients), viridans streptococci (one patient), *Histo-
plasma capsulatum* (one patient), and *E. coli* and *Bacteroides fragilis* (one patient) were isolated from the mycotic aneurysms at surgery or postmortem
examination. The two patients with *E. coli* infection had urinary tract infection
and positive blood cultures containing *E. coli*; the patient with polymicrobial
infection had a recent cholecystectomy and *E. coli* bacteremia. One patient
had IE (viridans streptococcal infection); the respiratory tract was the presumed
portal of entry in the patient with disseminated histoplasmosis.

Before the advent of antimicrobial therapy, approximately one-half of mycotic aneurysms were located intraabdominally (16). Intraabdominal mycotic
aneurysms were usually associated with bacteremia, often related to IE or intraabdominal surgery; the use of prophylactic antimicrobials for surgical proce-

dures and the prompt treatment of patients suspected of having bacteremia has reduced the frequency of intraabdominal mycotic aneurysms in the antimicrobial era.

In earlier reports, *Salmonella* species were the most common isolates from patients with intraabdominal mycotic aneurysm (10, 14, 72, 73); our experience and more recent reports indicate that the microbiologic spectrum is changing. Now *E. coli* and other Enterobactereaceae, *Staph. aureus*, anaerobes, and viridans streptococci constitute the majority of isolates from these patients (22, 69, 74, 75).

Diagnosis

Clinical signs Our experience with the clinical presentation of patients with intraabdominal mycotic aneurysm is similar to that reported elsewhere. These aneurysms are frequently associated with nonspecific or no symptoms until leakage or rupture occurs, at which time patients may develop localized abdominal or back pain or signs of an acute abdomen (76). While the presence of intraabdominal mycotic aneurysm is often unsuspected and is diagnosed at surgery or postmortem examination, a number of clinical signs may occur which suggest the diagnosis. The presence of a tender pulsatile abdominal mass in a patient with IE or bacteremia from other causes strongly suggests the diagnosis. However, because of the anatomic location, a pulsatile mass is often not apparent in these patients. Among our five patients, a clinical diagnosis of intraabdominal mycotic aneurysm was made in three. All five patients had fever; three had localized abdominal tenderness and a palpable pulsatile mass.

Patients with mycotic aneurysm of the hepatic artery may experience hematemesis, hematobilia, and jaundice (68, 77). Patients with splenic artery mycotic aneurysm may present as splenic abscess (78); renal artery mycotic aneurysm may be associated with arterial hypertension or hematuria (10, 74, 79). Rupture of mycotic aneurysm into the small or large bowel is usually associated with sudden onset of bloody, frequently massive, diarrhea (71).

Laboratory diagnosis Plain abdominal roentgenograms may reveal calcific aneurysms of the abdominal aorta. Noninvasive techniques such as B-mode echocardiography and computerized tomography may be helpful in defining intraabdominal masses, but angiography is the only procedure capable of confirming the diagnosis of intraabdominal aneurysm and of localizing the involved vessel or vessels. Arteriography should be performed promptly in all cases of suspected intraabdominal mycotic aneurysm.

Treatment and prognosis

Presumably, most, if not all, intraabdominal mycotic aneurysms will rupture if not excised. The use of appropriate antimicrobial agents preoperatively and identification and treatment of the underlying condition are important factors in therapy, but surgical excision of the infected tissue is essential.

Ideally, the infected arterial aneurysm should be ligated proximally and distally and excised. When the abdominal aorta is involved, revascularization must usually be established to preserve limbs and other vital structures. Collins et al. (80) reported a case of aortic mycotic aneurysm caused by *Candida* species treated successfully by ligation and resection alone. This procedure should be performed only if adequate collateral circulation has been demonstrated. In 1969 Mundth et al. (10) reported their experience with 13 patients with intraabdominal mycotic aneurysm. Ten of these 13 patients underwent surgery; all four with mycotic aneurysm that ruptured preoperatively died. Of the six patients whose aneurysm did not rupture, four survived from 2 to 9 years postoperatively. These four patients underwent resection of the aneurysm and interposition of an aortoiliac graft. Since 1969 there have been a few isolated reports of successful replacement of resected aortic mycotic aneurysm by an interposed synthetic graft (81, 82).

Two of our three surviving patients with intraabdominal mycotic aneurysm (Case 3 and the patient with *H. capsulatum* infection) were treated by excision of the aneurysm and interposition of a Dacron graft. The remaining surviving patient underwent ligation and excision of an infected iliac artery aneurysm. Collateral circulation in this patient was adequate to preserve the viability of the limb. Because the risk of reinfection of interposed aortic graft material is high, most authorities favor reestablishing circulation to the lower extremities through noninfected tissue planes, e.g., by using axillofemoral bypass grafts (76, 83, 84).

Mycotic aneurysm involving the superior or inferior mesenteric artery has been reported to have been treated successfully with ligation and excision (11, 65). Following superior mesenteric artery ligation, collateral circulation is frequently sufficient to maintain viability and function of the bowel (65, 85, 86). Should ischemic changes in the bowel occur following ligation, resection of the bowel should be delayed 24 h to allow ischemic changes to demarcate the line of viable intestine and thus preserve bowel length (65, 87). Successful vascular reconstruction of the superior mesenteric-celiac artery axis has been reported (11, 88), but because the risk of reinfection and rupture of the interposed venous or synthetic material is high, these patients should probably be treated with ligation and excision rather than reconstruction.

Postoperative therapy with antimicrobial agents administered parenterally should last at least 4 weeks. In patients who have a high risk of infection, e.g., those who have received interposed vascular grafts in infected areas, it may be desirable to administer indefinite suppressive oral antimicrobial therapy (Case 3).

The mortality among patients with intraabdominal mycotic aneurysm is high. Mortality for ruptured intraabdominal mycotic aneurysm approaches 100 percent (10, 23, 72). In 1974 Bob and Glassman (89) found reports of only 11 patients with intraabdominal mycotic aneurysm who had been treated successfully. Three of our five patients survived, but none of these survivors had a ruptured aneurysm. The two patients who died had rupture of an aortic aneurysm, and the diagnosis was made during postmortem examination.

PERIPHERAL MYCOTIC ANEURYSM

Of mycotic aneurysms, those which occur peripherally are the most accessible for diagnosis and treatment and are associated with the best prognosis.

Case 4

A 55-year-old male from Puerto Rico was admitted to Mayo Clinic hospitals in February 1970 with a 1-year history of fever. During childhood he had rheumatic fever and a cardiac murmur. His local physician treated him with ampicillin administered orally for 8 months, but the fever persisted; 2 weeks before admission to Mayo Clinic hospitals he noted the appearance of painful swelling in his left arm followed by a similar lesion in the right groin.

Pertinent physical findings on admission were temperature 39°C, a grade 3/6 holosystolic murmur of mitral incompetence, and tender pulsatile masses over the left brachial artery and the right femoral artery.

Abnormal laboratory tests included hemoglobin 10.6 g/dl, WBC 12,300 per cubic millimeter, and erythrocyte sedimentation rate 97 mm/h. Multiple blood cultures

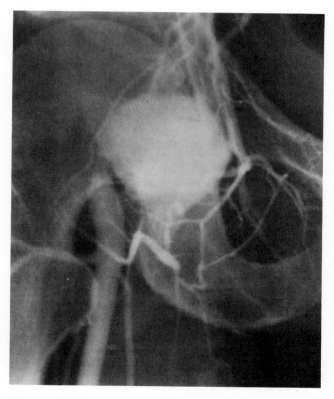

Figure 13   Pelvic arteriogram demonstrating 5-cm-diameter aneurysm of the distal right femoral artery.

yielded viridans streptococci. (MIC to penicillin was 0.09 μg/ml and MBC 0.78 μg/ml.) Treatment was initiated with intravenous penicillin (20 million units per day) and intramuscular streptomycin (500 mg twice daily). Peak SBT was 1:1024.

Pelvic arteriograms demonstrated a 5-cm-diameter aneurysm of the distal right femoral artery (Figure 13). The aneurysm filled and emptied slowly with contrast material. Left subclavian arteriogram demonstrated a 2-cm-diameter aneurysm of the left brachial artery which also filled and emptied slowly (Figure 14). Abdominal and thoracic aortograms and carotid angiograms failed to demonstrate additional aneurysms.

After 21 days of parenteral antimicrobial therapy, the patient underwent ligation and excision of the brachial artery aneurysm. The femoral artery aneurysm was ligated and excised with interposition of an autogenous venous graft. Gram-positive cocci were seen on a Gram stain of the brachial artery; postoperative cultures of the brachial and femoral artery aneurysms were negative. The histopathology of the specimens was consistent with mycotic aneurysm. Antimicrobial therapy with parenteral penicillin and streptomycin was continued postoperatively for 14 days. The patient was discharged in excellent condition. Follow-up blood cultures were negative, and the patient had no evidence of recurrence of infection 3 years postoperatively.

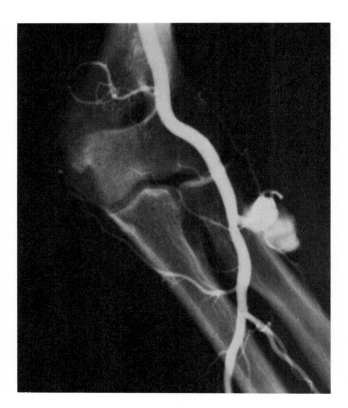

Figure 14 Subclavian arteriogram demonstrating 2-cm-diameter aneurysm of the left brachial artery.

Frequency, anatomic location, microbiologic etiology, and underlying conditions

The frequency of peripheral compared with other mycotic aneurysms depends on the patient population. Stengel (16) in 1923 reported that the majority of mycotic aneurysms primarily occur in the peripheral vessels. In our experience and that of others (10), the frequency of thoracic and intraabdominal mycotic aneurysms to peripheral is at least 3:1. Mycotic aneurysms located in the lower extremities are approximately three times as common as those in the upper extremities. Patient populations which include a substantial number of illicit drug abusers and those at high risk of vascular trauma demonstrate a preponderance of peripheral over aortic mycotic aneurysms (11, 22).

In our experience and earlier reports (16, 73, 90), most mycotic aneurysms which occur in the extremities are associated with IE. Of our six patients with peripheral mycotic aneurysm, five had IE. The remaining patient had mycotic aneurysm of the common carotid artery caused by a wound infection following radical neck surgery. The pathogenesis of mycotic aneurysm in the addict population is probably more often caused by direct trauma to peripheral arteries than by IE. Mycotic aneurysms in these patients commonly occur at sites of needle puncture, particularly in the antecubital fossa, groin, and wrist. Addicts may deliberately inject into an artery when superficial veins become thrombosed but, more commonly, intraarterial injection probably occurs inadvertently.

The microbiologic spectrum of peripheral mycotic aneurysms depends upon the patient population. In patients with IE, viridans streptococci is the most common isolate, and *Staph. aureus*, *Candida* spp., enterococci, gram-negative bacilli, and anaerobes are the most prevalent microorganisms isolated from addicts. In earlier reports, *Salmonella* spp. were frequent isolates from patients with peripheral mycotic aneurysms (14, 16).

Diagnosis

Clinical signs In most instances, on physical examination the diagnosis of a peripheral aneurysm is readily apparent. The presence of a tender pulsatile mass adjacent to a major blood vessel in an addict or in a patient with IE strongly suggests the diagnosis of mycotic aneurysm. The presence of mycotic aneurysm was suspected on physical examination in all six of our patients with peripheral lesions.

Laboratory diagnosis Because of the risk of uncontrolled bleeding, needle aspiration or incision and drainage of a pulsatile mass for diagnosis should be avoided. Arteriography should be performed promptly in all patients suspected of having peripheral mycotic aneurysm. Addicts may inject multiple intraarterial sites, and it may be desirable in these patients or in patients with IE to perform additional angiographic studies to exclude the possibility of occult mycotic aneurysms located in other peripheral arteries.

Treatment and prognosis

Appropriate antimicrobial therapy should be initiated promptly, and measures should be instituted to treat the underlying condition adequately. Some peripheral mycotic aneurysms may thrombose and undergo healing with antimicrobial therapy alone. The risk of rupture of untreated peripheral mycotic aneurysm is high, however, and surgical therapy of suspected mycotic aneurysm should not be delayed excessively.

The surgical treatment of choice for peripheral mycotic aneurysm is proximal and distal ligation and excision. The risk of bypass procedures in an attempt to prevent amputation of an extremity must be weighed carefully against the risk of potential exsanguination should the bypass become infected and rupture at the anastomosis. Anderson et al. (22) reported recurrent sepsis and bleeding in four patients with peripheral mycotic aneurysm treated with vein graft or suture repair of the aneurysm. All four patients subsequently underwent ligation procedures; two of these required limb amputation. The experience of Anderson et al. is similar to that of others (21, 23). Addicts frequently have extensive areas of necrosis and gross purulence in the soft tissues surrounding peripheral mycotic aneurysm, and the risk of recurrent infection following vascular reconstructive surgery in these patients is excessively high.

Frequently, collateral circulation provides adequate blood supply to an extremity following ligation of a major artery. The use of Doppler measurements of arterial pressure in an extremity may predict the likelihood of limb survival following arterial ligation. Doppler pressures measured in collateral arteries which are equal to 55 percent of those measured proximal to the ligated artery suggest that collateral circulation is sufficient to maintain limb viability (91). Most authorities believe strongly that ligation and excision is the treatment of choice for patients with peripheral mycotic aneurysm and that it is preferable to sacrifice the limb if necessary rather than the life of the patient.

Patients with mycotic aneurysm of the common carotid artery present a special problem. Ligation of the carotid artery without serious neurologic sequelae has been reported (92, 93). Establishment of extraintracranial arterial bypass around the aneurysm before ligation and excision may offer another surgical alternative. Our patient with common carotid artery aneurysm was treated successfully with ligation and excision and primary anastomosis. Patients with common carotid artery mycotic aneurysm should be considered individually. One must weigh the risk of neurologic complications following ligation and excision against the risk of reinfection of vascular reconstructed areas and potential rupture and fatal hemorrhage.

Among patients with mycotic aneurysm, those with peripheral mycotic aneurysm have the best prognosis (11, 22–23). The prognosis is especially favorable among patients treated with ligation alone. Anderson et al. (22) reported no deaths among nine patients with peripheral mycotic aneurysm; Yellin (11) observed no fatalities among four addicts with peripheral aneurysm. All six of our patients survived. Fatal cases of peripheral mycotic aneurysm are usually those which rupture before surgery or die of complications resulting from reinfection of arterial reconstruction.

REFERENCES

1 Goodhart JF: Cases of aneurysm from embolism. *Trans Pathol Soc Lond* 28:106, 1877.

2 Osler W: The Gulstonian lectures on malignant endocarditis, I, III. *Br Med J* 1:467, 577, 1885.

3 Eppinger H: Pathogenesis (Histogenesis und Aetiologie) der Aneurysmen einschliesslich des Aneurysma equi verminosum. *Pathol Anatom Studien Arch Klin Chir (Suppl Hft)* 35:1, 1887.

4 Lippincott SW: Abdominal aortic mycotic dissecting aneurysm. *Can Med Assoc J* 43:115, 1940.

5 Roach MR, Drake CG: Ruptured cerebral aneurysms caused by microorganisms. *N Engl J Med* 273:240, 1965.

6 Bell WE, Butler C: Cerebral mycotic aneurysms in children. Two case reports. *Neurology* 18:81, 1968.

7 Nakata Y et al: Pathogenesis of mycotic aneurysm. *Angiology* 19:593, 1968.

8 Molinari GF: Septic cerebral embolism. *Stroke* 3:117, 1972.

9 Molinari GF et al: Pathogenesis of cerebral mycotic aneurysms. *Neurology* 23:325, 1973.

10 Mundth ED et al: Surgical treatment of mycotic aneurysms and the complications of infection in vascular reconstructive surgery. *Am J Surg* 117:460, 1969.

11 Yellin AE: Ruptured mycotic aneurysm: A complication of parenteral drug abuse. *Arch Surg* 112:981, 1977.

12 Crane AR: Primary multilocular mycotic aneurysm of the aorta. *Arch Pathol* 24:634, 1937.

13 Blum L, Keefer EBC: Cryptogenic mycotic aneurysm. *Ann Surg* 155:398, 1962.

14 Revell STR Jr: Primary mycotic aneurysms. *Ann Intern Med* 22:431, 1945.

15 Singh H, Parkhurst GF: Bacterial aortitis. *NY State J Med* 72:2779, 1972.

16 Stengel A, Wolferth CC: Mycotic (bacterial) aneurysms of intravascular origin. *Arch Intern Med* 31:527, 1923.

17 Goadby HK et al: Mycotic aneurysm. *St Thomas Hosp Rep* 5:44, 1949.

18 Werner AS et al: Studies on the bacteremia of endocarditis. *JAMA* 202:199, 1967.

19 Belli J, Waisbren BA: The number of blood cultures necessary to diagnose most cases of bacterial endocarditis. *Am J Med Sci* 232:284, 1956.

20 Kaye D (ed): *Infective Endocarditis*. Baltimore, University Park Press, 1976.

21 O'Connor TW et al: Treatment of mycotic aneurysms. *Med J Aust* 2:1161, 1972.

22 Anderson CB et al: Mycotic aneurysms. *Arch Surg* 109:712, 1974.

23 Lawrence GH: Surgical management of infected aneurysms. *Am J Surg* 104:355, 1962.

24 Smith RF et al: Surgical treatment of mycotic aneurysms. *Arch Surg* 85:663, 1962.

25 Allcock J: Aneurysms, in Newton TH, Potts DG (eds): *Radiology of the Skull and Brain: Angiography*. St. Louis, Mosby, 1974, pp 2, 435–442, 489.

26 Roach M, Drake C: Ruptured cerebral aneurysms caused by microorganisms. *N Engl J Med* 273:240, 1965.

27 Olmsted WW, McGee TP; The pathogenesis of peripheral aneurysms of the central nervous system: A subject review from the AFIP. *Radiology* 123:661, 1977.

28 Bohmfalk GL et al: Bacterial intracranial aneurysm. *J Neurosurg* 48:369, 1978.

29 Jones HR et al: Neurologic manifestations of bacterial endocarditis. *Ann Intern Med* 71:21, 1969.

30 Gilroy J et al: Intracranial mycotic aneurysms and subacute bacterial endocarditis in heroin addiction. *Neurology* 23:1193, 1973.

31 Amine ARC: Neurosurgical complications of heroin addiction: brain abscess and mycotic aneurysm. *Surg Neurol* 7:385, 1977.

32 Bingham WF: Treatment of mycotic intracranial aneurysms. *J Neurosurg* 46:428, 1977.

33 Shibuya S et al: Mycotic aneurysm of the internal carotid artery. *J Neurosurg* 44:105, 1976.

34 Suwanwela C et al: Intracranial mycotic aneurysms of extravascular origin. *J Neurosurg* 36:552, 1972.

35 Adams RD et al: The clinical and pathological aspects of influenzal meningitis. *Arch Pediatr* 65:354, 1948.

36 Davis DO et al: Arterial dilatation in purulent meningitis: Case report. *J Neurosurg* 32:112, 1970.

37 Greitz T: Angiography in tuberculous meningitis. *Acta Radiol Diagn (Stock)* 2:369, 1964.

38 Wadia NH, Singhal BS: Vascular changes in tuberculous meningitis: An arteriographic study in 33 patients. *Proc Aust Assoc Neurol* 5:623, 1968.

39 Ahuja GK et al: Cerebral mycotic aneurysms of fungal origin. *J Neurosurg* 49:107, 1978.

40 Horten BC et al: Fungal aneurysms of intracranial vessels. *Arch Neurol* 33:577, 1976.

41 Schold C, Earnest MP: Cerebral hemorrhage from a mycotic aneurysm developing during appropriate antibiotic therapy. *Stroke* 9:267, 1978.

42 Cantu RC et al: The importance of repeated angiography in the treatment of mycotic-embolic aneurysms. *J Neurosurg* 25:189, 1966.

43 Katz RI et al: Mycotic aneurysm: Case report with novel sequential angiographic findings. *Arch Intern Med* 134:939, 1974.

44 **Hourihane JB:** Ruptured mycotic intracranial aneurysm. A report of three cases. *Vasc Surg* 4:21, 1970.

45 **Campbell E, Burklund CW:** Aneurysms of the middle cerebral artery. *Ann Surg* 137:18, 1953.

46 **Devadiga KV et al:** Spontaneous cure of intracavernous aneurysm of the internal carotid artery in a 14-month-old child. Case report. *J Neurosurg* 30:165, 1969.

47 **Michal JA, Coleman RE:** Localization of ^{67}Ga citrate in a mycotic aneurysm. *Am J Roentgenol* 129:1111, 1977.

48 **Shumacker HB:** Aneurysms of the aortic sinus of Valsalva due to bacterial endocarditis with special reference to their operative management. *J Thorac Cardiovasc Surg* 63:896, 1972.

49 **Gonzalez-Lavin L et al:** Mycotic aneurysms of the aortic root. *Ann Thorac Surg* 9:551, 1970.

50 **Danielson GK et al:** Successful treatment of aortic valve endocarditis and aortic root abscesses by insertion of prosthetic valve in ascending aorta and placement of bypass grafts to coronary arteries. *J Thorac Cardiovasc Surg* 67:443, 1974.

51 **Hatcher CR Jr et al:** Surgical aspects of endocarditis of the aortic root. *Am J Cardiol* 23:192, 1969.

52 **Odagiri S et al:** Ascending aorta–supraceliac abdominal aorta bypass. *Chest* 6:722, 1979.

53 **Crosby IK, Tegtmeyer C:** Mycotic aneurysm of the ascending aorta following coronary revascularization. *Ann Thorac Surg* 25:474, 1978.

54 **Oldham HN et al:** Surgical treatment of mycotic aneurysm associated with coarctation of the aorta. *Ann Thorac Surg* 15:411, 1973.

55 **Kieffer SA et al:** Mycotic aneurysm distal to coarctation of the aorta. *J Thorac Cardiovasc Surg* 42:507, 1961.

56 **Sellors TH:** Coarctation of the aorta associated with aneurysm. *Br J Surg* 43:365, 1956.

57 **Cossette R et al:** Ruptured aortic aneurysm in a 3½-year-old child with coarctation of the aorta. *Can Med Assoc J* 100:257, 1969.

58 **Crook BRM et al:** Mycotic aneurysms of coronary arteries. *Br Heart J* 35:107, 1973.

59 **Daoud AS et al:** Aneurysm of the coronary artery. *Am J Cardio* 11:228, 1963.

60 Kawasaki disease: *MMWR* 29:61, 1980.

61 **Kato H et al:** Coronary aneurysms in infants and young children with acute febrile mucocutaneous lymph node syndrome. *J Pediatr* 86:892, 1975.

62 **Yoshida H et al:** Mucocutaneous lymph node syndrome: A cross-sectional echocardiographic diagnosis of coronary aneurysms. *Am J Dis Child* 133:1244, 1979.

63 **Kato H et al:** Kawasaki disease: Effect of treatment on coronary artery involvement. *Pediatrics* 63:175, 1979.

64 **Parkhurst GF, Decker JP:** Bacterial aortitis and mycotic aneurysm of the aorta: A report of twelve cases. *Am J Pathol* 31:821, 1955.

65 **Mukerjee S et al:** Superior mesenteric artery aneurysm. *Br J Surg* 61:233, 1974.

66 **DeBakey ME, Cooley DA:** Successful resection of mycotic aneurysm of superior mesenteric artery: Case report and review of literature. *Am Surg* 19:202, 1953.

67 **Mojab K et al:** Mycotic aneurysm of the hepatic artery causing obstructive jaundice. *Am J Roentgenol* 128:143, 1977.

68 **Sukerkar AN et al:** Mycotic aneurysm of the hepatic artery. *Radiol* 124:444, 1977.

69 **Kyriakides GK et al:** Mycotic aneurysms in transplant patients. *Arch Surg* 111:472, 1976.

70 Case records of the Massachusetts General Hospital. *N Engl J Med* 292:1068, 1975.

71 **Shnider BI, Cotsonas NJ:** Embolic mycotic aneurysms, a complication of bacterial endocarditis. *Am J Med* 246:255, 1954.

72 **Zak FG et al:** Rupture of diseased large arteries in the course of enterobacterial (Salmonella) infections. *N Engl J Med* 258:824, 1958.

73 **Bennett DE, Cherry JK:** Bacterial infection of aortic aneurysms: A clinicopathologic study. *Am J Surg* 113:321, 1967.

74 **Kaufman SL et al:** Protean manifestations of mycotic aneurysms. *Am J Roentgenol* 131:1019, 1978.

75 **File TM et al:** *Campylobacter fetus* sepsis with mycotic aortic aneurysm. *Arch Pathol Lab Med* 103:143, 1979.

76 **Davies OG et al:** Cryptic mycotic abdominal aortic aneurysm. *Am J Surg* 136:96, 1978.

77 **Gupta S, Cope V:** Hepatic artery aneurysm as a cause of gastrointestinal bleeding. *Br J Radiol* 45:726, 1972.

78 **Jacobs RP et al:** Angiography of splenic abscesses. *Am J Roentgenol* 122:419, 1974.

79 **Clark RE et al:** Intrarenal mycotic (false) aneurysm secondary to staphylococcal septicemia. *Radiology* 115:421, 1975.

80 **Collins GJ et al:** Multiple mycotic aneurysms due to *Candida* endocarditis. *Ann Surg* 186:136, 1977.

81 **James EC, Gillepsie JT:** Aortic mycotic abdominal aneurysm involving all visceral branches: Excision and Dacron graft replacement. *J Cardiovasc Surg* 18:353, 1977.

82 **Riester WH, Serrano MD:** Infrarenal mycotic pseudoaneurysm. *J Thorac Cardiovasc Surg* 71:633, 1976.

83 **Blaisdell FW, Hall AD:** Axillary femoral

bypass for lower extremity ischemia. *Surgery* 54:563, 1963.

84 **Johnson WC et al:** Is axillo-bilateral femoral graft an effective substitute for aortic-bilateral iliac/femoral graft? An analysis of ten years' experience. *Ann Surg* 186:123, 1977.

85 **Laufman H:** Gradual occlusion of the mesenteric vessels: Experimental study. *Surgery* 13:406, 1943.

86 **Blalock A, Levy SE:** Gradual complete occlusion of the celiac axis, superior and inferior mesenteric artery, with survival of animals: Effects of ischemia on blood pressure. *Surgery* 5:175, 1939.

87 **Buchman RJ, Martin GW:** Management of mycotic aneurysm of superior mesenteric artery. *Ann Surg* 155:620, 1962.

88 **Vialago FC, Downs AR:** Ruptured atherosclerotic aneurysm of the superior mesenteric artery with celiac axis occlusion. *Ann Surg* 174:207, 1971.

89 **Bob HB, Glassman GI:** Management of mycotic aneurysm abdominal aorta. *Del Med J* 46:561, 1974.

90 **Barker WF:** Mycotic aneurysm. *Ann Surg* 139:84, 1954.

91 **Lennihan R Jr, Mackereth MA:** Ankle pressures in arterial occlusive disease involving the leg. *Surg Clin North Am* 53:657, 1973.

92 **Howell HS et al:** Mycotic cervical carotid aneurysm. *Surgery* 81:357, 1977.

93 **Moore O, Baker HW:** Carotid artery ligation in surgery of the head and neck. *Cancer* 8:712, 1955.

A review of "new" bacterial strains causing diarrhea

RANDALL J. RYSER
RICHARD B. HORNICK

The syndrome of diarrheal illness is a common worldwide medical problem. Functionally, the altered fecal mass represents the consequence of disturbed fluid secretion and/or absorption in the gastrointestinal tract. This physiological imbalance can be initiated by many microorganisms through a number of mechanisms. Clarification of the role of enterotoxins produced by *Vibrio cholerae* and *Escherichia coli* in the causation of increased fluid secretion in the small intestine has been a tremendous stimulus in discovering additional enterotoxin-producing microorganisms pathogenic for man. Invasion of mucosal lining by certain bacteria and the subsequent release of chemical mediators from the invoked inflammatory response may stimulate fluid secretion. The search for infectious agents which induce diarrhea by these and other means has spawned extensive efforts to investigate common as well as exotic microorganisms isolated from diarrheal stool specimens. These studies have extended the usual methods employed to isolate potential enteric pathogens. Highly selective media and/or unusual environmental conditions have been developed to identify newer diarrhea-producing bacteria. In this review we present a summary of accumulated information on some of the bacteria that have recently emerged as significant causes of diarrheal disease.

The organisms to be discussed were formerly unnamed, unclassified, or known as various *Vibrio* or *Yersinia* species. Three major groups will be discussed:

1 *Campylobacter fetus* (formerly *Vibrio fetus*) potentially may be the most common bacterial pathogen causing diarrhea in children.

2 *Yersinia enterocolitica* and *Yersinia pseudotuberculosis*, being isolated with increasing frequency, cause acute terminal ileitis and mesenteric lymphadenitis as well as enterocolitis in people.

3 *Vibrio parahemolyticus* is now recognized to be worldwide in its distribution and a major cause of foodborne acute diarrheal illness.

Other vibrios have been isolated, and some cause diarrheal illness. In this review, only a brief mention will be made since at present they do not appear to be significant causes of human diarrheal disease in the United States.

DIARRHEAL DISEASE ASSOCIATED WITH *CAMPYLOBACTER* SPECIES

Campylobacter is a thin, small, gram-negative curved or S-shaped rod. It has a single polar flagellum at one or both ends of the cell and moves in a characteristic rapid, darting, corkscrew pattern. It is a microaerophilic nonfermenter which uses the Krebs cycle intermediates and amino acids for energy. With the recent development of specific culture techniques, this thermophilic organism has been shown to be a significant cause of diarrheal disease worldwide.

Historical Background and Classification

Vibrios[1] have been associated with infections in animals since 1909, when they were noted to be related to abortions in sheep and cattle (1). The first possible cases of human vibrio infection were reported by Curtis in 1913 (2). Large numbers of curved, motile, gram-negative rods were noted in the vaginal discharges from two patients with puerpural infections. Microaerophilic vibrios were associated with acute diarrheal illness in people in 1946 (3). The organisms were seen microscopically in 42 percent of the stool specimens but were not cultured. However, 13 of 39 of these patients with diarrhea had vibrios isolated from their blood. Epidemiological evidence suggested contaminated milk as the common source in this outbreak. The following year V. *fetus* was isolated from the blood of a pregnant woman in France who had a grippelike illness and later delivered a stillborn infant with a necrotic placenta. In 1957 King noted that some strains had distinctly different growth characteristics and called them *related vibrios* (4). Sebald and Veron (1963) (5) performed DNA homology studies which showed that the related vibrios had a different nucleotide base content and proposed that these organisms should form a genus of their own in the family Spirillaceae. They chose the name *Campylobacter*, from the Greek for "curved rod." Several different subspecies have been isolated, but no definite classification has been agreed upon since the biotyping and serotyping of these organisms are still in their infancy. The genus is divided into two groups according to the ability of the organisms to produce catalase. The catalase-negative campylobacters (*C. sputorum* and *C. bubulus*) are not known to be pathogenic in human beings, although *C. sputorum* is part of the normal human oral flora found in the gingival crevices. The confusion arises with the catalase-positive organisms. Smibert has designated King's related vibrios as *Campylobacter fetus jejuni* (6), whereas Veron and Chatelain (7) feel that they are two separate species and list them as *C. jejuni* and *C. coli*. It has been proposed that, until further investigations determine whether there are multiple species, these or-

[1]In this section the term *vibrio* is employed for historical accuracy and is interchangeable with *campylobacter*.

ganisms simply be called related campylobacters. The only other organism in this group of human significance is *C. fetus intestinalis,* an opportunistic organism, isolated from patients with preexisting pathological conditions such as cirrhosis, diabetes, gastrectomy, cancer, leukemia, and immunosuppressive therapy. Therefore, the organisms most important in causing human illness are known variously as *C. fetus jejuni, C. coli/jejuni,* or related campylobacters. The first term has enjoyed the greatest use in the last few years.

Between 1957 and 1972 only 14 cases of related vibrio infection were reported in the literature (8). All those isolates were from blood or other body fluids. Some of the isolations (i.e., from blood cultures) were from patients with enteric illnesses, but vibrios were not isolated from the stools of these patients. Since blood cultures are infrequently done in patients with acute gastroenteritis, it can be surmised that the incidence of enteric infections was greatly underestimated. These organisms have peculiar growth requirements, and because of overgrowth by coliform organisms routine coproculture from patients with diarrhea usually failed to yield *Campylobacter.* In Australia in 1971 Cooper and Slee (9) reported the first selective methods for *Campylobacter* isolation, but work was not expanded. Dekeyser et al. in 1972 (10) developed a unique but cumbersome technique for isolation from stools. They took advantage of the organism's small size and filtered the supernate from homogenized stool specimens through a 0.65-μm Millipore filter. Further selectivity was provided by adding bacitracin, polymyxin, novobiocin, and actidione and incubating at 37°C for 3 days in an atmosphere of 95% N_2 and 5% CO_2. Subculturing was into thioglycolate broth at 42, 37, and 25°C. It was noted that the organisms grew best at 42°C. Campylobacters were finally successfully isolated from stools of patients with enteric illnesses. Screening of hospitalized patients for *Campylobacter* with this method was conducted in 800 pediatric patients and 100 adults with diarrhea and 1000 children without diarrhea (8). *Campylobacter* was isolated from the stools of 5 percent of the patients with diarrhea and 1.3 percent of those without diarrhea. This study clearly showed the importance of *Campylobacter* as a cause of acute gastroenteritis.

In 1977 a report by Skirrow (11) confirmed and extended the work of Butzler and Dekeyser in a series of 803 patients with diarrhea (*Campylobacter* isolated in 7.1 percent) and 194 persons without diarrhea (none with a positive culture for the organism). Additionally, a modified and more practical selection medium was developed. When 10 mg/liter of vancomycin, 2.5 IU/ml of polymyxin B, and 5 mg/liter of trimethoprim were added, the medium would select for *Campylobacter* without filtration. All the plates were incubated at 43°C in an atmosphere of 5% O_2, 10% CO_2, and 85% N. The motile campylobacters were readily detected after overnight incubation. This method is now widely employed to detect these bacteria.

Clinical Manifestations

Enteritis A composite characterization of *Campylobacter* enteritis can be summarized from the large series of published cases. The incubation period is relatively short (2 to 4 days). The onset of illness is sudden, with appearance of abdominal pain of variable intensity, nausea, anorexia, fever, malaise, headache, and myalgia. Diarrhea is almost always present; it may be one of the presenting manifestations, or it may not occur until several days after the onset of the other symptoms. The diarrhea is watery and is usually associated with more than eight bowel movements per day at its peak. Arthralgia, backache, vomiting, and rigors are less frequent. The illness *rarely* lasts longer than 1 week, but 25 percent of patients will have a relapse of symptoms, particularly the abdominal pain. The stools are often free of detectable *Campylobacter* at the time of this relapse.

Colitis   The illness appears to be localized to the upper GI tract because of the initial significant watery diarrhea. Furthermore, Cadronel et al. have recovered *Campylobacter* from the stomach, jejunum, and ileum of children with enteritis (12). However, many patients (from 14 to 92 percent in various studies) (13, 14) have progressively increasing abdominal pain which is cramping and which localizes in the periumbilical or lower quadrants. Since such patients have erythrocytes and leukocytes in their stools, colonic involvement is suggested. Sigmoidoscopy and rectal biopsies have been performed in patients with culture-proved *Campylobacter* enterocolitis (15, 16). Inflamed, friable, edematous mucosa was noted in all patients examined before resolution of the diarrhea. The biopsies showed decreased numbers of epithelial cells, irregular spacing, and loss of mucus production. Crypt abscesses and infiltration of the lamina propria with neutrophils, plasma cells, and lymphocytes were observed. In some cases the appearance was indistinguishable from that of acute ulcerative colitis. Electron-microscopic techniques demonstrated vibriolike structures in the mucosa. All these changes reversed completely with the resolution of the infection. Most were treated with erythromycin.

Other illnesses associated with *Campylobacter* infections   In addition to the enteritis and colitis with positive stool cultures, which is the most common human illness produced by *Campylobacter*, a wide variety of other syndromes have been associated with the isolation of *Campylobacter*. Skin pustules, erythema nodosum, Reiter's syndrome, arthritis, septicemia, endocarditis, pericarditis, meningitis, neurological abnormalities, lung abscesses, peritonitis, cholecystitis, urinary tract infections, abortions, and thrombophlebitis have all been reported (13, 17).

Infections associated with the gastrointestinal tract or associated manifestations of gastrointestinal infections such as reactive arthritis are usually due to C. *fetus jejuni* infections. Those not associated with the gastrointestinal tract or with severe illnesses such as septicemia are usually caused by C. *fetus intestinalis*. Human infections with C. *fetus intestinalis* are usually seen in immunosuppressed or otherwise compromised hosts (17). It is of interest to note that C. *fetus intestinalis* has a glycoprotein coat which has antiphagocytic properties (18), which may account for the ability of C. *fetus intestinalis* to survive in the blood and other body fluids outside the gastrointestinal tract. The subspecies *jejuni* lacks this glycoprotein coat.

Diagnosis

A strong suspicion of the presence of *Campylobacter* should be raised in patients with acute diarrheal illnesses who present with the clinical manifestations noted previously or who have been exposed to animals.

A rapid presumptive diagnosis can be made from phase contrast microscopy of a smear from a fresh diarrheal stool. Campylobacters can be recognized by their shape and characteristic rapid, darting, corkscrew motions (17).

A satisfactory holding medium contains thioglycolate broth, 0.16% agar, and the antibiotic and antifungal agents used in the isolation medium. The availability of a transportation medium that would allow for a transit time of up to 4 days at 18 to 37°C with an inoculum of 10^4 organisms has been reported (19). Culture of stools will yield the organism if appropriate selection media are used. Brucella agar plus 10 percent sheep erythrocytes and the inhibitory additives is recommended. Table 1 shows three combinations of inhibitory substances that have been useful in selective media. Incubation at 42°C in an atmosphere of 5% O_2, 10% CO_2, and 85% N_2 or H_2 is required. The plates should be checked at 24 and 48 h for gray, mucoid, nonhemolytic colonies that are oxidase- and catalase-positive. At this point, the organisms can usually be identified with phase microscopy because of the characteristic features noted above. With Gram stain a strong stain like 0.06% carbol-fuchsin should be used rather than safranin because *C. fetus jejuni* stains poorly with safranin. Serotyping is available and has epidemiological importance.

Serological diagnosis is possible, but antisera are not readily available. In one series 31 of 38 patients with positive stool cultures had elevated titers, and 10 showed a fourfold rise in titer (11). Antibodies have been characterized as IgG. Serological studies may be helpful to establish the diagnosis in symptomatic patients with negative stool cultures.

Pathogenesis of enteritis

No evidence of heat-labile toxin formation has been found to date, but some isolates produce a heat-stable toxin (17, 20). Tests for invasiveness in guinea pig conjunctivae (Sereny test) were negative, but tests for invasiveness using

Table 1 **Selective media for isolation of campylobacters**

Butzler et al. (8)	*Skirrow (11)*	*Blaser et al. (14)*
Bacitracin, 25 IU/ml	Vancomycin, 10 μg/ml	Vancomycin, 10 mg/liter
Novobiocin, 5 μg/ml	Polymyxin B sulfate, 2.5 IU/ml	Polymyxin B sulfate, 2500 IU/liter
Cycloheximide, 50 μg/ml		
Colistin, 10 μg/ml	Trimethoprim, 5 μg/ml	Trimethoprim, 5 mg/liter
Cefazolin, 15 μg/ml		Amphotericin B, 2 mg/liter
		Cephalothin, 15 mg/liter

Table 2 Incidence of organisms in stool specimens of 514 patients in Denver

Organism	No.	%	Organism	No.	%
Campylobacter	26	5.1	Candida albicans	2	0.4
Salmonella	19	3.7	Intestinal parasites	2	0.4
Shigella	13	2.5	C. fetus intestinalis	1	0.2
Giardia lamblia	4	0.8			

chicken embryos and 8-day-old chicks were positive in all strains tested. Evidence at present would imply at least two mechanisms, acting singly or in combination, by which *Campylobacter* cause watery diarrhea. First, by invasion and the mediators of fluid secretion associated with the subsequent inflammatory process; second, perhaps by a heat-stable toxin. In experimental salmonella infections in rabbits the inflammatory exudate has been shown probably to produce prostaglandins (21). These mediators can stimulate the energy systems in epithelial cells to secrete fluid and electrolytes. Administration of a potent prostaglandin inhibitor, indomethacin, will largely inhibit the fluid secretion in the experimental rabbit model. Presumably the method could be operative in other infections of the gut in which an inflammatory response occurs as a result of the invading pathogen. The colitis is presumably caused by the invasive propensity of the organism for epithelial cells of the colon. Further studies to clarify these pathogenic mechanisms are under way.

Epidemiology

The improved and rather simple methodology for isolation of the etiologic agent of this new diarrheal syndrome has stimulated screening for *Campylobacter* on a worldwide basis. The relative incidence of this infection as part of the etiological spectrum of diarrheal disease has been established. Thousands of cases from Belgium, Great Britain, Netherlands, Sweden, Australia, Rawanda, Zaire, South Africa, Canada, and the United States (13) have been reported, most of them between 1977 and 1979. In England and Wales in 1978, 6346 isolations were reported (17).

In a prospective study in 514 patients in Denver (14) the stool specimens were routinely processed to look for *Salmonella, Shigella, Candida, Staphylococcus aureus*, intestinal protozoa, and the ova and larvae of helminths. The results are given in Table 2.

The incidence of positive stool cultures for *Campylobacter* in several series of patients with gastroenteritis usually ranged from 5.0 to 14 percent. Almost universally, *Campylobacter* has been the most frequently isolated pathogen where screening for multiple agents has been performed. The number of patients with *Campylobacter*-induced enteritis has often outnumbered those from all other causes combined. In South Africa it was isolated from 30 percent of infants with acute gastroenteritis (22). Reports from the tropics indicate that the incidence of infection there may be higher than in the temperate zones (17). Worldwide, however, as of this time, it appears to be one of the most common, if not the most common, of all the bacterial pathogens isolated in patients with acute gastroenteritis.

The steps involved in the acquisition of *Campylobacter*-induced enteritis have not yet been clearly identified. A few epidemiological facts are known. The sex distribution seems to be about equal except for a higher incidence in males under 15 years old. In temperate climates the incidence of infection appears to be higher during the summer months. The few available reports from tropical climates indicate an even higher incidence there.

Several different modes of transmission have been proved or inferred (23).

Contact with animals   Campylobacters are widely distributed among mammals, but most of the animal strains are probably not pathogenic in human beings. This can be determined with certainty only as the classification, serotyping, and biotyping of campylobacters becomes more advanced. In Britain a high percentage of chickens are carriers of *Campylobacter* (91 percent of live chickens and 14 percent of freshly dressed chickens). There have been case reports of campylobacter enteritis involving butchers and poultry handlers (14). The *Campylobacter* in the chicken should not present a health hazard as long as the chicken is well cooked and uncooked food is not incidently cross-contaminated in preparing the chicken. Documented transmission of *Campylobacter* from dogs to people has been reported (24).

Contaminated food   Raw milk has been reported as a source of human infection involving single persons or outbreaks of multiple cases from the same raw milk source (23). The organisms probably gain access to the milk by fecal contamination.

Water   A large outbreak of campylobacter enteritis in Bennington, Vermont, was thought to be related to a contaminated water supply (25). Since the water supply was from a freshwater mountain stream, it is assumed that a wild animal had contaminated the water. The duration of this outbreak was about 2 weeks and involved about 2000 persons. In Southhampton, England, several cases of campylobacter enteritis were traced to contaminated natural water (26). Since coliform organisms were also found in the water, it was assumed that the presence of *Campylobacter* in the water represented fecal contamination.

Venereal transmission (23)   This is well documented in cattle, and it has been shown that bulls can develop an asymptomatic carrier state. No confirmed human case has been reported, but at least one instance of a *Campylobacter*-related septic abortion has been noted. The organism could not be cultured from the husband, but both he and his wife had elevated antibody titers.

Placental transfer at delivery   Several cases of C. *fetus* infections in fetuses and newborns are included in Reference 23.

Person-to-person spread by fecal oral route   The number of organisms required to cause disease in people can be inferred from one experimental observation (27). Campylobacter enteritis was induced by ingestion of 10^6 organisms. This inoculum size is comparable to doses required to cause human *E. coli* and salmonella infections. Organisms can be isolated from the stools of convalescent patients for as long as 1 month.

Animals appear to serve as reservoirs of this organism, and the spread of infection to human beings can occur directly from animals or animal products or by ingestion of water contaminated by animals.

Treatment

Most patients respond well to symptomatic treatment, and the illness lasts less than 1 week. Fluid replacement is the cornerstone of therapy. Ideally, an isotonic water-electrolyte solution should be used. The lack of a readily available solution for oral use precludes this approach. Therefore, in infants careful attention to fluid balance is required, and parenteral administration may be needed. Antidiarrheal agents probably should not be used because they may delay clearing of the stools and prolong symptoms (28). This has been inferred in some cases. Antibiotic treatment usually is not needed, but if it is necessary, erythromycin or tetracycline would be the drugs of choice. Reports of resistance to erythromycin have been noted in Belgium (29) and Sweden (30) but not in Great Britain or the United States. This varying susceptibility may be related to the prescribing practices of the veterinarians in these countries. For parenteral use, an aminoglycoside might be used. There has been one report suggesting that oral neomycin is useful for nonbacteremic infections.

Summary

C. fetus is a "new" pathogen whose significance in human infections has only recently been appreciated. It is worldwide in its distribution and is commonly found in cattle, sheep, and other animals. Among the presently known pathogens it appears to be the most frequent cause of acute bacterial gastroenteritis in children. A rapid, presumptive diagnosis can be made by identifying the comma-shaped, rapidly darting organism on phase microscopy.

Infection with this agent produces a characteristic clinical syndrome manifested by abdominal pain and diarrhea accompanied by fever, malaise, headache, myalgia, and nausea with little or no vomiting. Blood and leukocytes are often found in the stools when colitis is present. In some patients the colon may have an appearance indistinguishable from that of acute ulcerative colitis. The illness usually lasts less than 1 week and rarely requires more than symptomatic treatment. If antibiotics are deemed to be necessary, the oral drug of choice is either erythromycin or tetracycline.

DIARRHEAL DISEASE ASSOCIATED WITH *YERSINIA ENTEROCOLITICA*

Introduction

The genus *Yersinia* belongs to the family Enterobacteriaceae and at present contains the species *Y. pestis*, *Y. pseudotuberculosis*, and *Y. enterocolitica*. The devastating human illness that *Y. pestis*, the plague bacillus, produces has been known for centuries. *Y. pseudotuberculosis* has been known as a pathogen in animals since 1883 and in people since the early 1950s. *Y. enterocolitica*, first named in the mid-1960s, is now recognized as a significant pathogen in human enteric illness. The following discussion will deal with *Y. enterocolitica* with some references to *Y. pseudotuberculosis* as it relates to enteric disease. Several excellent recent reviews of *Y. enterocolitica* have appeared in the literature (31, 32).

Historical background

The genus *Yersinia* was first proposed in 1944 in honor of the French bacteriologist A. J. E. Yersin, who first isolated the plague bacillus in 1894 (33). The species of this genus, which were formerly included in the genus *Pasteurella*, were distinguished from other species of *Pasteurella* by being oxidase-negative. The genus designation *Yersinia* was not widely adopted for all species until the late 1960s and early 1970s. It was made official in the eighth edition of *Bergey's Manual* (1974), where these organisms were designated as *Yersinia* in the family Enterobacteriaceae.

Y. *pseudotuberculosis* was first isolated in 1883 from guinea pigs which had tuberculosis-like lesions (31). The organism became well recognized as a species of veterinary importance which caused epizootic disease in animals, especially rodents. The syndrome described was that of necrotizing granulomatous disease involving the liver, spleen, and abdominal lymph nodes. In 1953, Masshoff (34) described a purulent abscess-forming lymphadenitis in children who had been operated on for acute appendicitis. In the following year, he and Knapp were able to recover *Y. pseudotuberculosis* from patients with this entity and established the organism as a human pathogen (35).

The first description and report of isolation of *Y. enterocolitica* from human beings was in 1939 in New York State, where Schleifstein and Coleman described five cases (36). The name "*Bacterium enterocoliticum*" was coined in 1943 (37). Between that time and the 1960s, relatively few reports of isolations of this organism appeared. Reports from Europe were most frequent, and the organism was variously designated as *Pasteurella pseudotuberculosis* type B and *Pasteurella X*. In 1963 it was established that the strains isolated from both animals and people in Europe and America were similar (38). In 1964 Frederiksen proposed the name *Y. enterocolitica* for the organism (39). Case reports of infection with this new organism remained infrequent until the development of improved methods that permitted successful isolation with coproculture. The increased yield by these methods was reflected by the experience of Mollaret at the Pasteur Institute in Paris. The number of cases on file there grew from 642 in 1970 to 1000 in 1972. In 1974 the WHO designated the institute as an international referral center for *Y. enterocolitica*. By 1976 they had 5800 cases on file, and by 1977 the number was 6600.

Bacteriology

These organisms are relatively large (0.05 to 1.0 by 1 to 2 μm), facultatively anaerobic, oxidase-negative, and gram-negative asporogenic rods which display significant pleomorphism based upon the temperature, age of the culture, and media composition (31). Coccobacillary forms can be seen. The cells are immotile at 37°C, but at 22°C develop peritriochous flagella and become very motile.

Like *Y. pestis*, strains of *Y. pseudotuberculosis* are biochemically homogenous. *Y. enterocolitica* strains, however, differ substantially in their biochemical reactions, particularly to indole, esculin, rhamnose, xylose, and sucrose. At least five different biotypes have been recognized by most investigators. Because of this variability, it has been proposed that several new species be formed from the *Y. enterocolitica* subgroups. Some of the new names proposed are *Y. intermedia*, *Y. frederiksenii*, *Y. philomiragia*, and *Y. ruckeri* (40). Thirty-four O and nineteen H serotypes have been identified. The serotypes O3, O8, and O9 are most frequently found in human infection.

Yersinia grow well on enteric media and, on initial isolation, strongly resemble several other common Enterobacteriaceae (*Proteus*, *Shigella*, and *Providencia*) and are easily misdiagnosed. Several distinguishing features allow them to be recognized. They are lactose- and oxidase-negative gram-negative rods which do not produce hydrogen sulfide in triple sugar iron medium but are urease-positive.

Isolation from blood and body fluids that are usually sterile presents no problem because of the organism's ability to grow on ordinary media. Isolation from the feces, however, is more difficult because *Yersinia* grow slower than the other enteric organisms at 37°C. The abundant overgrowth plus the lack of a characteristic colony morphology makes recognition of *Yersinia* colonies difficult. The preferential growth at lower temperatures can be used to improve the yield of *Yersinia* from feces. Isolation rates are improved by incubating two sets of salmonella-shigella (SS) and MacConkey plates, one at room temperature (22 to 28°C) and one at 35 to 37°C. Optimum recovery of *Yersinia*, especially during the convalescent state, is achieved with the cold enrichment technique (41). Fecal specimens are suspended in saline buffered with 0.067 *M* phosphate at a pH of 7.6 and then incubated for 3 weeks at 4°C. Subplating onto SS and MacConkey agar is done at 1, 7, 14, and 21 days. *Yersinia* grow preferentially while the other enteric organisms do not survive or grow only minimally. Subsequent examination of the colonies with a stereomicroscope that gives oblique transillumination aids in the recognition of *Yersinia* colonies. On MacConkey agar the colonies have a light peach color (42). Cold enrichment has been used to isolate *Yersinia* from patients, animals, foods, and environmental sources (42).

Cold enrichment is currently the best method for isolating *Yersinia* from fecal specimens (43), but since it is cumbersome, simpler and faster selective techniques are needed. Recent reports have clarified the serotypes and clinical circumstances in which the use of cold enrichment is not necessary (44). The addition of novobiocin or carbenicillin to a broth used along with the standard MacConkey and SS plates allowed for the isolation without cold enrichment of 100 percent serotype O3 and O9 strains from infected patients. In that report, only the nonpathogenic biotype 1 strains were identified with cold enrichment alone (44). In the acute illness produced by serotype O3, when large numbers of organisms were being shed, direct plating alone was sufficient (45). In convalescent or asymptomatic patients with infection, a comparison study demonstrated that the direct plating method alone yielded the organisms in 66 percent of the cases. The remaining 34 percent were isolated by cold enrichment. Recovery of serotypes other than O3 was very poor without cold enrichment (46).

An innovative new selective medium for the direct isolation and presumptive identification of *Y. enterocolitica* has been evaluated (47). *Yersinia* has been noted to have pectinolytic activity. A pectin-containing agar was employed in which the colonies of *Yersinia* sank into the surface by 48 h and were thus readily discernable from those of other enteric organisms. The development of selective techniques like this or finding a suitable antibiotic mixture to add to the plates (as for isolation of *Campylobacter*) for increased selectivity will probably obviate the need for cold enrichment in the near future.

Antibody titers have been measured by agglutination or hemagglutination techniques. With infection, titers peak within 1 to 2 weeks and persist for 1 to 2 months after the illness. The serological diagnosis of serotype O9 infections may be complicated by the cross agglutination with *Brucella* species. Despite cross reactivity with some of the *Salmonella* species, no diagnostic interference has occurred. The ELISA (enzyme-linked immunosorbent assay) technique, which is ten- to a hundredfold more sensitive than the commonly used tube agglutination test, has detected previously unrecognized antigenic differences between *Yersinia* serotype O9 and *Brucella* spp. (48). The possibility now exists that this method may provide a reliable serological assay that can distinguish between *Yersinia* serotype O9 and *Brucella* infections in man. A radioimmunoassay for IgG and IgM antibodies to *Yersinia* has also been developed.

Clinical manifestations

Infection with *Yersinia* often produces either no symptoms or such a mild disturbance that it often goes unrecognized. Symptomatic infection in young children manifests as fever, abdominal pain, and diarrhea. In teenage children and adults abdominal pain can be prominent enough to mimic a clinical picture consistent with acute appendicitis. At laparotomy an acute terminal ileitis and mesenteric adenitis are usually discovered in these patients. Most infections occur in children under 10 years of age, and the diarrheal illness they manifest is identical to that produced by other enteric pathogens.

In a prospective study of children with acute gastroenteritis, *Y. enterocolitica* was isolated from 2.8 percent, *Salmonella* from 4.4 percent, and *Shigella* from 1.1 percent (46). Illness was mild in the majority of patients, and medical consultation was not obtained until after the diarrhea had been present for almost a week (median 8 days and range 2 to 43 days). The symptoms most frequently noted were diarrhea (98 percent), fever (68 percent), abdominal pain (64.5 percent), and vomiting (38.5 percent). The diarrhea was characterized by five to ten greenish but not malodorous stools of variable consistency during the first week of the illness. The mean duration of the diarrhea was 14 days (range 1 to 46 days). Blood was noted in the stools of 26 percent of the patients. Abdominal pain was cramping and persistent, although usually relieved by defecation. This symptom was continual for a median of 7.7 days with a range of 2 to 28 days. In some of the older patients, the pain localized to the right lower quadrant, and one patient had an appendectomy. The fever lasted a mean of 4 days; the vomiting, 2.4 days. Only 4 percent of the patients had to be admitted for dehydration, bloody stools, or prolonged diarrhea. The stools remained positive for Yersinia from 4 to 79 days (mean 27 days) after the resolution of symptoms. In adults, the most frequent symptoms noted were abdominal pain (84 percent), diarrhea (78 percent), fever (43 percent), anorexia (22 percent), nausea (13 percent), and vomiting (8 percent) (49). About 2.5 percent of adult patients developed accompanying erythema nodosum or arthritis. These complications were not seen in children. The abdominal pain was localized in the right iliac fossae in 40 percent of the patients, was diffuse in 24 percent of the patients, and periumbilical in 8 percent. Epigastric and hypogastric pain were infrequent. The pain was usually described as colicky. The symptoms were usually present for 1 to 2 weeks before the diagnosis was established. In five cases the symptoms were present for several months before the diagnosis was established. Endoscopic evaluation demonstrated changes consistent with acute colitis in several of the patients, and two were found to have mucosal ulcers. Radiologic evaluation of the bowel revealed involvement of the terminal 10 to 20 cm of the ileum in 88 percent of the patients. Several different radiological patterns were observed and correlated with the stage of the illness (50). During the first 10 to 14 days thickening of the bowel wall, presence of large nodules (up to 1 cm in diameter), and narrowing of the lumen were observed. The nodules decreased in size during the second and third weeks with coincidental improvement in the bowel wall. During the fourth and fifth weeks, a diffuse edematous stage with loss of mucosal folds was noted. Finally, during the fifth through eighth weeks after the onset of the symptoms, the valvulae conniventes started to reappear but were distorted. Some small nodules and edema were still present at this stage. The abnormalities finally disappeared altogether after 10 weeks.

The pathological findings in patients found to have acute terminal ileitis at laparotomy are unique to Yersinia infection. Mesenteric adenopathy is present, and the nodes may be matted together, suggesting a mass. The terminal ileum is usually thickened and inflamed for a variable distance. The operative appearance may be identical to that of Crohn's disease, but there is no documented cultural or serological evidence to date implicating Yersinia in the pathogenesis of Crohn's disease (51). Lymph node biopsies should be obtained for histological evaluation and culture in patients with a history compatible with yersiniosis; an ileal biopsy is not necessary and will only enhance the opportunity of complications (52). The histological examination of a lymph node fails to reveal microabscesses, which are often found in patients infected with Y. pseudotuberculosis (31).

A variety of extraintestinal manifestations accompany the enteric infection of Y. enterocolitica, including nonsupurative arthritis or arthralgia, erythema nodosum, uveitis, Reiter's syndrome, carditis, thyroiditis, ophthalmitis, acute glomerulonephritis, hepatitis, pancreatitis, and hemolytic anemia (31). Since the enteric infection may be mild or asymptomatic, patients may present with any of the above manifestations as primary problems. One case of persistent fever due to Yersinia infection has been reported (53). Infection with Yersinia has been documented in seven patients with recent onset of sarcoidosis (54).

Many patients with thyroid disease have been found to have antibodies to Y.

enterocolitica (55). There is evidence of specific increased cellular immune activity initiated by *Yersinia* in patients with thyroid disease (56). What role these organisms have in the pathogenesis of thyroid disease is unclear at present.

The arthritis is an oligoarthritis that usually involves the knees, ankles, and wrists and produces very painful, swollen, and warm joints accompanied by an elevated erythrocyte sedimentation rate, C-reactive protein, and white blood cell count (57). The serum protein electrophoresis pattern is also abnormal. The arthritis usually persists for 4 to 6 months but in some patients may become chronic (58). Several patients who were positive for HLA-B27 have developed ankylosing spondylitis or Reiter's syndrome (59). *Yersinia* infection may also present with a syndrome which is indistinguishable from acute rheumatic fever (60). *Y. enterocolitica* has been suggested as an etiologic agent for that entity. Although patients with acute *Yersinia* infection have changes consistent with carditis, the relatively recent association of the organism with this disease entity does not permit adequate follow-up to determine whether valvular damage will result (58).

In cases of septicemia, the opportunity to develop metastatic foci is present, and the following have been noted: hepatic and intraabdominal abscesses, septic arthritis, osteomyelitis, meningitis, peritonitis, and lung abscess. An erysipelas-like skin disease and furuncles have been reported and may represent primary inoculation in the skin or be spread via the bloodstream from an enteric source.

Almost all patients who presented with *Y. enterocolitica* septicemia have had some underlying disease, particularly cirrhosis (31). Their presenting symptoms were fever, headache, malaise, abdominal pain, nausea, and vomiting. The mortality in these patients was about 50 percent. Those with cirrhosis had a greatly increased mortality, and with hemachromatosis the outcome is universally fatal. Laboratory studies with mice have demonstrated increased pathogenicity of *Y. enterocolitica* in the presence of increased iron. The healthy liver seems to play a critical role in the resistance of the host to *Y. enterocolitica* infection.

Pathogenicity

Study of the pathogenesis of *Yersinia* infections has been hampered by the lack of a suitable animal model. Current investigations use mice, rabbits, and monkeys, in which mesenteric adenitis as well as diarrheal disease can be produced. The mechanisms implicated in the production of human diarrhea may well be related to the toxogenicity as well as invasive characteristics of the organism.

The enterotoxin is heat-stable and similar to that produced by *E. coli* (61). It has given positive results in both the infant mouse and the rabbit ileal loop assay. The enterotoxin is produced by many strains, but its production is much more prevalent in strains which are pathogenic for humans. Only 10 percent of the largely nonpathogenic rhamnose-positive strains produced enterotoxin. The toxin is produced in significant quantities only at 25°C (62). This would suggest that patients who developed diarrhea must ingest a sufficient dose of preformed enterotoxin or that the diarrhea is mediated by other processes initiated by *Yersinia*.

Invasiveness has been clearly demonstrated in HeLa cells, HEp-2 cells, peritoneal macrophages, and rabbit ileal loop inoculation (62). Only strains which are pathogenic for human beings, namely O3, O5B, O8, and O9, were shown to invade HeLa cells. The organisms not only penetrate cells but multiply within them, including macrophages. The injection of 10^8 organisms into the duodenal lumen of rabbits revealed that the virulent strains rapidly penetrated the epithelial cells of the intestinal mucosa and migrated into the lamina propria (63). The avirulent strains did not penetrate and were rapidly excreted from the intestine without producing any symptoms. The organisms that penetrated to the lamina propria were able to reach the regional lymph nodes, apparently by carriage in phagocytes, but were not killed as they continued to multiply. The accumulation of mononuclear phagocytes resulted in granuloma formation. The rapid multiplication within the cells produced necrobiotic changes in the central areas of the granulomata, which became hemorrhagic and ulcerated. These inflammatory changes in the gut wall and perhaps elsewhere could contribute to the diarrheal state by releasing mediators to stimulate fluid secretion (21). Furthermore, these findings would also explain the colitis sometimes seen in patients with this infection.

Immunization with heat-killed *Yersinia* was shown to produce an effective immune response to subsequent intravenous challenge (64). The challenge dose was quickly cleared in the immunized mice, and no *Yersinia* were detectable in the liver or spleen 24 h after a challenge. It was demonstrated that the immune serum enhanced opsonization, resulting in effective phagocytosis and clearing of the *Yersinia* by the reticuloendothelial system.

Epidemiology

Y. enterocolitica has been isolated from many locations throughout the world (65). The isolates have been from people and a variety of domestic and wild animals. The mammals from which they have most frequently been isolated include swine, cattle, goats, sheep, horses, dogs, cats, rabbits, hares, chinchillas, deer, and elk. They have been isolated from a variety of birds, including chickens. Rodents, including household rats, have also been noted to be infected. Isolations from oysters and some freshwater fish have similarly been reported. They have been found in surface and well waters, lakes and streams, and drinking water. Some of the foods that have been found to be contaminated are meat (fresh and vacuum-packed), milk, cheese, ice cream, mussels, and oysters (65–67).

The oral route is the predominant portal of entry in human beings. Several outbreaks related to a common infected food source or water supply have been reported (65, 68). Person-to-person spread has been suggested by an intrafamilial outbreak and two reports of outbreaks in hospitals (69, 70). In one of the hospital outbreaks an incubation period of 10 days was noted (71). Spread to others in the family occurred in 47 percent of the cases in a recent prospective study of *Y. enterocolitica*–related gastroenteritis (46). Data on the infectious dose requirements for inducing disease in human subjects are meager. One experiment involving a volunteer indicated that a large dose of organisms (3.5×10^9) was required to produce infection (72). The ability of the organism to multiply at room temperature, to survive for long periods (18 months) at 4°C in distilled water or on meat, and to grow in tap water suggests that *Yersinia* can be ubiquitous (42). Once an environment is contaminated, persistence of *Yersinia* is likely.

The ability of *Yersinia* to grow at low temperatures also makes it an important source of food contamination; 10^2 to 10^3 organisms per gram were found in 3.8 percent of vegetables sampled (65). The incidence of infected swine may be as great as 8 percent (73). In a sampling of 300 pork samples, 1.3 percent were found to be contaminated with Y. *enterocolitica*, as were 4 percent of 150 ham slices (74). Large increases in the number of organisms in raw or cooked beef and pork occurred when the meat was stored at 7°C for 10 days or at 25°C for 24 h (75). Peak seasonal incidence of yersiniosis during the summer and winter months in some European countries coincides with the domestic slaughtering of pigs for festive occasions.

Only a few of the 34 O and 19 H serotypes have been shown to be pathogenic for human beings. The localization of specific serotypes to various areas of the world and not elsewhere is an epidemiological fact which has not been explained. In Europe types O3 and O9 are primarily implicated; in the United States a wide variety have been identified but most commonly type O8, a unique American pathogen. The organisms found in eastern Canada are type O3 (not type O8, found in nearby New York State). Serotype O3 is also found in Japan and South Africa. The O3 strains in Canada are a different phage type from those in Europe. In Europe the pig harbors the same strain of Y. *enterocolitica* which is usually isolated from infected patients. The strain is serotype O3, biotype 4, and bacteriophage type 8.

The incidence of *Yersinia* infection in patients with acute enterocolitis ranges from 2.0 to 5 percent. Prospective determinations of recorded incidences are New York State 2.3 percent, Canada 2.8 percent, Belgium 4.6 percent, and Germany 5 percent. In Sweden 2.5 percent of asymptomatic persons have significant Y. *enterocolitica* antibody titers. Screening 4411 German patients for antibodies against Y. *enterocolitica* and Y. *pseudotuberculosis* revealed significant titers in 6.71 and 4.58 percent, respectively (76).

Treatment and control

The infection is usually mild and self-limited and requires only symptomatic treatment. Whether antibiotics will shorten the diarrheal illness remains to be proved. In patients with extraintestinal disease or septicemia, the use of antibiotics seems appropriate. The organisms have been shown to be sensitive in vitro to gentamicin, chloramphenicol, tetracycline, and trimethoprim-sulfamethoxazole. They are resistant to penicillin and cephalothin due to the production of a β-lactamase. Their sensitivity to erythromycin is variable (Table 3).

Table 3 Antibiotic sensitivities

	Yersinia	Campylobacter	Vibrio parahaemolyticus
Penicillin	R	R	R
Ampicillin	V	I	R
Carbenicillin	I	S	I
Cephalothin	R	R	S
Tetracycline	S	S	S
Erythromycin	V	S*	V
Chloramphenicol	S	S	S
Clindamycin	R	S	I
Gentamicin	S	S	S
Kanamycin	S	S	I
Sulfa	S		V
TMP-SMZ†	S	I	
Metronidazole		S	

* Variable sensitivity (some resistant strains).
† Trimethoprim-sulfamethoxazole.
NOTE: S = sensitive, I = intermediate, V = variable, R = resistant.

Because of the likelihood of person-to-person spread by a fecal to oral route, hand-washing and stool-isolation precautions should be enforced. Since small numbers of *Yersinia* continue to be excreted in the stools for 3 to 4 weeks after the resolution of symptoms, continued awareness of possible contamination should be stressed to the responsible family member to prevent intrafamilial spread.

Summary

Y. enterocolitica is a recently recognized enteric pathogen that has an important role in human disease. Its unique growth characteristics make it not only difficult to isolate but also a potential major cause of food poisoning. Prospective studies and serologic surveys indicate that its incidence is similar to that of salmonella and shigella and only somewhat less than that of *Campylobacter*. It should be considered and looked for in any young person with acute enterocolitis and in adults with acute or subacute abdominal pain and evidence of infection. Stool cultures should be obtained, and if a laparotomy is performed, the mesenteric lymph nodes should be biopsied and cultured. *Y. enterocolitica* infection should also be considered in the differential diagnosis of patients presenting with other illnesses such as fever of undetermined origin, acute rheumatic fever, arthritis, Reiter's syndrome, uveitis, erythema nodosum, thyroiditis, and perhaps sarcoidosis.

DIARRHEAL DISEASE ASSOCIATED WITH VIBRIO PARAHAEMOLYTICUS

V. parahaemolyticus is a relatively recently discovered halophilic vibrio known to be a major cause of acute gastroenteritis in persons living in or visiting coastal areas. Illness with this organism has been related to exposure to seawater and the consumption of raw or improperly prepared seafoods.

Historical background

In Japan it is customary to eat uncooked seafood and shellfish. In 1950 an outbreak of food poisoning occurred in Osaka that was related to consumption of *shirasuboshi* (semidried young sardines); 272 persons became ill, 20 of them fatally. Fujino isolated a bacterium, which he named *Pasteurella parahaemolytica*, from the stools of patients and the intestinal contents obtained at autopsy (77). Several other outbreaks of gastroenteritis attributable to this organism were reported in the 1950s and early 1960s. In 1963 Sakazaki and his associates recognized the organism to be a vibrio and published the first definitive description of the morphological characteristics, growth requirements, biochemical properties, and taxonomy of this new organism which they named V. parahaemolyticus (78). Further epidemiological investigations established that V. parahaemolyticus was the leading cause of foodborne gastroenteritis in Japan.

Subsequently, the organism was found to be indigenous to coastal and estuarial waters throughout the world (79). The first isolation of V. parahaemolyticus in the United States was from sediment of the Puget Sound in Washington State in 1967 (80). Since then, the organism has been isolated from almost all the coastal areas of the United States (81, 82). Since the late 1960s and early 1970s, many outbreaks of acute gastroenteritis related to seafood ingestion have been attributed to V. parahaemolyticus in the United States (79, 83).

Bacteriology

V. parahaemolyticus is a gram-negative, halophilic, motile, facultative anaerobe which has a single polar flagellum. It is lactose-negative and oxidase-positive. The organism grows in 3 percent salt solution, accounting for its isolation in coastal and estuarial seawater. It inhabits the sediments during the cold winter months; as the water temperature rises during the spring, the bacteria leave the sediment and populate the water above (84). A direct correlation between the ambient water temperature and the abundance of the organism has been demonstrated. During the warmer months, marine life is colonized and V. parahaemolyticus has been recovered from a variety of seafoods, particularly crustaceans (81).

Since the organism is halophilic, it will not grow on the usual enteric isolation media. On media selective for vibrios, round, smooth colonies 3 to 5 mm in diameter with green and blue centers appear. Generation time is rapid (10 min). Usually the organism can readily be recognized by its morphology, motility, and biochemical characteristics (84). Serotyping has been done, but it is not a routine procedure. All strains share a serologically identical H flagellar antigen. Eleven O and fifty-two K cell wall antigen types have been recognized, but they are not entirely specific since other marine vibrios agglutinate in the presence of V. *parahaemolyticus* anti-O and anti-K antisera (79, 81).

In 1963 Sakazaki divided the species into two subgroups based on biochemical and growth characteristics (78). Subgroup 1 was felt to be pathogenic, whereas subgroup 2 was avirulent. The subgroup 2 organisms have since been designated as a separate species and given the name V. *alginolyticus*. They do not cause gastroenteritis but have been associated with wound infections and otitis. The large majority of isolates from coastal waters belonged to subgroup 2, whereas almost all isolates from persons with acute gastroenteritis belonged to subgroup 1. In 1968, hemolysin production by subgroup 1 organisms was described (85). Investigators at the Kanagawa Prefectural Public Health Laboratory in Yokohama noted that pathogenic strains exhibited hemolysis in media containing human blood. Since then it has been demonstrated that the *Kanagawa phenomenon* correlated with the pathogenicity of a given strain of V. *parahaemolyticus*. In one series in Japan, 96 percent of 2720 isolates from patients with gastroenteritis were Kanagawa-positive, while only 1 percent of 650 isolates from seawater and seafood were Kanagawa-positive (86). None of the 15 volunteers given 10^9 organisms that were Kanagawa-negative became ill (86).

Clinical features

Infection with V. *parahaemolyticus* usually produces a gastroenteritis which is self-limited. Occasionally severe or prolonged illness will require hospitalization. Extraintestinal disease definitely related to V. *parahaemolyticus* has not been described. Several cases of septicemia and/or wound infections have been reported but have since been shown to be related to V. *alginolyticus* or a related vibrio, the lactose-positive vibrio.

The gastroenteritis has an incubation period of 10 to 20 h, but it can vary between 2 and 48 h. This variation depends upon the number of organisms ingested, the nature of the food, and the acidity of the stomach (87). The severity of the subsequent illness is probably also related to these factors, as it has been shown that a much more toxic illness resulted in volunteers who ingested quantitatively more organisms (88). The manifestations of the gastroenteritis are as follows: an explosive watery diarrhea (98 percent), cramping abdominal pain (82 percent), nausea (71 percent), vomiting (52 percent), headache (42 percent), fever (27 percent), and chills (24 percent) (79). When present, the fever rarely exceeded 102°F (89). The diarrhea can be profuse, and about 15 stools during the first 24 h is common (89). However, hypotension due to fluid loss is uncommon (89). A striking leukocytosis of 20,000 cells per cubic millimeter is often seen. Blood and mucus are frequently observed in stained smears of stool. Sigmoidoscopy has demonstrated small superficial mucosal ulcerations in one patient (89). The disease as a rule is self-limited; as in cholera, the organisms are excreted in large numbers during the acute illness, but the number falls off rapidly as clinical recovery becomes manifest. Therefore, the stools should be examined as soon as possible. The duration of the illness can vary between 2 and 10 days, but most patients are improved or their symptoms resolve completely in 2 to 3 days (79). Fatigue will usually persist for several days.

Pathogenesis

V. *parahaemolyticus*, like *Campylobacter, Yersinia, Shigella*, and invasive *E. coli*, can produce watery diarrhea and/or a dysentery syndrome. Since most strains that induce large volume liquid stools can be shown to produce enterotoxins, much effort has been expended in attempting to identify similar enterotoxins from V. *parahaemolyticus*. Initially, the enterotoxogenic activity of the hemolysins were extensively studied (86). These hemolysins have been shown to have cardiac toxicity in mice and to be cytotoxic in certain tissue culture cell lines (90). Early results indicated that purified, concentrated (by freeze-drying) hemolysins caused fluid accumulation in the animal model systems (91). Further investigations demonstrated that these results were not due to postulated enterotoxin activity but that the fluid secretion was secondary to the high saline content of the resuspended freeze-dried hemolysin (92). In those animal systems an osmotic effect on fluid and electrolyte movement was precipitated by an intraluminal salt concentration of 3 to 5 percent and greater. Better controlled experiments subsequently demonstrated a correlation between some Kanagawa-positive strains and a positive reaction in a rabbit ileal loop system (93). This toxic factor could account in part for the fluid production in patients, but no direct human data on this point are available.

The colitis that occurs in patients infected with V. *parahaemolyticus* may be a consequence of the invasive capabilities of this organism (91). In infected rabbits, rapid epithelial cell penetration occurs, resulting in bacteremia; fluorescent antibody studies have identified penetration of the vibrios into the lamina propria similar to the localization of salmonella in the same region of experimental animals (94). Inflammation is a consequence of this invasive process. These cells may be responsible for the febrile reaction of the host as well as contributing prostaglandins which could promote fluid secretion (21). In human beings the presence of sheets of white cells in methylene blue–stained stool smears attests to the colitis established in the distal colon by V. *parahaemolyticus*. In most cases of human disease these findings are attributed to the Kanagawa-positive strains. In the experimental animal, some Kanagawa-negative strains elicit similar findings. Whether these latter strains have unique toxins rather than hemolysins or use other mechanisms to invade cells is unknown. It is important to study these strains further because they may account for 3.5 to 11 percent of isolates from human patients suffering from vibrio gastroenteritis (86).

Epidemiology

V. *parahaemolyticus* has been found in coastal waters throughout the world. The bulk of the epidemiological data comes from Japan, where the incidence of food poisoning is highest because of the custom of eating raw seafood. However, isolated outbreaks have been investigated and reported elsewhere in the world, including the United States.

As noted previously, not all strains are pathogenic. Classification in subgroup 1 or demonstration of the Kanagawa phenomenon has been shown to correlate with pathogenicity. Either Kanagawa-positive or subgroup 1 strains are found in a high proportion of patients with acute enteritis during the summer months in Japan. Since they can account for up to 70 percent of the foodborne illness during the months of June to October, the term *Japanese summer diarrhea* was coined. The organism is not isolated during other months of the year.

One of the popular foods in Japan is *sushi*, made of cooked rice, raw fish, and shellfish. One study examined the food materials and utensils of 50 randomly selected sushi cooks in Tokyo (95). V. *parahaemolyticus* was never isolated from any of the specimens during the winter, but in summer it was isolated from 88.6 percent of the food and 82.3 percent of the utensils. Significantly though, 86 percent of the strains isolated belonged to nonpathogenic subgroup 2. During the summer 2000 healthy hotel workers were examined (95), and 0.8 percent were found to have V. *parahaemolyticus* in their stools, two-thirds of the strains isolated belonging to subgroup 2. The following January, 1000 of these same workers were examined, and all their stools were negative for V. *parahaemolyticus*. Additionally, 200 symptom-free sushi cooks were examined during the summer (95); 7 percent had V. *parahaemolyticus* in their stools, and again about two-thirds of the strains isolated belonged to subgroup 2. The isolation rate in the cooks was about nine times that of the hotel employees. When the same 200 cooks were examined again the following February, all stools were negative.

In the United States and other parts of the world, many outbreaks of acute gastroenteritis related to eating seafood, particularly shellfish, have been reported. Several occurred on cruise ships or airplanes, where detailed epidemiologic investigations were permitted (87, 96). In most cases the outbreaks could be attributed to improper handling of food. Usually it was demonstrated that the food had been cross-contaminated by the same cooks handling both raw and cooked food. The cooked food had been replaced in the same container in which raw food had been shipped or the raw and cooked food had been placed together in the same storage areas or refrigerators. Inadequate refrigeration or leaving the food at room temperatures too long was also implicated. In one of the cruise ships, washing down the galley with seawater apparently caused the contamination of surfaces where food was prepared (96).

The organism is sensitive to heat and disinfection. It will not survive heating for 15 min at 60°C (97). Refrigeration at 4°C and freezing at −20°C were both shown to be sublethal. When crabs were inoculated with 0.1 ml of a broth culture and then boiled in water for 5 min, V. *parahaemolyticus* was subsequently recovered from the center flesh, claws, meat, and inside surface of the shells (87), but adequate cooking will sterilize most other seafood. The organism's generation time of 10 min can permit it to grow rapidly at room temperatures. If left out in the open or poorly refrigerated, contaminated food may develop enough organisms to induce disease. Such food appears normal and has no unusual taste. Raw food that has been refrigerated or frozen should not be allowed to stand at room temperature for long periods before consumption. Scrupulous care must be given to avoid cross contamination. Food should never be put back into the original delivery container once cooked, and those handling the raw food should not touch the cooked food.

If outbreaks do occur, all potential food sources should be cultured. Special enrichment techniques are available that allow recovery of the bacteria from refrigerated or frozen food (98).

Summary of epidemiological features of *V. parahaemolyticus* infections

1 V. *parahaemolyticus* is not found in food or people during the cold months of the year. It achieves infectious levels only between June and October in temperate climates. In warmer climates, the incidence may be more constant throughout the year.

2 More than 80 percent of seafood, particularly shellfish, will be contaminated with V. *parahaemolyticus* during the summer months. The utensils used to prepare the food are also similarly contaminated.

3 In spite of the high prevalence of V. *parahaemolyticus* in the food supply, only about 14 percent of the strains are pathogenic, and the occurrence and severity of acute gastroenteritis due to food poisoning depends upon the dose of pathogenic organisms ingested.

4 Healthy subjects who eat seafood during the summer may transiently have non-pathogenic V. *parahaemolyticus* as part of their intestinal flora. A small number of subjects will be colonized with apparently pathogenic strains and yet remain healthy.

5 There is no chronic carrier state. As soon as a person stops ingesting contaminated food, the stools clear. No subject in Japan has been found to have V. *parahaemolyticus* in the stool during the winter.

6 No secondary cases or person-to-person transmission has been documented.

7 The organisms multiply rapidly, and infected raw food can quickly contaminate containers, utensils, or food handlers. Infection in cooked foods is due to cross contamination.

Treatment

Because the illness is usually self-limited, treatment with antibiotics is seldom warranted. Symptomatic treatment and maintaining fluid balance are the usual therapeutic measures. One study demonstrated that patients treated with chloramphenicol, tetracycline, or kanamycin cleared their stools in 5 days, as opposed to 15 days in those not treated (84). However, no mention of the clinical response was noted in that study. Occasionally it will be necessary to treat with antibiotics. The organism has been uniformly sensitive to gentamicin and chloramphenicol (Table 3). It also responds well to tetracycline. It is resistent to penicillin and ampicillin and variably sensitive to erythromycin and cephalosporins.

Summary

V. *parahaemolyticus* is an organism that has a worldwide distribution and is a major cause of foodborne acute gastroenteritis in coastal areas or isolated outbreaks elsewhere related to eating seafood. Person-to-person transmission and secondary cases have not been reported. Because of the decreased numbers of the organism in coastal waters during the colder months, the seafood-borne illness that is produced is seen only between June and October in temperate climates. Only a small percentage of the strains are pathogenic, and there is good correlation between a hemolytic activity known as the Kanagawa phenomenon and the pathogenicity of a particular strain. The acute gastroenteritis that is produced is usually self-limited, and mortality is very rare.

DIARRHEAL DISEASE ASSOCIATED WITH MISCELLANEOUS *VIBRIO* SPECIES

Noncholera vibrios

In addition to the classical V. *cholerae* and El Tor V. *cholerae*, another group of organisms is serologically distinct from V. *cholerae* but still included in the taxonomic group V. *cholerae*. These organisms are commonly referred to either by the misnomer *nonagglutinating vibrios* (NAGs) or the confusing term *noncholera vibrios* (NCVs).

Although these organisms have been associated with isolated cases as well as outbreaks of diarrheal illness, the duration of the diarrhea and the volume of fluid excreted rarely approach those seen with classical V. *cholerae* infection. Furthermore, in contrast to classic cholera, they have also been associated with infections outside the GI tract, and leukocytes have been noted in the stools of some of these patients. Thus, they appear to produce disease by different pathogenic processes.

They have rarely caused infection in the United States but are isolated with a greater frequency than V. *cholerae*. In the 3-year period between 1972 and 1975, 26 cases referred to the CDC in Atlanta were analyzed (99). Thirteen of these (50 percent) had NCV isolated from their stools and had an acute illness characterized by diarrhea, abdominal cramps, nausea, and vomiting. Four (15 percent) had NCV isolated from the biliary or other upper gastrointestinal sites. In none of these patients was there an acute illness that could be attributed to the presence of NCVs. Nine (35 percent) had NCV isolated from body tissues or fluid at other sites. Four of these patients died. All who died were over 50 years old and had other underlying illnesses.

Of the 26 patients, 19 lived in the coastal states (99). Many of those patients with acute diarrhea had a history of recent shellfish ingestion or foreign travel. Some of those with systemic infection due to NCV had a history of recent occupational or recreational exposure to salt water. It is of significance to note that NCVs have been isolated from coastal waters, for example, Chesapeake Bay (81), when sought.

Asymptomatic intestinal infection has been reported, and, as noted above, these organisms have been isolated from the biliary tract. An asymptomatic carrier state is likely to exist.

In studies of their pathogenicity, some strains have been shown to produce an enterotoxin which is identical to that produced by V. *cholerae*. However, in rabbit ileal loops most strains produce less fluid accumulation than the classical cholera agent (100). Other experiments have shown them to have both toxic and invasive properties.

The nomenclature and taxonomy of these organisms are perplexing problems. They are identical to V. *cholerae* in every way except that they do not agglutinate with O group I antiserum and, as noted previously, produce different clinical syndromes. They share the same DNA content and H antigens and produce the same proteases and alkaline phosphatases. The distinction between them is further confused by the fact that agglutinable strains of V. *cholerae* have been shown to lose the group I antigen entirely and NCVs have been reported to gain the ability to agglutinate with group I antiserum (101).

Nonagglutinating vibrios is a misnomer because they do agglutinate in homologous antiserum. Noncholera vibrios is confusing because of the other pathogenic vibrios discussed elsewhere in this paper; the term is not specific.

In 1972 the International Committee on Systemic Bacteriology Subcommittee on Taxonomy of Vibrios met and decided to use the designation V. *cholerae* for both the agglutinating and nonagglutinating strains. This was taxonomically correct for the reasons mentioned previously but created a real problem for those who have to deal with quarantine for cholera disease. As previously noted, the nonagglutinating cholera vibrios produce a clinical syndrome that is usually less severe than that of the classical V. *cholerae*. They have also been found in significant numbers in coastal waters whereas V. *cholerae* has not. To institute the same public health measures for both would be unwarranted (101).

There are several ways to deal with the present problem in nomenclature. The simplest would be to amend the sanitary regulations to apply only to those isolations of V. *cholerae* associated with strains that do agglutinate in type I antisera. Another possibility would be to give the nonagglutinating V. *cholerae* strains their own species name. V. *enteritidis* has been proposed for this purpose.

In summary, not all isolates that are reported as V. *cholerae* are classical V. *cholerae*, and some may be associated with quite different clinical syndromes. They may assume a role of greater clinical importance in the future as the number of immunosuppressed patients grows. Their nomenclature may also change in the next few years as their distribution in nature and clinical effects become better known.

Vibrio cholerae

The classic strain of V. *cholera* has been isolated from a patient with severe diarrhea in Texas and from patients and water samples in Louisiana. These recent isolations of an organism that has not been isolated for several decades in the United States is an unexplained epidemiological surprise. Of great interest is the phage typing results of these isolates. Type 17, Maidstone classification, was found; it is unique in the United States, not having been identified as yet in any other country. It is unlikely that cholera will spread and become a public health hazard in the United States, but the physician faced with the treatment of a patient with unexpected cholera disease should have no trouble if he applies the basic premise needed for all diarrheal states. The replacement of fluid and electrolyte losses is the key to successful therapy.

Other halophilic vibrios

The efforts to isolate pathogenic vibrios from salt water have identified other organisms which are pathogenic for human beings but do not appear to cause diarrheal diseases. The first is the lactose-positive vibrio (102), sometimes called V. *vulnificus* (103). This organism has been shown to cause severe life-threatening human septicemic disease. It seems to select debilitated individuals and can cause rapid death. V. *alginolyticus*, which is biologically similar to V. *parahaemolyticus* and V. *vulnificus* (104), rarely infects man. The usual manifestations are skin ulcers, cellulitis, and otitis. Other vibrios have been identified from these same sources, but their importance as human pathogens is unknown.

REFERENCES

1 **Smith T:** Spirilla associated with disease of the fetal membranes in cattle. *J Exp Med* 28:701, 1918.

2 **Curtis AH:** A motile curved anaerobic bacillus in uterine discharges. *J Infect Dis* 12:165, 1913.

3 **Levy AJ:** A gastroenteritis outbreak probably due to a bovine strain of vibrio. *Yale J Biol Med* 18:243, 1946.

4 **King EO:** Human infections with *Vibrio fetus* and a closely related vibrio. *J Infect Dis* 101:119, 1957.

5 **Sebald M, Vernon M:** Teneur en bases de l'ADN et classification des vibrions. *Ann Inst Pasteur Lille* 105:897, 1963.

6 **Smibert RM:** The genus *Campylobacter*. *Ann Rev Microbiol* 32:673, 1978.

7 **Veron M, Chatelain R:** Taxonomic study of the genus *Campylobacter*. *Int J Sys Bacteriol* 23:122, 1973.

8 **Butzler JP et al:** Related vibrio in stools. *J Pediatr* 82:493, 1973.

9 **Cooper IA, Slee KJ:** Human infection by *Vibrio fetus*. *Med J Aust* 1:1263, 1971.

10 **Dekeyser P et al:** Acute enteritis due to related vibrio: First positive stool cultures. *J Infect Dis* 125:390, 1972.

11 **Skirrow MB:** *Campylobacter* enteritis: A "new" disease. *Br Med J* 2:9–11, 1977.

12 **Cadranel S et al:** Enteritis due to "related vibrio" in children. *Am J Dis Child* 126:152, 1973.

13 **Rettig PJ:** *Campylobacter* infections in human beings. *J Pediatr* 94:855, 1979.

14 **Blaser MJ et al:** *Campylobacter* enteritis: Clinical and epidemiological features. *Ann Intern Med* 91:179, 1979.

15 **Lambert ME et al:** *Campylobacter* colitis. *Br Med J* 1:857, 1979.

16 **Blaser MJ et al:** Acute colitis caused by *Campylobacter fetus s.s. jejuni*. *Gastroenterology* 78:448, 1980.

17 **Butzler JP, Skirrow MB:** *Campylobacter* enteritis. *Clin Gastroenterol* 8:737, 1979.

18 **McCoy EC et al:** Superficial antigens of *Campylobacter* (*Vibrio*) *fetus*: Characterization of an antiphagocytic component. *Infect Immun* 11:517, 1975.

19 Winter AJ, Caveney NT: Evaluation of a transport medium for *Campylobacter* (*Vibrio*) *fetus*. *J Am Vet Med Assoc* 173:472, 1978.

20 Guerrant RL et al: Campylobacteriosis in man: Pathogenic mechanisms and review of 91 bloodstream infections. *Am J Med* 65:584, 1978.

21 Gots RE et al: Indomethacin inhibition of *Salmonella typhimurium*, *Shigella flexneri* and cholera-mediated rabbit ileal secretion. *J Infect Dis* 130:280, 1974.

22 Bokkenheuser VD et al: Detection of enteric campylobacteriosis in children. *J Clin Microbiol* 9:227, 1979.

23 Taylor P et al: *Campylobacter fetus* infection in human subjects: Association with raw milk. *Am J Med* 66:779, 1979.

24 Blaser MJ et al: *Campylobacter enteritis* associated with canine infection. *Lancet* 2:979, 1978.

25 Waterborne *Campylobacter gastroenteritis*—Vermont. MMWR 27:207, 1978.

26 Knill M et al: Environmental isolation of heat-tolerant *Campylobacter* in the Southhampton area. *Lancet* 2(8097):1002, 1978.

27 Steele TW, McDermott S: *Campylobacter enteritis* in South Australia. *Med J Aust* 2:404, 1978.

28 Dupont HL, Hornick RB: Clinical approach to infectious diarrhea. *Medicine* 52:265, 1973.

29 Vanhoof R et al: Susceptibility of *Campylobacter fetus subsp. jejuni* to twenty-nine antimicrobial agents. *Antimicrob Agents Chemother* 14:553, 1978.

30 Walder M, Forsgren A: Erythromycin resistant campylobacters. *Lancet* 2:1201, 1978.

31 Bottone EJ: *Yersinia enterocolitica*: A panoramic view of a charismatic microorganism. *CRC Crit Rev Microbiol* Jan 1977, p 211.

32 Kohl S: *Yersinia enterocolitica* infections in children. *Ped Clin N Am* 26:433, 1979.

33 van Loghim JJ: The classification of the plague bacillus. *Antonie van Leeuwenhoek* 10:15, 1944.

34 Masshoff W: Eine neuartige Form der mesenterialen Lymphadenitis. *Dtsch Med Wochenschr* 78:532, 1953.

35 Knapp W, Masshoff W: Zür Aetiologie der abszerdierenden Retikulo zvtaren Lymphadenitis. *Dtsch Med Wochenschr* 79:1266, 1954.

36 Schleifstein JI, Coleman MB: An unidentified microorganism resembling *B. lignieri* and *Pasteurella pseudotuberculosis* and pathologic for man. *NY State J Med* 39:1749, 1939.

37 Schleifstein JI, Coleman MB: *Bacterium enterocoliticum*. *Div Lab Res, NY State Dept Health, Annal Rep* Albany, 1943, p 56.

38 Knapp W, Thal E: Untersuchungen über die kulturell biochemischen serologischen, tierexperimentallen und immunologischen Eigenschaften einer vorlaufig "Pasteurella X" benannten Bakterienart. *Zentralbl Bakteriol Orig A* 190:472, 1963.

39 Fredericksen W: A study of some *Yersinia pseudotuberculosis*–like bacteria ("Bacterium enterocoliticum" and "Pasteurella X"). *Proc 14th Scand Congr Pathol Microbiol*, Oslo, Universiteits forlaget Trykningssentral, Oslo, 1964, p 103.

40 Brenner DJ: Speciation in *Yersinia*. *Contr Microbiol Immunol* 5:33, 1979.

41 Eiss J: Selective culturing of *Yersinia enterocolitica* at a low temperature. *Scand J Infect Dis* 7:249, 1975.

42 Highsmith AK et al: *Yersinia enterocolitica*: A review of the bacterium and recommended laboratory methodology. *Health Lab Sci* 14:253, 1977.

43 Weissfeld AS, Sonnenwirth AC: *Yersinia enterocolitica* in adults with gastrointestinal disturbances: Need for cold enrichment. *J Clin Microbiol* 11:196, 1980.

44 Van Nogen R et al: Nonvalue of cold enrichment of stools for isolation of *Yersinia enterocolitica* serotypes 3 and 9 from patients. *J Clin Microbiol* 11:127, 1980.

45 Pai CH et al: Efficacy of cold enrichment techniques for recovery of *Yersinia enterocolitica* from human stools. *J Clin Microbiol* 9:71, 1979.

46 Marks MI et al: *Yersinia enterocolitica* gastroenteritis: A prospective study of clinical bacteriologic and epidemiologic features. *J Pediatr* 96:26, 1980.

47 Bowen JH, Kominos SD: Evaluation of a pectin agar medium for isolating *Yersinia enterocolitica* in 48 hours. *Am J Clin Pathol* 72:586, 1979.

48 Carlsson HE et al: Enzyme-linked immunosorbent assay (ELISA) for titration of antibodies against *Brucella abortus* and *Yersinia enterocolitica*. *Acta Path Microbiol Scand C* 84:168, 1976.

49 Vantrappen G et al: *Yersinia* enteritis and enterocolitis: Gastroenterological aspects. *Gastroenterology* 72:220, 1977.

50 Ekberg O et al: Radiological findings in *Yersinia* ileitis. *Radiology* 123:15, 1977.

51 Persson S et al: Studies on Crohn's disease. *Acta Chir Scand* 142:84, 1976.

52 Gurry JF: Acute terminal ileitis and *Yersinia* infection. *Br Med J* 2:264, 1974.

53 Bliddal J, Kaliszan S: Prolonged monosymptomatic fever due to *Yersinia enterocolitica*. *Acta Med Scand* 210:387, 1977.

54 **Agner E, Larsen JH:** Yersinia enterocolitica infection and sarcoidosis—A report of seven cases. *Scand J Resp Dis* 60:230, 1979.

55 **Shenkman L, Bottone EJ:** Antibodies for *Yersinia enterocolitica* in thyroid disease. *Ann Intern Med* 85:735, 1976.

56 **Bech K et al:** Cell mediated immunity to *Yersinia enterocolitica* serotype 3 in patients with thyroid diseases. *Allergy* 33:82, 1978.

57 **Winblad S:** Arthritis associated with *Yersinia enterocolitica* infections. *Scand J Infect Dis* 7:191, 1975.

58 **Kalliomaki JL, Leino R:** Follow-up studies of joint complications in Yersiniosis. *Acta Med Scand* 205:521, 1979.

59 **Laitinen O et al:** Relation between HLA-B27 and clinical features in patients with Yersinia arthritis. *Arth Rheum* 20(5):1121, 1977.

60 **Laitinen O et al:** Rheumatic fever and *Yersinia* arthritis: Criteria and diagnostic problems in a changing disease pattern. *Scand J Rheum* 4:145, 1975.

61 **Robins-Browne RM et al:** The pathogenesis of *Yersinia enterocolitica* gastroenteritis. *Contr Microbiol Immunol* 5:324, 1979.

62 **Feeley JC et al:** Detection of enterotoxigenic and invasive strains of *Yersinia enterocolitica*. *Contr Microbiol Immunol* 5:329, 1979.

63 **Une T, Zen-Yoji H:** Investigations on the pathogenicity of *Yersinia enterocolitica* by experimental infections in rabbits and cultured cells. *Contr Microbiol Immunol* 5:304, 1979.

64 **Carter PB et al:** Host responses to infection with *Yersinia enterocolitica*. *Contr Microbiol Immunol* 5:346, 1979.

65 **Mollaret HH et al:** Summary of the data received at the WHO Reference Center for *Yersinia enterocolitica*. *Contr Microbiol Immunol* 5:174, 1979.

66 **Morris GK, Feeley JC:** *Yersinia enterocolitica*: A review of its role in food hygiene. *Bull WHO* 54:79, 1976.

67 **Black RE et al:** Epidemic *Yersinia enterocolitica* infection due to contaminated chocolate milk. *N Engl J Med* 298(2):76, 1978.

68 **Eden KV et al:** Waterborne gastrointestinal illness at a ski resort—Isolation of *Yersinia enterocolitica* from drinking water. *Publ Health Rep* 92:245, 1977.

69 **Gutman LT et al:** An interfamilial outbreak of *Yersinia enterocolitica* enteritis. *N Engl J Med* 288:1372, 1973.

70 **Kist M et al:** Ausbreitung einer Yersinia-enterocolitica-Infektion im Krankenhaus. *Dtsch Med Wochenschr* 105:185, 1980.

71 **Toivanen P et al:** Hospital outbreak of *Yersinia enterocolitica* infection. *Lancet* 1:801, 1973.

72 **Szita MI et al:** Incidence of *Yersinia enterocolitica* infection in Hungary. *Contr Microbiol Immunol* 2:106, 1973.

73 **Hurvell B et al:** Isolation of *Yersinia enterocolitica* from swine at an abattoir in Sweden. *Contr Microbiol Immunol* 5:243, 1979.

74 **Asakawa Y et al:** Investigations of source and route of *Yersinia enterocolitica* infection. *Contr Microbiol Immunol* 5:115, 1979.

75 **Hanna MO et al:** Isolation and characteristics of *Yersinia enterocolitica*-like bacteria from meats. *Contr Microbiol Immunol* 5:234, 1979.

76 **Knapp W:** Akute Enteritiden mit "neuen" Erregern. *Munch Med Wochenschr* 121:239, 1979.

77 **Fujino T et al:** On the bacteriological examination of shirasu food poisoning. *Med J Osaka Univ* 4:299, 1953.

78 **Sakazaki R et al:** Studies on the enteropathic, facultatively halophilic bacterium *Vibrio parahaemolyticus*. *Jap J Med Sci Biol* 16:161, 1963.

79 **Dadisman TA Jr et al:** *Vibrio parahaemolyticus* gastroenteritis in Maryland. *Am J Epidemiol* 96:414, 1973.

80 **Baross J, Liston J:** Isolation of *Vibrio parahaemolyticus* from the northwest Pacific. *Nature* 217:1263, 1968.

81 **Colwell RR et al:** *Vibrio cholerae, Vibrio parahaemolyticus* and other vibrios: Occurrence and distribution in Chesapeake Bay. *Science* 198:394, 1977.

82 **VanderZant C et al:** Isolation of *Vibrio parahaemolyticus* from Gulf Coast shrimp. *J Milk Food Technol* 33:161, 1970.

83 **Barker WH Jr:** *Vibrio parahaemolyticus* outbreaks in the United States. *Lancet* 1:551, 1974.

84 **Barker WH Jr, Gangarosa EJ:** Food poisoning due to *Vibrio parahaemolyticus*. *Ann Rev Med* 25:75, 1974.

85 **Miyamoto Y et al:** In vitro hemolytic characteristic of *Vibrio parahaemolyticus*: Its close correlation with human pathogenicity. *J Bacteriol* 100:1147, 1969.

86 **Sakazaki R et al:** Studies on the enteropathic facultatively halophilic bacteria, *Vibrio parahaemolyticus*: III. Enteropathogenicity. *Jap J Med Sci Biol* 21:325, 1968.

87 **Peffers ASR et al:** *Vibrio parahaemolyticus* gastroenteritis and international air travel. *Lancet* 1:143, 1973.

88 **Takikawa I:** Studies on pathogenic halophilic bacteria. *Yokohama Med Bull* 9:313, 1958.

89 **Bolen JL et al:** Clinical features in enteritis

due to *Vibrio parahaemolyticus*. *Am J Med* 57:638, 1974.

90 **Honda T**: Identification of lethal toxin with thermostable direct hemolysin produced by *Vibrio parahaemolyticus*, and some physico-chemical properties of the purified toxins. *Infect Immun* 13:133, 1976.

91 **Sakazaki R et al**: Studies on the enteropathogenic activity of *Vibrio parahaemolyticus* using ligated gut loop models in rabbits. *Jap J Med Sci Biol* 27:35, 1974.

92 **Johnson DE, Calia FM**: False positive rabbit ileal loop reactions attributed to *Vibrio parahaemolyticus* broth filtrates. *J Infect Dis* 133:436, 1976.

93 **Brown DF et al**: Enteropathogenicity of *Vibrio parahaemolyticus* in the ligated rabbit ileum. *Appl Environ Microbiol* 33:10, 1977.

94 **Boutin BK et al**: Demonstration of invasiveness of *Vibrio parahaemolyticus* in adult rabbits by immunofluorescence. *Appl Environ Microbiol* 37:647, 1979.

95 **Zen-Yoji H et al**: Epidemiology, enteropathogenicity and classification of *Vibrio parahaemolyticus*. *J Infect Dis* 115:436, 1965.

96 Gastroenteritis caused by *Vibrio parahaemolyticus* aboard a cruise ship. *MMWR* 27:65, 1978.

97 **Thomas PM, Howell DJ**: *Vibrio parahaemolyticus* gastroenteritis associated with international air travel. *Med J Aust* 2:823, 1976.

98 **Ray B et al**: Method for detection of injured *Vibrio parahaemolyticus* in seafood. *Appl Environ Microbiol* 35:1021, 1978.

99 **Hughes JM et al**: Non-cholera vibrio infections in the United States: Clinical, epidemiologic and laboratory features. *Ann Intern Med* 88:602, 1978.

100 **Carpenter C**: More pathogenic vibrios. *N Engl J Med* 300:39, 1979.

101 **Smith HL**: Serotyping of non-cholera vibrios. *J Clin Microbiol* 10:85, 1979.

102 **Hollis DG et al**: Halophilic vibrio species isolated from blood cultures. *J Clin Microbiol* 3:425, 1976.

103 **Farmer JJ**: *Vibrio ("Beneckea") vulnificus*, the bacterium associated with sepsis, septicemia, and the sea. *Lancet* 2:903, 1979.

104 **Pezzlo M et al**: Wound infections associated with *Vibrio alginolyticus*. *Am J Clin Pathol* 71:476, 1979.

Endocarditis complicating parenteral drug abuse

JOHN N. SHEAGREN

INTRODUCTION

Scope of the problem

Drug use in America The history of parenteral drug use in the United States is a long one. Scattered instances of individuals abusing opiates go back to the nineteenth century, but communitywide drug use, especially in urban areas, has become a problem only during the last several decades (1). Data from the National Institute of Drug Abuse indicate that at the time of World War II drug use became widespread, especially in cities, and the illicit drug industry began to proliferate. Through the 1950s and 1960s with acceleration during the Vietnam War, parenteral drug use increased dramatically. Drug use has always been commonplace among young men in military action; on their return home, continued drug use has been the rule (2).

The traffic in heroin now involves several billion dollars per year. It is estimated that the income of someone smuggling drugs into this country can be as high as several hundred thousand to several million dollars per year. After the dealer cuts and sells the narcotic, individual pushers in cities repackage the product and themselves make several hundred thousand dollars per year (3). The interrelationship between dealers and pushers in the industry is complex and violent, but the financial rewards are enormous. Thus, it seems highly likely that the use of illicit parenteral drugs will continue, if not increase.

Type of parenteral drug use While opiates (especially heroin) are the principal parenteral drugs publicized in the media and the primary source of financial gain to the drug dealer, other types of parenteral drugs are commonly abused. The most commonly used nonopiate drugs are the amphetamines (4). Many

Support provided through Merit Review Funds from the Veterans Administration Research Service.

other types of drugs and substances are prepared and injected in individuals seeking different types of "highs." These run the gamut from paregoric to antihistamines and other types of cold pills to a variety of amphetamine and analgesic tablets.

Methodology of drug preparation and injection   It is important to understand how parenteral drug abusers prepare and inject the substances used. Heroin, the most commonly used substance, is purchased on the street in small packets that are usually wrapped in glassine or aluminum foil. The purchase price of a packet ranges from 10 to 20 dollars based on the ability of the dealer or pusher to convince the purchaser of the quality (purity) of the product. The user may then cut (dilute) the heroin further if he believes that the opiate content is high. To prepare a dose for injection, the powdery material is placed in a screw-off type bottle cap (called a "cooker"), a small amount of an appropriate liquid is added (usually tap water, but saliva or toilet bowl water may be substituted if no clean water is available), and the material is mixed while gently being heated with a match. The user aims to dissolve as much material as possible. The semidissolved mixture is then either drawn directly into a syringe (or eye dropper) or filtered roughly through some cotton, a piece of gauze, or other cloth material before being drawn into the syringe. Preparation of the site to be injected is usually minimal. The injector places a belt or some other tourniquetlike device around the upper arm, clenches the fist until veins appear, and sometimes rubs some saliva on the skin before inserting the needle. The user then enters a small vein with the syringe, draws some blood back into it, and injects the material. The same needle and syringe are often shared by a colleague. Often, at the end of the injection, more blood is drawn back into the syringe and is reinjected in order to "wash out" residual drug. The syringe, needle, and bottle cap are then rinsed with tap water, wrapped in a handkerchief or placed in some other carrying device, and put back in the pocket. Commonly, a small amount of blood remains in the syringe; this is a perfect medium for bacterial growth as well as a potential inoculum of one drug user's blood into another person if the needle and syringe are shared.

Oral medications (pills and capsules) are prepared similarly; the proper amount of the pill to be injected (for example, a tablet like Preludin[1]) is crushed on a counter- or tabletop. The crushed powder is carefully scraped together and dropped into a cooker, and a small amount of fluid is added over low heat in an attempt to dissolve the material. Many insoluble bits and pieces of the carrying agent contained in the pill remain undissolved. In order to obtain the maximum return from the crushed pill, the particulate matter is often injected directly into the vein.

Cutting agents used for heroin and other opiates vary widely. Commonly used materials include a variety of sugars (such as mannitol, lactose, etc.) and quinine, which is presumed by the drug user to enhance the effect of the opiate. Although other types of soluble sugars are sometimes used, in the rush of

[1] Brand name of Boehringer-Ingelheim Ltd. for phenmetrazine hydrochloride.

cutting a newly arrived batch of heroin any white substance that appears to be appropriate may be used. No attempt to maintain sterility is made by either the dealer or pusher, and obviously the final percentage of opiate in a given packet of heroin varies. The average bag of cut "heroin" weighs about 90 mg (5), of which 0 to 10 percent is pure heroin. Occasionally, a drug dealer under pressure to sell a large amount of heroin will inappropriately increase the amount in a packet, and overdoses will result.

Infectious complications of parenteral drug abuse *Acute narcotism* (drug overdose) is the major cause of death in narcotic abusers. Infection is uncommon as a cause of death, accounting for less than 5 percent of cases evaluated by the Medical Examiner in New York City (5). On the other hand, acute infections account for over 58 percent of hospital admissions of drug addicts (6). In the survey of 200 addict admissions by White (6), 30.5 percent were admitted with acute hepatitis and 27.5 percent with other infections. Only 2 of the 200 were noted to have endocarditis; yet 6 other patients were "bacteremic without an obvious focus," and an unknown number of the 16 admitted for "pulmonary infection" had "pulmonary abscesses" and/or "septic emboli." Thus, probably about 5 percent of those 200 patients had endocarditis on admission to the hospital. This percentage is similar to the estimate of Banks et al. (7), who calculated that 8 percent of drug abusers admitted to the District of Columbia General Hospital had bacterial endocarditis. Thus, it seems reasonable to estimate that 25 percent of all hospital admissions of parenteral drug abusers are primarily for septic complications of drug abuse, and about 1 in 4 of those are for endocarditis.

IMMUNOLOGIC ALTERATIONS IN PARENTERAL DRUG ABUSERS

Effects of injected drugs on the immune system

For the purposes of this discussion, the immune system is classified into three components: (1) the nonspecific immune system (encompassing those elements of immunity not requiring prior contact with the organism), (2) the specific humoral immune system, and (3) the cell-mediated immune system. The nonspecific system consists of the barrier systems (skin and mucous membranes), the complement system, the polymorphonuclear neutrophils (PMNs), and, to some extent, the macrophages.

The major impairment in host defenses in the parenteral drug abuser is the consequence of breeching the barrier system. The drug abuser constantly disrupts the skin by injecting foreign materials into his subcutaneous tissues and veins. It is easy to understand how superficial, subcutaneous, and deep soft tissue infections develop. The effect of the various intravenously injected drugs on the function of the PMNs or the complement system has not been systematically studied. It is possible that opiates, amphetamines, or mixing agents have some effect locally on the adherence, migration, or even bactericidal capabilities of the PMNs. In concentrations commonly reached in people, alcohol has some deleterious effects on PMN function (8).

The most commonly found abnormality of the humoral immune system in the habitual parenteral drug abuser is hyperglobulinemia (9). The total levels of immunoglobulins are increased, and selective increases in IgM are demonstrable in these individuals (10). There is no known quantitative or qualitative defect in the ability of these antibodies to interact with antigens, and it is assumed that the increased levels of immunoglobulins are polyclonal in nature. Specific antibodies against the wide variety of bacteria present in street heroin and on the needles and syringes used by drug abusers are presumably present (11). Other causes of the increase in polyclonal immunoglobulins are relevant in parenteral drug users and probably are the major reason for such abberations. For example, parenteral drug users frequently abuse alcohol as well and also have an extremely high incidence of viral hepatitis. Thus, many develop some form of either alcoholic or viral chronic active liver disease, often producing elevations in serum globulin levels.

A variety of autoantibodies, such as rheumatoid factor and those causing positive Coombs' tests, have been described in parenteral drug abusers (9). Again, these are probably the immunologic concomitants of chronic hyperimmunization along with an almost certain lack of suppressor cell control of B cell and/or plasma cell function which occurs in patients with chronic liver disease and malnutrition (12). In these latter conditions, autoantibodies are common.

As regards cellular immune function, although no studies of the direct effect of heroin or amphetamines on T lymphocytes have been performed, it is unlikely that any demonstrable specific T lymphocyte defects are directly related to the injected drugs. It is far more likely, as suggested above, that secondary diseases influence T lymphocyte function. As a result of T lymphocyte malfunction, not only does hyperactivity of the B cell system occur but specific defects in T effector cell function may be demonstrable. For example, in patients chronically malnourished or with underlying chronic liver disease, there is suppression of delayed hypersensitivity. In that setting, an increased incidence of infections with certain organisms (mycobacteria, fungi, and certain viruses) may occur; such infections are uncommon in drug abusers and, when present, do not disseminate more often than when they occur in normal persons. The common denominator may well be protein-calorie malnutrition (12). While an occasional instance of generalized lymphadenopathy may be seen in the drug addict (13), there is probably no increase in neoplastic diseases other than those associated with other attendant risk factors, such as use of tobacco and alcohol.

Inflammatory and/or immunologic syndromes in parenteral drug abusers

A variety of confusing clinical syndromes described in parenteral drug abusers are often accompanied by fever; differentiation from infection, and especially from endocarditis, may be difficult.

Pyrogenic reactions to injected materials Drug abusers may occasionally present with chills and high fever, altered mentation, and, in some cases, decreased blood pressure; however, they may be found after evaluation not to have an infection. The specific materials among the injected substances that trigger these pyrogenic reactions are not known. Either contaminating bacteria themselves (11) or free endotoxins interact with white blood cells to produce the pyrogenic response. The typical syndrome consists of the following: shortly after injecting, the addict develops a shaking chill, may become hypotensive, and when brought to the emergency room is found to have a high fever (103 to 105°F). The pathogenesis of this syndrome most likely involves the release of endogenous pyrogen by PMNs, like the mechanism of fever following injection of purified bacterial endotoxins (14). Whether activation of complement, kinin, or prostaglandin is involved in this reaction, as it is in patients with the syndrome of septic shock (15), is unclear.

Hepatitis and its immunologic sequelae As stated above, the parenteral drug abuser is constantly at risk of acquiring hepatitis (usually type B, although the incidence of non-A–non-B is also probably high). As a manifestation of the immunologic reactions to the virus, febrile, multiorgan system syndromes may appear which may mimic endocarditis. The prodromal stage of viral hepatitis may present with fever (16), which is sometimes quite high and associated with chills. As discussed below, the febrile drug user must be admitted to the hospital, appropriate cultures must be obtained, and the patient must be treated with antibiotics. After 2 or 3 days blood cultures are found to be negative; subsequently, clinical and laboratory evidence of hepatitis develops. Similarly, some drug abusers with known chronic active liver disease may develop intermittent fevers, chills, arthralgias, etc.; at each episode, such patients require thoughtful reassessment for underlying systemic infection. Other immune manifestations of active hepatitis can be very confusing. For example, a patient may develop frank arthritis as an initial manifestation of immune complex disease sometimes observed in the early stages of type B hepatitis (17); differentiation from septic arthritis may be difficult. Some individuals with hepatitis may develop skin lesions or a rash which resembles the dermal manifestations of endocarditis (18). In all these settings the possibility of endocarditis cannot be ruled out until appropriate evaluations of blood and joint fluid cultures are made. Severe bacterial sepsis may also lead to fairly dramatic alterations in liver function. Thus, a drug user may present with fever and chills, be noted to be jaundiced, and be sent home with the diagnosis of viral hepatitis when, in fact, the patient has a bacteremia.

Disseminated vasculitis A bizarre multiorgan syndrome associated with fever has been described in patients using amphetamines (19, 20) and has been shown by biopsy, angiography, and postmortem examination to be a disseminated vasculitis (19). Whether it is related to amphetamine abuse per se or is simply another immunologic manifestation of hepatitis is unclear. Hepatitis B–related immune complexes have been associated with a polyarteritis nodosa–like syndrome (21). Such a vasculitis is more likely to be related to immune reactions to viral or bacterial products than to amphetamine itself. Furthermore, to the author's knowledge, additional patients suffering from such a disease have not been described recently; thus, the specific amphetamine-related syndrome may not exist.

Heroin nephropathy   Some patients with a history of chronic parenteral drug abuse are found to have proteinuria along with elevated blood pressure and varying degrees of renal failure (22). While many of these patients are asymptomatic, some may initially present with an intercurrent febrile reaction, probably not related to the underlying chronic renal disease. At that point, when a patient is found to have proteinuria and an active urine sediment, sometimes with hematuria, one must consider the diagnosis of endocarditis. In patients with bacterial endocarditis (and more frequently in those with bacterial endocarditis due to *Staphylococcus aureus*), classic, immune complex glomerulitis may be seen (23). Such patients present with fever and chills; at the time of admission, the BUN and creatinine are rising, and an active urine sediment is present. Staphylococci are grown from the bloodstream (and frequently from the urine sediment as well). The syndrome resolves promptly with antibiotic therapy.

How the relatively asymptomatic and almost certainly immunologically mediated *heroin nephropathy* relates to heroin use is unclear. It is probable that the syndrome results from chronic immunologic stimulation with the variety of bacteria and fungi present in injected heroin, unsterile needles, and syringes (11). The resulting hyperimmunization probably produces immune complex formation and ultimately glomerulonephritis. This syndrome must be differentiated from the glomerulonephritis associated with hepatitis B infection (24) and from amyloidosis which has recently been described in drug abusers (25).

Other immunologic syndromes   Occasionally, a parenteral drug abuser will present with diffuse lymphadenopathy with or without splenomegaly, and on biopsy the lymph node shows reactive hyperplasia (13). Whether these individuals are suffering an illness like serum sickness or have intercurrently become infected with cytomegalovirus or Epstein-Barr virus is unclear. Some of these patients are found to be in the early phases of hepatitis. When fever accompanies this syndrome and splenomegaly is present, the distinction from bacterial endocarditis must be made. The approach to such patients should include obtaining cultures and initiation of antimicrobial therapy if the patients are febrile, with reassessment of the situation again after 24 to 48 h.

PATHOGENESIS OF INFECTIVE ENDOCARDITIS IN PARENTERAL DRUG ABUSERS

Types and sources of organisms

The most common organism responsible for this syndrome continues to be *Staph. aureus* (26). The next most common organisms vary in differing series but are streptococci and/or gram-negative enteric bacilli. Other, more unusual organisms, for example, *Bacillus* spp., probably cause more infections than have been recognized in the past (27, 28). Fungal endocarditis is presently uncommon.

The source of *Staph. aureus* is clearly the addict himself. Studies of cultured street heroin, injection needles, and paraphernalia have revealed that *Staph. aureus* is *not* present in these materials (11); however, the organism is carried in the nose and throat in a much higher percentage of drug users than in normal control subjects (29). For some reason, needle use in general predisposes to increased nasopharyngeal carriage of *Staph. aureus* in a variety of patient populations. This is an occurrence not only in the drug addict but also in the patient with diabetes (30), the patient on hemodialysis (31), and even the allergic patient initially receiving injections for desensitization (32). No explanation for this interesting phenomenon is presently available, but it is this author's opinion that it may have something to do with microcolonization by *Staph. aureus* of the small skin defects created by needle use. This occurrence would parallel the phenomenon of *Staph. aureus* skin microcolonization which occurs in patients with atopic dermatitis (33). Subsequent inoculation of the organism into the nose and throat then occurs, and it seems logical that, once carried in the nose and throat, the organism can contaminate the skin before injection. From the skin, the organism probably gains access to the bloodstream during drug injection; the phage type of *Staph. aureus* strain in the nose and throat of drug addicts entering the hospital with *Staph. aureus* endocarditis always is the same as that of the organism isolated from the blood (34).

The source of organisms other than *Staph. aureus* is probably the external environment. Studies of cultured heroin and paraphernalia, while not showing the presence of *Staph. aureus*, did reveal a large number of other organisms (11). The most common bacteria present both in heroin and on injection apparatus were *Bacillus* spp. followed in frequency by coagulase-negative staphylococci (on paraphernalia) and *Aspergillus* spp. (in heroin). *Clostridium perfringens* and enteric gram-negative bacilli were common on injection paraphernalia. A wide variety of fungi were found in the heroin samples, but *Candida* spp. were not.

The probable source of the gram-negative bacteria causing endocarditis in drug users is the water used to dilute the injected mixture. For example, in the Detroit area, *Pseudomonas* was for a time the second most common organism to cause endocarditis in drug abusers (*Staph. aureus* was the major cause) (35, 36); in the San Francisco area, *Serratia marcescens* was reported to be the second most common cause (37). Both these organisms survive in water. Occasionally, multiple organisms grow from the bloodstream, and in at least one instance toilet bowl water had been used to mix the injected drug (38).

Other organisms commonly causing endocarditis in drug abusers are streptococci (26). Occasionally alpha-hemolytic (viridans-like) streptococcus is isolated from both heroin and injection paraphernalia (11). Viridans streptococci and enterococci most probably originate from the addicts' normal flora, as do the streptococci causing the syndrome of subacute bacterial endocarditis in non-drug users. Presumably, these types of streptococci have a greater ability to adhere to heart valves than other organisms of the normal human flora (especially gram-negative bacilli). This may explain their increased frequency in bacterial endocarditis (39, 40). In such cases (as is true in the non-drug user), it is expected that known organic valve lesions will be more common. In addition, some young drug abusers may have asymptomatic cardiac valve lesions (aortic or mitral), which may explain why most cases of streptococcal endocarditis in addicts involve predominantly the left side of the heart (41).

There are clearly two syndromes of endocarditis in the drug abuser. One is predominantly caused by *Staph. aureus* and involves the tricuspid valve. This is the syndrome of right-sided endocarditis (although on occasion, there is spill-over to left-sided valves). The left-sided syndrome is caused by less virulent organisms, often streptococci. The left-sided valves in these cases have probably been previously damaged or deformed. Differences between the syndromes of right- and left-sided endocarditis are outlined in Table 1.

Presumed effects of injected materials on the tricuspid valve

Since the syndrome of endocarditis in the individual with entirely normal valves before the episode is due almost solely to *Staph. aureus* and almost always starts on the right side of the heart, it has been presumed that repeated intravenous injections of drugs must produce a lesion of some sort on the tricuspid valve (26). It is quite likely that the regular injection of particulate material somehow scarifies the tricuspid valve, leading to endothelial cell disruption and deposition of small platelet and fibrin clots. Thereafter, organisms inoculated into the blood during the course of drug injection adhere to, and multiply in, the small clot and result in the vegetation. The postulated sequence of events causing this syndrome is outlined in Table 2. As clearly demonstrated in experimental animals (42), any area of disruption on the endothelial surface results in a platelet thrombus and becomes a site on which bacteria in the bloodstream may readily seed (43).

Table 1   Differences between the syndromes of right- and left-sided endocarditis associated with parenteral drug abuse

Category	Right-sided	Left-sided
Clinical syndrome	Acute with pulmonary emboli	Subacute with systemic emboli
Causative organisms	*Staph. aureus* (90%) > gram-negative bacilli (5%)	Streptococci ≥ *Staph. aureus*
Surgery required	Rarely	Commonly
Outcome	Excellent	Fair

**Table 2   Pathogenesis of right-sided
endocarditis syndrome in parenteral drug abusers**

Event	*Outcome*
Repeated injections of illicit drugs	Increased nasopharyngeal carriage of *Staph. aureus* with skin contamination Increased likelihood of bacteremia with gram-negative bacilli, especially water contaminants Endothelial disruption on tricuspid valve with platelet thrombus formation
Intermittent bacteremia with *Staph. aureus* or gram-negative bacilli (*Pseudomonas* or *Serratia* spp.)	Seeding of bacteria to platelet thrombus on tricuspid valve, causing vegetation of bacterial endocarditis
Tricuspid valve endocarditis	Fever, chills, pleuritic chest pain; nodular cavitating densities on chest roentgenogram
Neglect of symptoms and/or misdiagnosis by physicians	Multiple organ abscess formation Involvement of left-sided heart valves Septic shock syndrome Death

How injected materials cause endothelial disruption of the tricuspid valve is not clear. These materials may mechanically traumatize the valve; frequent injections of large amounts of particulate materials probably disrupt the valve's endothelial surface physically (26), and increases in pulmonary arterial pressure produced by the injection of particulate material may be an additional predisposing factor. Administration of epinephrine, resulting in transient increases in systemic blood pressure, predisposes experimental animals to left-sided endocarditis (44). It is possible that the same mechanism may obtain in the pathogenesis of left-sided endocarditis in drug users; amphetamines produce an increase in systemic blood pressure along with tachycardia, which in the presence of bacteremia may predispose to the development of endocarditis. It is this author's impression that endocarditis is a more common complication of amphetamine abuse than of heroin abuse.

Involvement of other valves

After a vegetation develops on the tricuspid valve, the ensuing bacteremia is continuous. Thus, there is an increasing risk that other normal valves will become involved subsequently. The longer the patient goes without receiving treatment, the more likely it will be that the normal left-sided valves will become secondarily involved. The likelihood of metastatic abscess formation and/or the development of the septic shock syndrome certainly increases (Table 2). Of course, individuals with preexisting abnormalities of the aortic or mitral valves are at high risk of developing primary left-sided endocarditis with what-ever organism is injected into the blood stream. The pathogenesis of left-sided valve involvement is outlined in Table 3.

THE CLINICAL SYNDROMES OF ENDOCARDITIS IN PARENTERAL DRUG ABUSERS

The drug abuser with endocarditis classically presents with the abrupt onset of fever and chills. *All other physical findings of endocarditis may be absent at the time of presentation.*

The classic triad of the right-sided endocarditis syndrome

Since most cases of drug associated endocarditis involve *Staph. aureus* and occur on the tricuspid valve, a classic syndrome has emerged (45). Often, physi-

Table 3 Pathogenesis of left-sided endocarditis syndrome in parenteral drug abusers

Event	Outcome
Repeated injections of illicit drugs by person with preexisting minor aortic and/or mitral valve lesions (rheumatic, congenital, etc.)	Injections of large inocula of bacteria contaminating heroin, (e.g., *Bacillus* spp.) Skin contamination by normal mouth flora (e.g., streptococci, *Staph. epidermidis,* etc.)
Constant small endothelial disruptions of organic, left-sided valvular lesions lead to platelet thrombus formation	Bacteria seed to platelet thrombi forming vegetations of bacterial endocarditis
Endocarditis develops on aortic or mitral valves	Fever and systemic embolization occur; valve malfunction may occur
Malfunction of left-sided valves leads to congestive heart failure	Surgical valve replacement may be required Increased likelihood of second episode of endocarditis
	or
Right-sided endocarditis with prolonged *Staph. aureus* bacteremia due to neglect of symptoms or misdiagnosis by physicians	Prolonged tachycardia and "stress" leading to endothelial disruption on aortic and/or mitral valves with platelet thrombus formation Seeding of *Staph. aureus* to platelet thrombus forming vegetation.
Endocarditis develops on aortic and/or mitral valves	Sequence of events as outlined in endocarditis and malfunction of left-sided valves (see above)

cal evidence of regular drug use may be present in the form of injection tracks or scarified veins. The patient will report having had either a chilly sensation or frank shaking chills several days earlier. If the patient's temperature is *carefully* taken at the time of presentation, a fever will almost invariably be present. Fever may be quenched, however, by the use of antipyretics or antibiotics; self-medication with antibiotics is not infrequent in the drug community. The final element in the triad (in addition to the history and signs of drug abuse and the presence of fever) is pleuritic chest pain. Since the classic syndrome is that of right-sided endocarditis, embolic phenomena result in recurrent pulmonary emboli with pleuritic pain and, sometimes, hemoptysis. As described below, individuals with these symptoms almost always show on chest radiographs the classical findings of septic pulmonary emboli, i.e., multiple patchy densities which frequently cavitate (46). The *majority* of such patients either do not have an audible murmur or have an insignificant murmur that is considered to be a functional or a flow murmur (26, 45). Later, most patients develop a definite, though often transient, murmur of tricuspid insufficiency.

The presence of *fever* is all that is required to make a presumptive diagnosis of endocarditis in the patient with a known history of drug abuse (47, 48). Even occasional "afebrile" drug users presenting to the physician with a history of a chill and fever (especially those with chest discomfort and/or a pulmonary infiltrate) must be presumed to have endocarditis. Usually the temperature will become elevated if observed long enough. Most individuals, however, are febrile at the time of evaluation. Cultures must be obtained from all such individuals; they should be admitted to the hospital for initiation of therapy, despite the absence of any other finding. This means that many individuals without endocarditis will be admitted and started on antibiotics. If after a day or two in the hospital the blood cultures are negative and the patient has no clinical signs of illness, antibiotics can be stopped and the patient can be discharged. Among the few drug abusers this author has seen die early after admission to the hospital with widespread metastatic abscess formation have been several who had been seen earlier in other hospitals and in whom the diagnosis was missed.

The full-blown endocarditis syndrome

Relationships exist between the causative organism, the valve involved, and the clinical syndrome with which the patient presents.

The right-sided endocarditis syndrome This is the classic syndrome seen in the drug abuser with endocarditis of the tricuspid valve due to *Staph. aureus.* Over the last decade, this syndrome has emerged as the predominant one observed in the United States (26, 45). Other organisms occasionally involved (in perhaps 5 percent of cases) include *Pseudomonas* spp. (35, 36) and *Serratia marcescens* (37), which also probably colonize platelet thrombi on the tricuspid valve just as *Staph. aureus* does. Case histories indicate that the clinical illness begins with fever and chilly sensations (45). After a variable period, pleuritic chest pain and cough develop as small septic emboli begin to involve the lungs. The murmur of tricuspid insufficiency is usually absent or faint on admission and only later emerges in recognizable form. In most patients with right-sided endocarditis who are drug abusers, the murmur disappears completely by the end of 4 weeks of therapy (45). Anyone with *Staph. aureus* endocarditis is generally very ill and may be suffering from malfunction of multiple additional organ systems. For example, such patients may present after only several days of generalized symptoms (headache, stiff neck, and disorientation), having developed either meningitis that is blood-borne or a consequence of rupture of a small parameningeal abscess into the subarachnoid space. Other common symptoms include pain and tenderness over bony prominences, especially the sacrum, hips, and long bones. Septic arthritis may be present. Disseminated intravascular coagulation can develop in the course of this sometimes fulminant illness (49).

The left-sided endocarditis syndrome This syndrome is seen in patients who develop vegetations on the aortic or mitral valves. While many of these cases are caused by *Staph. aureus*, many are due to other organisms, especially streptococci (41). Usually these individuals have either had known underlying valvular heart disease or previously unrecognized lesions. They may present with an especially fulminant syndrome if *Staph. aureus* is the causative organism. In this situation the setting is that of "superacute" endocarditis, often with rapidly ensuing deterioration of valve function. Heart murmurs are prominent in these patients, and the diagnosis of endocarditis is rarely missed. Embolic phenomena are likely to occur early in these cases, and true Janeway lesions are more often seen with *Staph. aureus* endocarditis than in endocarditis due to other organisms.

Complications

The mortality rate for endocarditis in the otherwise healthy group of young drug users is low. Almost all the patients with the syndromes of right-sided endocarditis who come to the hospital early enough do well (50). Mortality rates vary from 5 to 15 percent in this group; the major problems are secondary involvement and destruction of the aortic valve with the onset of left-sided congestive heart failure and isolated incidences of central nervous system infection (for example, rupture of a brain abscess into the subarachnoid space). Mortality is much higher in patients whose left-sided valves are primarily involved with *Staph. aureus*; in individual series, it has been reported that 20 to 50 percent of such patients ultimately expire, usually of heart failure and/or complications during the perioperative period. Other complications of both left- and right-sided syndromes are rarely fatal and include brain abscess, meningitis, septic pulmonary emboli, osteomyelitis, septic arthritis, renal cortical abscesses, multiple skin abscess formation, and major peripheral arterial emboli (26). Glomerulonephritis occurs frequently in patients with *Staph. aureus* endocarditis and may lead to rapidly deteriorating renal function, sometimes requiring hemodialysis. If the organism is a gram-negative rod like *Pseudomonas* or *Serratia* (even if the vegetation is on the tricuspid valve), the mortality rate is much higher (35). Patients infected with these organisms may require surgery for eradication of the infection (51), although occasionally such patients will respond to antibiotic therapy alone.

DIAGNOSIS OF INFECTIVE ENDOCARDITIS IN PARENTERAL DRUG ABUSERS

Although the febrile drug abuser coming to the emergency room or the physician's office presents a wide variety of possible problems, very simple diagnostic choices merit consideration. All that is required to make the presumptive diagnosis of endocarditis is fever along with the history of parenteral drug abuse.

The appropriate clinical evaluation

Three blood cultures, each culture consisting of two bottles, one aerobic and one anaerobic, should be obtained through three separate venipunctures as rapidly as dictated by the clinical situation. The three blood cultures could be obtained over a 5- to 10-min period if the patient appears critically ill, and antimicrobial therapy can be initiated immediately. No patient is ever so sick that the physician should forgo an appropriate evaluation (including cultures of the blood and all other potentially infected body cavities) before instituting antimicrobial therapy. A history and physical examination are rapidly performed to detect signs of metastatic infection or early signs of consumption coagulopathy and septic shock. If there is any alteration of mental status and/or a stiff neck, the cerebrospinal fluid should be examined with culture and Gram-stained smear of the spun sediment. In the presence of localized pain, swelling, and fluctuance, the involved area should be aspirated, and Gram-stained smears and cultures should be made. Gram-stained smears of the peripheral blood can be performed; it has been reported that up to 50 percent of patients with endocarditis have organisms visible within the glass-adherent PMNs from a single drop of unanticoagulated peripheral blood (52). A careful urine analysis should be performed to detect cellular elements and casts.

The problem of culture-negative endocarditis

The most important factor influencing whether or not blood cultures will be positive is previous antibiotic administration. Despite prior ingestion of antibiotics, the blood cultures still are usually positive; but since bacterial growth may be delayed, it is important that the microbiology laboratory be requested to incubate the cultures for 2 weeks or longer.

Blood cultures are almost uniformly positive if no antibiotics have been taken previously. In our series of 40 cases of endocarditis in drug abusers due to *Staph. aureus*, 253 blood cultures were obtained and 246 (97 percent) were positive (45). Even in endocarditis in non-drug users, if antibiotics have not been administered within the 2-week period before hospitalization, the vast majority (over 95 percent) of all blood cultures drawn are positive (53). Thus, under usual circumstances, negative blood culture results are strong evidence *against* the diagnosis of endocarditis. Problems arise not only when individuals have taken antibiotics but also when certain organisms are difficult to grow. For example, anaerobic bacteria are clearly more likely to cause endocarditis when toilet bowl water is used as a diluent for the injected narcotics. *Bacteroides fragilis* and other more fastidious anaerobes are readily isolated from the commonly employed blood culture media. Some fungi grow poorly in blood cultures (43), but at present they rarely occur in cases of endocarditis in drug abusers. *Aspergillus* spp. (very difficult to isolate from blood) have not been reported as a cause of endocarditis in the drug abuser who has not undergone cardiac surgery (26).

A negative blood culture report on the second or third day after admission of the febrile patient who had *not* received prior antibiotic therapy and who exhibited no other findings that support the diagnosis of endocarditis may reasonably lead to discontinuation of antibiotic therapy. The patient may be discharged from the hospital after two additional days of observation. The occasional individual with endocarditis for whom antibiotics have been inappropriately discontinued will almost invariably develop a fever and bacteriologic relapse within 24 to 48 h (54). Those with a history of antibiotic use and findings that make the diagnosis of endocarditis likely should be continued on parenteral therapy for 10 to 14 days until teichoic acid antibody analyses (see below) have been completed. It is most probable that an individual who has a relatively small staphylococcal vegetation on the tricuspid valve, who has been treated for several days with antibiotics, and who has *no other signs or symptoms of metastatic abscess formation* and no teichoic acid antibodies at 14 days after admission has been cured.

Additional studies which may shed light on culture-negative cases are echocardiography (55) and angiography (56). Especially helpful is the new two-dimensional ultrasound technology. If vegetations are demonstrated, the diagnosis is essentially confirmed despite the absence of positive blood cultures. Also, patients who develop embolic phenomena, new murmurs, or metastatic abscesses also require continuation of antibiotic therapy.

Diagnostic serologic methods

Serologic methods are available to assist in clinical decision making in endocarditis caused by two organisms, *Staph. aureus* and *Pseudomonas aeruginosa*. The presence of antibodies against the cell wall teichoic acids of *Staph. aureus* correlates strongly with deep, serious staphylococcal infections, especially endocarditis. In fact, the validity of this correlation was confirmed in drug abusers with endocarditis (57). Crowder and White first described the high percentage of patients with endocarditis due to *Staph. aureus* who have elevated levels of antibodies to cell wall teichoic acids (58). Subsequently, it has been found that in excess of 90 percent of parenteral drug users who have the syndrome of endocarditis due to *Staph. aureus* develop increases in such antibodies (59). About one-third of such patients do not have measurable antibodies on admission to the hospital (59); as one might suspect, these individuals have a shorter duration of symptoms at the time of hospitalization than those with antibodies. Those without antibodies on admission will develop a rise in titer by the tenth or

fourteenth day (59, 60). In some patients in whom blood cultures remain negative, especially in those who have taken antibiotics before coming to the hospital, the rising antibody titer will firmly establish the diagnosis of endocarditis due
to *Staph. aureus* (59). It is unusual, however, for such individuals to have
negative blood cultures. Thus, although the antibody titer is not especially
helpful in the diagnosis of this syndrome, it is extremely useful in following
individuals who have deep metastatic complications not clinically recognized.
For example, we have seen several patients whose titer failed to decrease after 4
to 6 weeks of antibiotic therapy and who presented some weeks later with
osteomyelitis or other foci of recrudescent infection. Also, individuals in whom
infection relapses shortly after discontinuing therapy will develop a rise in antibodies if the clinical relapse is due to *Staph. aureus* (57).

Pseudomonas endocarditis has also been associated with a rise in antibodies
to that organism. In fact, there was a high level of correlation between a high
level of IgM antibody to the *Pseudomonas* cell wall polysaccharide and an
active infection (61).

It is beyond the scope of this review to discuss the serologic diagnosis of viral
hepatitis. Nonetheless, one should be aware of the fact that either antecedent or
concomitant hepatitis B infections have occurred or may be occurring in a
patient with a complex, febrile illness.

Other serologic techniques possibly of use in the febrile drug abuser relate to
the occasional development of autoantibodies. For example, 25 percent of the
drug abusers with *Staph. aureus* endocarditis develop rheumatoid factors (62).
Thus, in a patient (who does not have rheumatoid arthritis) whose blood cultures remain negative but whose rheumatoid factor is rising, the diagnosis of
endocarditis becomes more likely. It is important to look for changes in titers in
such situations rather than simply for the presence or absence of a given type of
antibody; other workers have reported rheumatoid factor to be positive in many
asymptomatic drug abusers (9).

MANAGEMENT

Antibiotic choices

Choices of antibiotics are outlined in Table 4.

Antibiotics for the presumptive case   Before any microbiologic data are available, an antistaphylococcal antibiotic must be included in the therapeutic program. With no history of penicillin allergy, nafcillin or oxacillin are the drugs of
choice. If the patient is allergic to penicillin, either a cephalosporin (in the
absence of a history of anaphylaxis) or vancomycin should be substituted. While
all the penicillinase-resistant penicillins are approximately equal in efficacy
against *Staph. aureus*, nafcillin has been shown to be less toxic than methicillin
(63). Although oxacillin has not yet been compared directly with nafcillin or
methicillin, it is probably fair to say that oxacillin and nafcillin are comparable
both in efficacy and in side effects. While all the penicillins may produce typical
"fever and rash" reactions, certain of them are associated more commonly with

Table 4   Antibiotic management of parenteral drug abusers with presumed or defined endocarditis

Clinical situation*	Antibiotics	
	First choice	*Second choice*
Before culture data available	Nafcillin + tobramycin	Cefazolin or vancomycin + gentamicin
Staph. aureus	Nafcillin	Cefazolin or vancomycin
Pseudomonas	Ticarcillin or carbenicillin + tobramycin or gentamicin or amikacin	None
Serratia	Same	None
Enterococcus	Ampicillin or penicillin + tobramycin	Vancomycin + gentamicin
Fungus	Amphotericin B + surgical valve replacement (to be performed as soon as possible)	None

* In blood cultures.

a given toxicity. The specific toxicity of nafcillin is the rare development of neutropenia (64). For oxacillin, the peculiar toxic reaction is a mild form of hepatitis (65). The major toxicity of methicillin lies in its tendency to produce an interstitial nephritis (66), rarely, if ever, seen with nafcillin or oxacillin. Since, at present, the vast majority of both community- and hospital-acquired *Staph. aureus* strains are resistant to penicillin, a penicillinase-resistant drug must always be used from the outset.

Since some areas in the country experience a higher incidence of gram-negative bacteria as the etiology of endocarditis in drug abusers, an aminoglycoside should also be used in initial therapy. Either gentamicin or tobramycin would be a reasonable choice. Tobramycin is becoming favored because it appears to be somewhat less nephrotoxic.

Therapy is initiated in the non-penicillin-allergic patient with nafcillin, 12 g per day, plus full doses of tobramycin. One must be alert to the rapid changes in renal function which occur in this group of patients and adjust the dose of aminoglycoside accordingly.

Antibiotics for the defined case   If *Staph. aureus* is isolated from the blood, the aminoglycoside can be stopped and nafcillin can be continued to complete a

4-week course of therapy. While *Staph. aureus* is synergistically killed by the combination of nafcillin plus an aminoglycoside in vitro (67) and in the rabbit endocarditis model (68), there is no added clinical benefit in continuing the combination beyond the first several days (69). If *Pseudomonas* spp. or *Serratia marcescens* is isolated from the blood, the aminoglycoside must be continued, and high doses of carbenicillin (for example, 36 g in 24 h) or ticarcillin (for example, 18 g in 24 h) must be added. Such combination therapy is optimal for treating these infections and, occasionally, antibiotic therapy alone will result in a cure (35, 37, 70). However, such infections due to gram-negative bacilli, even on the tricuspid valve, are very difficult to treat successfully with antibiotics alone, and surgery is often required to eradicate the infection. Following excision of the tricuspid valve, a prosthetic valve is often not required because of the low pressures on the right side of the heart and the ability of young, healthy individuals to tolerate free tricuspid insufficiency if the cardiac status is normal otherwise. Several such cases have been reported (71–73). Valve replacement in the presence of active endocarditis, even on left-sided valves, is successful in over one-half of the cases (74).

If the enterococcus is isolated from blood cultures, therapy with nafcillin can be discontinued, the aminoglycoside can be continued, and high-dose ampicillin or penicillin can be added as for other cases of enterococcal endocarditis (43). Synergy studies are required in such cases, as are serial serum bactericidal assays, to optimize therapy. Occasionally, other bacteria and fungi will be identified. Specific appropriate antibiotic regimens will need to be tailored to the special situation. Therapy with amphotericin B plus surgery (as soon as possible) will be required to cure fungal endocarditis (26, 41).

Antibiotic management when blood cultures remain negative In most instances of suspected endocarditis in drug abusers with negative blood cultures, it is unlikely that endocarditis is present. In such cases, measurement of teichoic acid antibodies and echocardiographic studies may be helpful in diagnosis. Results of such studies will dictate whether antibiotics should be continued. For the patient who defervesces, apparently in response to the initial administration of antibiotics, but who has previously received antibiotics it seems reasonable to continue parenteral antibiotic therapy for 14 days. At that time, the level of teichoic acid antibodies is helpful for decision making. If such antibodies are absent and the patient is otherwise doing well, therapy can be discontinued and the patient can be discharged after a 3- to 4-day observation period. It is presumed in such cases that

1 Endocarditis was actually not present.

2 If the patient had endocarditis, it was caused by a penicillin-sensitive organism (such as the viridans type of streptococcus) and therefore 2 weeks of therapy sufficed (in such instances, the patient can be discharged on oral penicillin or dicloxacillin).

3 The patient had endocarditis due to *Staph. aureus* without a change in teichoic acid antibody titers.

It is not only difficult to keep these patients in the hospital for prolonged periods of time, but in the above instances the likelihood of endocarditis is so low that a

2-week course of parenteral antibiotics followed by several weeks of oral therapy seems a reasonable compromise. Other variables that might cause the clinician to be more conservative include the obvious presence of left-sided organic valve lesions (even if no changes in the murmur occur) or the development of new left-sided valve lesions during the initial period of observation. Individuals relapsing under such circumstances will be at much higher risk of developing the more serious complications (as noted below) of congestive heart failure (usually requiring surgery) as well as of major embolic phenomena.

Antibiotics for the patient allergic to penicillin   At the outset, it seems reasonable to use either a cephalosporin (cefazolin is, in the author's opinion, the cephalosporin of choice) or vancomycin (see Table 4). Either drug will be effective against *Staph. aureus*. For long-term therapy of patients with documented endocarditis, cefazolin is probably easier to use than vancomycin; after several days or weeks of treatment, cefazolin can be given intramuscularly for brief periods to rest the already overworked veins. Venous access in these patients usually becomes very difficult.

Parenteral versus oral antibiotic therapy

The syndrome of right-sided endocarditis due to *Staph. aureus* is easily treated, and the vast majority of patients do extremely well. Given that situation, at least one infectious disease group (which cares for large numbers of such patients) has reported that 2 weeks of parenteral therapy seems sufficient (75). Their regimen consists of 2 weeks of parenteral therapy, and the patient is then placed on oral dicloxacillin. Serum bactericidal levels against the patient's staphylococcus are obtained (peak and trough) after administering an oral dose of the drug. For most patients, a 500-mg to 1-g dose is sufficient to generate satisfactory serum bactericidal levels, and the patient can be discharged on such a dose given four times daily. Again, the problem of venous access and/or individual patient preference may force such a course in some patients who are unwilling to stay for intramuscular cefazolin therapy.

Duration of therapy

While patients with the syndrome of right-sided endocarditis due to responsive organisms (*Staph. aureus* or streptococci) can probably be satisfactorily treated parenterally for 2 weeks and then placed on oral therapy, the majority of experts in infectious diseases treat such patients by the intravenous route for 4 to 6 weeks if the patient is willing to remain in the hospital. For patients with endocarditis due to gram-negative bacilli (*Pseudomonas* or *Serratia*), at least 6 weeks of therapy is indicated. Combination antibiotic therapy at full doses will probably eradicate many such infections. In cases in which enterococcus is the etiologic agent, if sufficiently high serum bactericidal levels can be obtained with combined antibiotic therapy, 4 to 6 weeks of therapy is probably sufficient.

Surgical intervention

The need for surgical intervention in drug abusers with endocarditis is the same as that in non-drug users (43) and is outlined in Table 5. Surgical intervention is most frequently required for patients with left-sided valve involvement who develop significantly compromised hemodynamic function. One should look for signs of early left ventricular failure in patients with aortic or mitral lesions and consider surgery early if left-sided failure begins to develop (76). The presence of leftsided vegetations large enough to be seen by echocardiogram is associated with increased morbidity and mortality (77). It is unreasonable to consider individuals with such vegetations for valve replacement, especially if hemodynamic alterations are also developing. Thus, the presence of echocardiographically demonstrable vegetations adds incentive to intervene surgically earlier rather than later.

The presence of recrudescent or antibiotic-resistant right-sided endocarditis, usually caused by *Pseudomonas* or *Serratia* spp., is an indication for operating to remove the valve (37). Operation in this setting is aimed at cure of the infection and not at support of hemodynamic function. In such cases, the tricuspid valve can be excised and no prosthesis need be inserted if the patient is otherwise hemodynamically normal (71–73). Results of surgery are good (74), even in patients with active endocarditis who have been on full-dose antimicrobial therapy for only a few days. Approximately 50 to 75 percent of such individuals will survive surgery without residual infection in or around the newly inserted prosthetic valve(s). How long such individuals should be treated after surgery is unknown. It seems reasonable to give four additional weeks of parenteral antimicrobial therapy followed by prolonged oral suppressive therapy (if an effective oral drug is available). For example, a patient with endocarditis due to *Staph. aureus* on the aortic valve who requires cardiac surgery will usually have received several days of therapy before the operation and should be treated for 4

Table 5 Indications for cardiac surgery in parenteral drug abusers with endocarditis

Valve involved	Indication
Left-sided	Onset of congestive heart failure* More than one systemic embolic event; possibly with just echo-demonstrable vegetations
Right-sided	Uncontrollable infection (usually with gram-negative bacilli)
Either	Infection on a previously inserted prosthetic valve
	Fungal endocarditis

* Surgery indicated at the earliest sign of failure with aortic valve involvement or if failure uncontrollable with mitral valve involvement.

weeks postoperatively with nafcillin. That patient can then be switched to oral dicloxacillin, serum bactericidal levels can be evaluated, and the patient can be followed closely in the clinic. The dose of dicloxacillin can be reduced by half 2 to 3 months after discharge and discontinued entirely at 6 months.

The problem of continued drug use

One of the biggest problems with managing drug abusers with endocarditis is that of continued drug injection. The basic personality defect(s) which foster the development of the drug habit are rarely altered either by a life-threatening infection or cardiac surgery. Thus, continued drug use following surgery is common. Such people are at extremely high risk of infecting their newly acquired prosthetic valve, usually with potentially disastrous results. Second and third valve replacements have occasionally been required in such people, despite the increased risk of failure with each additional replacement.

A separate ethical issue is whether or not such patients, having demonstrated continued narcotic use following valve replacement, should be permitted to undergo second and third valve replacements. The cost of valve replacement including hospital and physician fees averages $20,000 per episode. The majority of drug users do not have insurance coverage; thus, the entire cost is borne either by the hospital or by the state. Some institutions have developed an institutional policy denying surgical support to drug abusers with second episodes of drug-associated endocarditis on previously inserted prosthetic valves.

Prevention of endocarditis in parenteral drug abusers

This may seem an incongruous topic for this chapter, but it is worth considering. It is not unreasonable to think about educating the drug community about endocarditis and its genesis with a view toward prevention. For example, given that *Staph. aureus* is by far the most common etiologic agent of episodes of endocarditis in drug abusers, one might suggest to the drug dealers that a dose of nafcillin or oxacillin be mixed with the heroin in the hope that the dose of antibiotic might prevent implantation of *Staph. aureus* on heart valves. Such an approach is successful in preventing staphylococcal infection during the implantation of prosthetic valves. One would, of course, also need to educate drug abusers about the problem of anaphylaxis.

It also would seem reasonable to suggest that oral dicloxacillin or cephalexin be used earlier rather than later when fever occurs for more than a brief period following drug injection. The presence of chills and fever, possibly indicating bacteremia and seeding of the tricuspid valve, could almost certainly be treated if dicloxacillin were given for several days in full doses beginning on the day of the initial episode.

REFERENCES

1 **Chambers CD, Hunt LG:** Epidemiology of drug abuse, in Pradhan SN, Dutta SN, (eds): *Drug Abuse: Clinical and Basic Aspects.* St. Louis, Mosby, 1977, p 11.

2 **Peterson GC, Wilson MR:** A perspective on drug abuse. *Mayo Clin Proc* 46:468, 1971.

3 **Stimmel B:** The socioeconomics of heroin dependency. *N Engl J Med* 287:1275, 1972.

4 **Dutta SN, Kaufman E:** Multiple drug

abuse, in Pradhan SN, Dutta SN (eds): *Drug Abuse: Clinical and Basic Aspects*. St. Louis, Mosby, 1977, p 303.

5 **Baden MN:** Pathology of the addictive states, in Richter RW (ed): *Medical Aspects of Drug Abuse*. Hagerstown, Md, Harper & Row, 1975, p 189.

6 **White AG:** Medical disorders in drug addicts. *JAMA* 223:1469, 1973.

7 **Banks et al:** Infective endocarditis in heroin addicts. *Am J Med* 55:444, 1973.

8 **Smith FE, Palmer DL:** Alcoholism, infection and altered host defenses. *J Chron Dis* 29:35, 1976.

9 **Sheagren JN, Tuazon CU:** Immunological aspects, in Pradhan SN, Dutta SN (eds): *Drug Abuse: Clinical and Basic Aspects*. St. Louis, Mosby, 1977, p 321.

10 **Cushman P:** Persistent increased immunoglobulin M in treated narcotic addiction. *J All Clin Immunol* 52:122, 1973.

11 **Tuazon CU et al:** The microbiologic study of street heroin and injection paraphernalia. *J Infect Dis* 129:327, 1974.

12 **Law DK et al:** Immunocompetence of patients with protein-calorie malnutrition. *Ann Intern Med* 79:545, 1973.

13 **Geller SA, Stimmel B:** Diagnostic confusion from lymphatic lesions in heroin addicts. *Ann Intern Med* 78:703, 1973.

14 **Dinarello CA, Wolff SM:** Pathogenesis of fever in man. *N Engl J Med* 298:607, 1978.

15 **Ulevitch RJ, Cochrane EG:** Role of complement in lethal bacterial lipopolysaccharide-induced hypotensive and coagulative changes. *Infect Immun* 20:204, 1978.

16 **Hoofnagle JH:** Acute hepatitis, in Mandell GL et al (eds): *Principles and Practice of Infectious Diseases*. New York, Wiley, 1979, p 1043.

17 **Wands JR et al:** The pathogenesis of arthritis associated with acute hepatitis-B surface antigen–positive hepatitis. *J Clin Invest* 55:930, 1975.

18 **Weiss TD et al:** Skin lesions in viral hepatitis. *Am J Med* 64:269, 1978.

19 **Citron BP et al:** Necrotizing angiitis associated with drug abuse. *N Engl J Med* 283:1003, 1970.

20 **Stafford CR et al:** Mononeuropathy multiplex as a complication of amphetamine angiitis. *Neurology* 25:570, 1975.

21 **Fye KH et al:** Immune complexes in hepatitis B antigen–associated periarteritis nodosa. *Am J Med* 62:783, 1977.

22 **Thompson AN, Guha A:** Renal complications, in Pradhan SN, Dutta SN (eds): *Drug Abuse: Clinical and Basic Aspects*. St. Louis, Mosby, 1977, p 400.

23 **Gutman RA et al:** The immune complex glomerulonephritis of bacterial endocarditis. *Medicine* 51:1, 1972.

24 **Kohler PF et al:** Chronic membranous glomerulonephritis caused by hepatitis B antigen–antibody immune complexes. *Ann Intern Med* 81:448, 1974.

25 **Meador KH et al:** Renal amyloidosis and subcutaneous drug abuse. *Ann Intern Med* 91:565, 1979.

26 **Cannon NJ, Cobbs CG:** Infective endocarditis in drug addicts, in Kaye DK (ed): *Infective Endocarditis*. Baltimore, University Park Press, 1976, p 111.

27 **Weller PF et al:** The spectrum of *Bacillus* bacteremias in heroin addicts. *Arch Intern Med* 139:293, 1979.

28 **Tuazon CU et al:** Serious infections from *Bacillus* species. *JAMA* 241:1137, 1979.

29 **Tuazon CU, Sheagren JN:** Increased rate of carriage of *Staphylococcus aureus* among narcotic addicts. *J Infect Dis* 129:725, 1974.

30 **Tuazon CU et al:** *Staphylococcus aureus* among insulin-injecting diabetic patients—An increased carrier rate. *JAMA* 231:1272, 1975.

31 **Kirmani N et al:** *Staphylococcus aureus* carriage among patients on chronic hemodialysis. *Arch Intern Med* 138:1657, 1978.

32 **Kirmani N et al:** Carriage of *Staphylococcus aureus* among patients receiving allergy injections. *Ann Allergy*, in press.

33 **Bibel DJ et al:** *Staphylococcus aureus* and the microbial ecology of atopic dermatitis. *Can J Microbiol* 23:1062, 1977.

34 **Tuazon CU, Sheagren JN:** Staphylococcal endocarditis in parenteral drug abusers: Source of the organism. *Ann Intern Med* 82:788, 1975.

35 **Reyes MP et al:** *Pseudomonas* endocarditis in the Detroit Medical Center. *Medicine* 52:173, 1973.

36 **Archer G et al:** *Pseudomonas aeruginosa* endocarditis in drug addicts. *Am Heart J* 88:570, 1974.

37 **Mills J, Drew D:** *Serratia marcescens* endocarditis: A regional illness associated with intravenous drug abuse. *Ann Intern Med* 84:29, 1976.

38 **Child JA et al:** Mixed infective endocarditis in a heroin addict. *J Med Microbiol* 2:293, 1969.

39 **Ramirez-Ronda CH:** Adherence of *Streptococcus mutans* to normal and damaged canine aortic valve. *Clin Res* 25:382A, 1977.

40 **Scheld WM et al:** Bacterial adherence in the pathogenesis of endocarditis. *J Clin Invest* 78:1394, 1978.

41 **Reiner NE et al:** Enterococcal endocarditis in heroin addicts. *JAMA* 235:1861, 1976.

42 **Durack DT, Beeson PB:** Experimental bacterial endocarditis: I. Colonization of a sterile vegetation. *Br J Exp Pathol* 53:44, 1972.

43 **Scheld WM, Sande MA:** Endocarditis and intravascular infections, in Mandell GL et al (eds): *Principles and Practice of Infectious Diseases*. New York, Wiley, 1979, p 653.

44 **Highman B, Altland PD:** Streptococcal and staphylococcal endocarditis and renal lesions in rats after epinephrine in oil and dibenamine. *Proc Soc Exp Biol Med* 120:819, 1965.

45 **Tuazon CU et al:** Staphylococcal endocarditis in drug users: Clinical and microbiological aspects. *Arch Intern Med* 135:1555, 1975.

46 **Jaffe RB, Koschmann EB:** Septic pulmonary emboli. *Radiology* 96:527, 1970.

47 **Tuazon CU, Sheagren JN:** Septic complications in Pradhan SN, Dutta SN (eds): *Drug Abuse: Clinical and Basic Aspects.* St. Louis, Mosby, 1977, p 332.

48 **Sheagren JN:** Drug abuse and infection, in Mandell GL et al (eds): *Principles and Practice of Infectious Diseases.* New York, Wiley, 1979, p 2284.

49 **Murray HW et al:** Staphylococcal septicemia and disseminated intravascular coagulation: *Staphylococcus aureus* endocarditis mimicking meningococcemia. *Arch Intern Med* 137:844, 1977.

50 **Menda KB, Gorbach SL:** Favorable experience with bacterial endocarditis in heroin addicts. *Ann Intern Med* 78:25, 1973.

51 **Carruthers MN, Kanokvechayant R:** *Pseudomonas aeruginosa* endocarditis. *Am J Med* 55:811, 1973.

52 **Powers DL, Mandell GL:** Intraleukocytic bacteria in endocarditis patients. *JAMA* 227:313, 1974.

53 **Werner AS et al:** Studies on the bacteremia of bacterial endocarditis. *JAMA* 202:199, 1967.

54 **Tuazon CU, Sheagren JN:** Relapse of staphylococcal endocarditis after clindamycin therapy. *Am J Med Sci* 269:145, 1975.

55 **Sheikh MU et al:** Right sided infective endocarditis: An echocardiographic study. *Am J Med* 66:283, 1979.

56 **Harris CN et al:** Forward angiography in the identification of vegetations in tricuspid endocarditis. *Chest* 71:218, 1977.

57 **Nagel JG et al:** Teichoic acid serologic diagnosis of staphylococcal endocarditis. *Ann Intern Med* 82:13, 1975.

58 **Crowder JG, White A:** Teichoic acid antibodies in staphylococcal and nonstaphylococcal endocarditis. *Ann Intern Med* 77:87, 1972.

59 **Tuazon CU, Sheagren JN:** Teichoic acid antibodies in the diagnosis of serious infections with *Staphylococcus aureus*. *Ann Intern Med* 84:543, 1976.

60 **Tuazon CU et al:** *Staphylococcus aureus* bacteremia, relationship between formation of antibodies to teichoic acid and development of metastatic abscesses. *J Infect Dis* 137:57, 1978.

61 **Reyes MP et al:** *Pseudomonas* endocarditis: Hemagglutinating antibodies to *Fisher-Devlin-Gnabasik* immunotypes in sera. *J Lab Clin Med* 83:845, 1974.

62 **Sheagren JN et al:** Rheumatoid factor in acute bacterial endocarditis. *Arthr Rheum* 19:887, 1976.

63 **Kancir LM et al:** Adverse reactions to methicillin and nafcillin during treatment of serious *Staphylococcus aureus* infections. *JAMA* 138:909, 1978.

64 **Sandberg M et al:** Neutropenia probably resulting from nafcillin. *JAMA* 32:1152, 1975.

65 **Onorato IM, Axelrod JL:** Hepatitis from intravenous high-dose oxacillin therapy. *Ann Intern Med* 89:497, 1978.

66 **Bowder WA et al:** Antitubular basement membrane antibodies in methicillin-associated interstitial nephritis. *N Engl J Med* 291:381, 1974.

67 **Tuazon CU et al:** In vitro nafcillin-gentamicin synergism against pathogenic strains of *Staphylococcus aureus*. *Curr Ther Res* 23:760, 1978.

68 **Sande MA, Courtney KB:** Nafcillin-gentamicin synergism in experimental staphylococcal endocarditis. *J Lab Clin Med* 88:118, 1976.

69 **Sande MA et al:** Comparison of nafcillin with nafcillin plus gentamicin in the treatment of addicts with *Staphylococcus aureus* endocarditis. *19th ICAAC abst* no. 362, 1979.

70 **Yoshikawa TT et al:** Endocarditis due to *Pseudomonas aeruginosa* in a heroin addict: Successful treatment with trimethoprim sulfamethoxazole mixture plus colistin. *Chest* 72:794, 1977.

71 **Graham DY et al:** Infective endocarditis in drug addicts: Experiences with medical and surgical treatment. *Circulation* 47:37, 1973.

72 **Wright JS, Glennie JS:** Excision of tricuspid valve with later replacement in endocarditis of drug addiction. *Thorax* 33:518, 1978.

73 **Simberkoff MS et al:** Two-stage tricuspid valve replacement for mixed bacterial endocarditis. *Arch Intern Med* 133:212, 1974.

74 **Stenson EB et al:** Operative treatment of active endocarditis. *J Thor Cardiovasc Surg* 71:659, 1976.

75 **Parker RH, Fossieck BE:** Oral antimicrobics in the treatment of staphylococcal endocarditis. *16th ICAAC Abstr* no. 222, 1976.

76 **Mann T et al:** Assessing the hemodynamic severity of acute aortic regurgitation due to infective endocarditis. *N Engl J Med* 293:108, 1975.

77 **Mintz GS et al:** Survival of patients with aortic valve endocarditis: The prognostic implications of the echocardiogram. *Arch Intern Med* 139:862, 1979.

ADDITIONAL READINGS

Cannon NJ, Cobbs CG: Infective endocarditis in drug addicts, in Kaye DK (ed): *Infective Endocarditis*. Baltimore, University Park Press, 1976, p 111.

Louria DB: Infectious complications of non-alcoholic drug abuse. *Ann Rev Med* 25:219, 1974.

McLeod R, Remington JS: Postoperative fungal endocarditis, in Duma RJ (ed): *Infections of Prosthetic Heart Valves and Vascular Grafts: Prevention, Diagnosis, and Treatment*. Baltimore, University Park Press, 1977, p 163.

McLeod R, Remington JS: Fungal endocarditis, in Rahimtoola SH (ed): *Infective Endocarditis*. New York, Grune & Stratton, 1978, p 211.

Sheagren JN: Drug abuse and infection, in Mandell GL et al (eds): *Principles and Practice of Infectious Diseases*. New York, Wiley, 1979, p 2284.

Sheagren JN, Tuazon CU: Immunologic aspects, in Pradhan SN, Dutta SN (eds): *Drug Abuse: Clinical and Basic Aspects*. St. Louis, Mosby, 1977, p 321.

Stimmel B, Dack S: Infective endocarditis in narcotic addicts, in Rahimtoola SH (ed): *Infective Endocarditis*. New York, Grune & Stratton, 1978, p 195.

Tuazon CU, Sheagren JN: Septic complications, in Pradhan SN, Dutta SN (eds): *Drug Abuse: Clinical and Basic Aspects*. St. Louis, Mosby, 1977, p 332.

The cephalosporins and cephamycins: a perspective

WILLIAM L. HEWITT

This perspective of the therapeutic usefulness of the cephalosporins available to practicing physicians in the United States in April 1980 is necessarily personal and may emphasize certain aspects which seem particularly important to me. It is intended to be a balanced evaluation of the merits of these agents. Other cephalosporins undergoing current clinical trials will be mentioned briefly but should be similarly considered when relevant clinical data become more extensive. Sufficient basic information will be presented so that physicians other than infectious disease specialists can understand the perspective; however, an exhaustive review of these data is not intended nor is a consideration of the relationship of the cephalosporins to other antimicrobials, especially the penicillins, since this has been recently and comprehensively dealt with by others (1).

Cephalothin (Keflin) became available in 1964 approximately 20 years after the discovery that a fungus, *Acremonium brotzu*, produces this antibacterial substance. Over the subsequent 15 years seven antibiotics, three of which were formulations for oral use, became available and were designated *first-generation cephalosporins* (Table 1). They differed in a practical sense only in their routes of administration and pharmacokinetic characteristics rather than in microbiological properties, effectiveness, or toxicity (except for cephaloridine). Two additional compounds under current investigation also fall in this group. Three antibiotics with somewhat broadened spectra, designated *second-generation celphalosporins*, were introduced in the last 2 years; at least five third-generation agents with activity against *Pseudomonas aeruginosa* are under active clinical investigation in the United States at the present time. Extensive research into the relationships between structure and activity has resulted in the preparation of derivatives under current laboratory study which are numerous enough to tax the imagination.

234

Table 1   The major cephalosporins and cephamycins

First generation	Second generation	Third generation
Cephalothin (Keflin)	Cefamandole (Mandole)	Cefotaxime
Cephaloridine (Loridine)	Cefoxitin (Mefoxin)†	Cefoperazone
Cephapirin (Cefadyl)	Cefaclor (Ceclor)	Moxalactam†
Cefazolin (Ancef, Kefzol)	Cefuroxime*	Cefsulodin
Cephalexin (Keflex)		Ceftizoxime†
Cephradine (Anspor, Velosef)		
Cefadroxil (Duricef)		
Ceforanide*		
Cefonicid*		

* Still investigational or not available in the United States.
† Cephamycins.

MECHANISM OF ACTION

The penicillins and cephalosporins contain a unique beta lactam ring structure, the integrity of which is necessary for antimicrobial activity (Figure 1). It is curious that this unique ring structure is essentially confined in nature to these antibiotic substances. They also have a sulfur-containing ring which is characteristically different for the two classes of compounds, respectively termed 6-aminopenicillanic acid and 7-aminocephalosporanic acid. Enzymes classified as β-lactamases (penicillinases, cephalosporinases) hydrolyze the β-lactam ring and destroy the antimicrobial activity of the compound. The addition of a methoxy group to the cephalosporin nucleus prevents access of the enzymes to the β-lactam ring. The parent cephalosporins of this series of compounds are produced by a *Streptomyces* spp. instead of *Acremonium* and have been referred to as *cephamycins*. The Food and Drug Administration has ruled, however, that they are to be regarded as cephalosporins.

The cephalosporins, like the penicillins, act against susceptible bacteria by interfering with a terminal step in cell-wall synthesis which requires cross-linking of peptidoglycan strands. This process normally ensures rigidity of the bacterial cell wall and provides the characteristic shape of the cell. Tomasz has recently reviewed new evidence on how the β-lactam antibiotics kill and lyse bacteria and how they may attack different target enzymes and in different sequences (2). The major mechanism of bacterial resistance to the cephalosporins is the ability of the bacterial cell to produce a β-lactamase. These enzymes may be secreted extracellularly, as in *Staphylococcus*, or may be cell-bound, like the β-lactamases of gram-negative bacteria. The cephalosporins as a group are quite resistant to the β-lactamases secreted by staphylococci and are variably resistant to the β-lactamases of gram-negative bacilli. At least 11 enzymes with different properties and bacterial distribution have been described, some of which are normally specific to a single type of organism such as *P. aeruginosa*

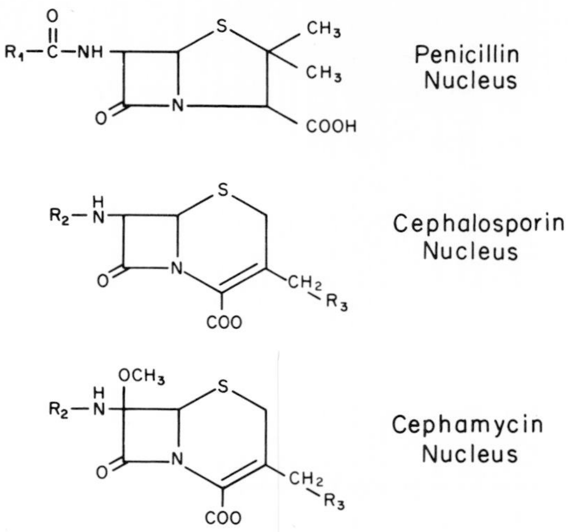

Figure 1   Basic molecular configuration of the penicillins and cephalosporins.

(3). Since the majority of these enzymes are plasmid-mediated, the genetic mechanism for conferring them on a particular bacterial cell can be transferred between bacteria of the same or different species. The various cephalosporins differ in their susceptibility to the different types of β-lactamases; clinically useful enzyme resistance must be essentially total and to one or several of the commonly occurring enzymes. Although the first-generation cephalosporins vary in their susceptibility to staphylococcal β-lactamase, there is no evidence that this fact is of any clinical significance (4). The first-generation cephalosporins are quite susceptible to the common β-lactamases of gram-negative bacteria. Although cephalexin and cephradine are somewhat less susceptible than the first-generation parenteral cephalosporins, any optimistic claims about the therapeutic advantages of this property for these agents or any of the other oral cephalosporins remains to be proved. Cefoxitin (like cefuroxime) is quite stable to β-lactamases, as are the third-generation cephalosporins. The resistance of cefamandole is considerably more restricted than that of cefoxitin; accordingly the antibacterial activity of cefamandole against cephalothin-resistant strains of gram-negative bacteria is generally influenced unfavorably by a high inoculum of bacteria in susceptibility testing, and a marked difference is observed between bacteriostatic and bactericidal concentrations (5). The β-lactamase resistance of a compound may be reflected by its activity on bacteria producing the enzymes (i.e., such bacteria would be susceptible), but since mechanisms other than β-lactamases also play a role in bacterial resistance, the resistance of a cephalosporin to β-lactamase does not ensure its antibacterial activity. Impermeability of the cell wall may be an important factor and may act concurrently with cell-bound lactamases by regulating the amount of antibiotic which gains access to the cell relative to the quantity capable of neutralization by the β-lactamase produced. In the case of *Pseudomonas*, impermeability is probably the most important mechanism of resistance. The dichotomy between cephalosporin resistance to β-lactamases and antibacterial activity is also well illustrated by the much greater β-lactamase resistance of cefoxitin than of cefamandole despite the inactivity of cefoxitin against *Haemophilus influenzae*. In fact, both cefamandole and cefaclor are relatively good substrates for some β-lactamases. The activity of a compound is thus the net result of its resistance to β-lactamase, its ability to penetrate the bacterial cell, and its effectiveness in competing with the enzymes responsible for cell-wall synthesis (6).

The newer, third-generation cephalosporins are a heterogeneous group with respect to chemical structure and antibacterial activity. Some are exceedingly active, inhibiting the majority of the Enterobacteriaceae and *Proteus* at one-tenth the concentration of cefazolin, cefamandole, or cefoxitin; several have activity against *P. aeruginosa* at attainable serum concentrations.

IN VITRO ACTIVITY

Any discussion of in vitro activity should begin with the understanding that composition of the culture medium and size of the bacterial inoculum used for susceptibility testing affect the result. Standardized methodology proposed by an international collaborative group represents an attempt to overcome this problem (7). Even so, technical variability persists, and valid comparisons are best reserved for simultaneous testing of different agents in a specific experimental setting. Susceptibility tests performed on solid agar medium in plates using various dilutions of antibiotic incorporated in the medium often show a higher degree of susceptibility than when the same organism is tested simultaneously in serial broth dilutions. This may be related to a lower inoculum commonly inherent in agar dilution testing or to the presence of a very small number of mutants which can survive and grow in broth but which would go unnoticed in the plate method.

The in vitro characteristics of the first-generation cephalosporins are similar. Although in some reports the differences may appear considerable, no evidence exists to impart clinical relevance to these observations. For example, cefazolin is reported by several investigators to be more active on a weight basis against *Escherichia coli* and *Klebsiella* than cephalothin and cephalexin, and the blood levels with usual doses are considerably higher than are characteristic for the latter two agents; however, cefazolin is more highly protein-bound, and if the susceptibility tests are done using serum as a diluent instead of broth, the antibacterial activity is reduced tenfold. Thus, a somewhat different clinical implication might be achieved from in vitro data, depending on the emphasis given to differences in methodology. All the cephalosporins are quite active against all gram-positive cocci except for group D enterococci (*Streptococcus bovis*, a nonenterococcal group D streptococcus is susceptible) and methicillin-resistant *Staphylococcus aureus*. The cephalosporins are also more regularly active than the penicillins against *Staph. epidermidis*. The first-generation cephalosporins are active against the majority of strains of *E. coli*, *K. pneumoniae*, *Proteus mirabilis*, *Salmonella*, and *Shigella*. Although occasional strains of *Enterobacter*, *Serratia*, *Acinetobacter*, *Citrobacter*, and indole-positive *Proteus* may be susceptible to these agents, for practical purposes they should be regarded as resistant unless the contrary has been proved. *P. aeruginosa* is also regularly resistant to the cephalosporins commercially available at present. Despite their activity against some anaerobic gram-negative bacilli, anaerobic cocci, and *Clostridium*, the resistance of *Bacteroides fragilis*, so commonly present in anaerobic infections, speaks against their usefulness for infections due to anaerobes generally.

The second-generation cephalosporins are somewhat less active against gram-positive cocci (probably of no clinical significance) and have extended activity against gram-negative bacilli. They are active against a large number of ampicillin- and cephalothin-resistant isolates, cefoxitin having the most reliable activity in our experience.

The primary in vitro advantage of cefamandole significant to physicians is greater activity against *Enterobacter* spp. and *H. influenzae*. The activity of cefamandole against *H. influenzae* and *H. parainfluenzae* is roughly comparable to that of ampicillin. Ampicillin-resistant strains are also susceptible to cefamandole, but the range of sensitivity is greater and some strains are relatively resistant. Since one-third of ampicillin-resistant strains were found resistant to cefamandole by one group, confidence in this agent must be based on susceptibility testing (8). The significance of the enhanced activity against *Enterobacter* is uncertain, because for most strains such activity can be demonstrated only by agar (not by broth) susceptibility testing methods (9). This discrepancy is due to the frequent presence of variants resistant to readily achievable blood levels that are not detected by agar dilution methods. Some of the cefamandole-resistant variants can inactivate the antibiotic whereas others do not. The clinical significance of this relatively high mutation rate to cefamandole resistance can be determined only by the bacteriological and clinical results of treatment in patients with infection due to these organisms (10). Similar observations have been made in connection with the susceptibility of *Klebsiella* to the first-generation cephalosporins (11). Although cefamandole is also more active against indole-positive *Proteus*, *Citrobacter*, and *Providencia*, marked variability in susceptibility is noted, depending upon inoculum size; the usefulness of this agent for infections caused by these bacteria must await adequate clinical experience. Reports of the activity of cefamandole against *B. fragilis* are quite variable, possibly reflecting methodological differences, but there is sufficient evidence to conclude that this organism is much more resistant to cefamandole than to cefoxitin.

Cefoxitin, at least partially as a result of its high resistance to β-lactamases, has a wider antibacterial spectrum than the first-generation agents and has good activity against enzyme-producing strains of *E. coli*, *Klebsiella*, indole-positive *Proteus*, *Citrobacter*, and *Providencia*. It is also active against somewhat less than half of the strains of *Serratia marcescens*, which is important because of the frequent resistance of this organism to carbenicillin. *Neisseria gonorrhoeae*, including the penicillin-resistant organisms, is also susceptible. The most unusual activity of cefoxitin is against *B. fragilis*, over 90 percent of strains being inhibited by easily achievable blood levels. It is also active against *Legionella pneumophila*. *Enterobacter* and *H. influenzae* are relatively resistant. Cefoxitin is relatively inactive against *Clostridium difficile*. Cases of pseudomembranous enterocolitis have been associated with cefoxitin administration.

Cefaclor is remarkable for its activity against both ampicillin-susceptible and β-lactamase–producing isolates of *H. influenzae*, although some strains of the latter may be resistant to usually achievable blood levels. Gray and Dillon (8) reported 17 of 27 ampicillin-resistant strains to be resistant to cefaclor. It is more active on a weight basis against some gram-negative bacilli than other oral first-generation cephalosporins, but this difference is not striking. *B. fragilis* is resistant. Cefaclor has good activity against gram-positive cocci. The instability of this compound in agar or buffer may render susceptibility results unreliable unless properly performed. Cefaclor is relatively susceptible to the β-lactamases of gram-negative bacteria.

PHARMACOKINETICS

For agents like the penicillins and cephalosporins which (except for such compounds as procaine penicillin and benzathine penicillin) are highly water-soluble with rapid renal clearance, the peak blood level is mainly a function of the dose, the rapidity of the administration, and the half-life of the compound. Attachment to binding sites on bacteria in a susceptible phase of cell-wall synthesis occurs rapidly and irreversibly. It is generally accepted that the peak blood level should be some small multiple of the minimum inhibitory concentration (MIC) of the infecting organism. The exact duration of the peak level or how often it should occur in patients with normal or compromised host defenses in order to affect patient outcome favorably is not clear. Some such relationship must exist, however. From a practical standpoint, it is of some importance because of the need to answer the question: What is a susceptible organism? A class of bacteria is usually regarded as susceptible if the majority of the individual representatives of that class are inhibited in standardized susceptibility testing procedures by readily achievable serum concentrations.

Although the susceptibility of bacteria to an antimicrobial agent and its peak blood levels are obviously important in the treatment of infection, the major determinants of patient outcome are host factors less readily measurable. The response of patients to therapy may not simplistically reflect the activity of a drug in vitro and its pharmacokinetics. Recently there has been considerable discussion regarding the importance of the minimal concentration of an antibacterial substance which shows a measurable effect on bacterial growth. Concentrations of antimicrobial substances below the level required to inhibit or kill may produce structural alterations in bacteria and can quite markedly reduce the number of bacteria in vitro compared with a population not similarly exposed. Host defense factors may also operate more favorably against bacteria exposed to subinhibitory concentrations, which are often as low as one-tenth of the conventional bacterial susceptibility, i.e., the MIC (12).

Conventional pharmacokinetic parameters include half-life, peak serum concentration, protein binding, extent of metabolism, and routes of excretion. Although serum levels are extensively used for predicting likelihood of a therapeutic response, it should be noted that only the free, non-protein-bound portion of the total serum concentration is microbiologically active and available for diffusion to the extravascular compartments. Both the protein binding of the different cephalosporins and the reported values for the specific agents vary widely. Thus, the protein binding of cephalothin has been reported by various authors to be 65 to 79 percent, of cefazolin 73 to 92 percent, of cephalexin 12 to 38 percent, and of cephradine 6 to 30 percent. Cefamandole and cefoxitin are 65 to 75 percent protein-bound. The role of protein binding in the ultimate distribution of a penicillin or cephalosporin to tissue compartments is still unsettled. The relationship of protein binding to therapeutic efficacy is even more controversial. The complexity of the problem is illustrated by the lack of a straight-line relationship between the localization of an antibiotic to plasma by protein binding (Table 2) and the effect of repeated administration and prolonged half-life on tissue concentrations (13–15). The apparent volume of distribution for all the cephalosporins indicates that at least 75 percent of the drug is located outside the vascular system, but this does not provide any information about localization in particular tissues. Direct measurements of drug concentrations in tissues are necessary to obtain this information, and the first- and second-generation agents (except possibly cefuroxime) do not exhibit significant differences in this regard.

All the oral cephalosporins are readily absorbed from the gastrointestinal tract, yield similar blood levels, manifest delayed absorption in the presence of food (resulting in lower and delayed peak serum levels), and appear rapidly in urine with 60 to 80 percent excretion within 6 h. The half-life of these agents

Table 2   The relation between plasma protein binding and amount of drug localized to plasma

Plasma protein binding, %	Drug amount in plasma, % of total
0	6.7
50	12
60	15
70	19
80	26
90	42
95	59
98	78
99	88
100	100

SOURCE: From Reference 13.

is quite similar except for that of cefadroxil, which is significantly prolonged. Although several studies have suggested less urinary recovery of cefaclor, this may be a reflection of the instability of the compound during collection and assay of the specimen. The metabolic degradation of cefaclor to inactive fragments in the presence of serum may contribute to this lowered recovery. The latter process also prevents accumulation of cefaclor even in the presence of markedly depressed renal function; even with a creatinine clearance of less than 10 ml/min, the half-life is only 2.5 to 2.8 h. The protein binding of cephalexin and cephradine is essentially identical; that of cefadroxil, slightly greater; and that of cefaclor, significantly higher.

The differences between the oral cephalosporins are small, with the possible exception of cefaclor because of its activity against *Haemophilus*. Since they are employed for mild or moderately severe illnesses, no differences have been demonstrated in their clinical performances. A prolonged half-life, as in the case of cefadroxil, might suggest dosing at less frequent intervals, but little critical data exist on this question for the cephalosporins individually or as a group. Cefadroxil is promoted mainly for urinary tract infections, with claims for successful treatment with once-a-day dosage or even a single dose. It is highly likely that the majority of uncomplicated lower tract infections in young adult females would respond similarly to any of the much less expensive older oral cephalosporins and even to a single dose of other still less expensive oral active agents. Comparative studies are lacking and would be of interest.

The pharmacokinetic parameters of cephalothin and cephapirin are essentially identical except for somewhat lower protein binding with the latter. They are also very similar for cefamandole and cefoxitin except that cefamandole has a slightly longer half-life with slightly higher mean peak serum levels after comparable doses intravenously. The dosage recommendations in the package inserts for cephalothin and cefamandole are very similar, and I have the impression (as was true for cephalothin during the early period of its use) that many physicians believe 4.0 g per day (1 g every 6 h) is adequate for the treatment of serious infections, which is what the package insert would imply. I am reasonably sure most infectious disease specialists would not support this practice and would prefer a daily dose of at least 6 g, and preferably 8 to 12 g, divided into four hourly doses. The dosages in the package insert for cefoxitin are more clearly presented and conform to the higher recommendations just stated.

The half-life of cefazolin is significantly longer than that of any of the other parenteral cephalosporins (except cefuroxime), and peak blood levels with comparable doses are correspondingly significantly higher. Adequate serum concentrations are also more prolonged. Cefazolin can therefore be administered at a dosage of 4.0 g per day, and in fact this dose need not be exceeded. This, combined with administration every 6 h for the treatment of serious infections, makes it highly cost-effective. Cephalothin and cephapirin are desacetylated in various tissues and body fluids to relatively inactive compounds. However, since the usual daily doses are higher than for cefazolin, it is not clear whether this has any therapeutic disadvantage. The urinary recovery of the parenteral cephalosporins is 80 to 85 percent, except for cephalothin and cephapirin, for which recovery is approximately 50 percent due to the excretion of inactive metabolites.

The cephalosporins are actively secreted into bile. Among the first-generation cephalosporins, cefazolin produces the most reliable levels; both cefamandole and cefoxitin produce biliary concentrations far in excess of those necessary to inhibit most bacteria present in the infected biliary tree. The relative importance in the treatment of biliary tract infections of biliary concentrations compared with those in the tissues of the biliary tract and liver is unknown. None of the cephalosporins achieve reliable concentrations in the common bile duct or gallbladder bile in the presence of biliary tract obstruction.

The cephalosporins diffuse well into serous cavities but penetrate poorly into the vitreous and aqueous humor and prostatic tissue. They are secreted in low concentrations in nursing mother's milk and cross the placenta with fetal serum concentrations roughly 10 percent of those of the mother. The cephalosporins penetrate poorly into the cerebrospinal fluid and are not acceptable choices for the treatment of central nervous system infections if other effective agents are available.

The protein binding and serum half-life of the third-generation cephalosporins under current investigation display wide differences, which, together with their antimicrobial variability, may create significant benefits in terms of frequency of administration and daily dosage. Even central nervous system infection may become amenable to cephalosporin treatment.

THERAPEUTIC INDICATIONS AND PROPHYLACTIC USES

Since the introduction of the cephalosporins, the therapeutic indications for them have been controversial. To some extent this may be related to their historical relationship to the penicillins, with which their properties so overlap (as well as to their overuse and cost). The major abuse of the cephalosporins consists of their use in categorical infections such as those of the urinary tract and respiratory tract for which other equally effective, safe, and certainly less expensive agents are available. The most reprehensible use is as a substitute for thoughtful clinical judgment and careful diagnostic studies in patients with fever of obscure origin. Another major abuse consists of their unnecessarily prolonged use for antimicrobial prophylaxis, but peer review and surgical education have reduced this practice substantially. *The Medical Letter* no longer states that "the cephalosporins are rarely the initial drugs of choice for any infection unless other antibiotics are unsuitable because of allergy or toxicity." It now gives several choices for the initial management of life-threatening bacteremia, including concurrent use of a cephalosporin with gentamicin or tobramycin (16). It nonetheless fails to indicate any cephalosporin as the drug of *first* choice for any infection while listing them as alternative drugs for 21 diseases caused by different bacteria. (In six of these diseases an aminoglycoside as a single agent is listed as the drug of first choice for patients not severely ill since for the severely ill patients "some consultants would add a penicillin or a cephalosporin.") It is therefore somewhat of an anachronism that the cephalosporins should account for 200 million dollars annually in drug sales in the United States and constitute 25 percent or greater of the average hospital pharmacy budget. It is often said that 80 percent of this use is for antimicrobial prophylaxis; here, *The Medical Letter* gives the cephalosporins roughly equal billing with the penicillins and with reasonably good foundation since the majority of controlled comparative trials concerned with prophylactic uses related to surgery have involved one or another of the cephalosporins (17). Much of the popularity of the first-generation cephalosporins in outpatient and surgical infections of mild or moderate severity is related to the belief that they have a broader spectrum of activity and are relatively free from adverse effects compared with other easily administered agents. Such a belief is obviously more compelling when a precise bacteriologic diagnosis is unavailable, which otherwise might enable the physician to tailor the antimicrobial therapy more specifically. Whether or not it is proper to treat these infections without culture, the fact remains that many, if not the majority, are treated in this fashion. If cultures were performed, results would often reveal a mixed bacterial flora, the most frequent components being staphylococci, streptococci, and Enterobacteriaceae. In 9000 isolates of gram-positive cocci over a 16-month period at UCLA, *Staph. aureus* accounted for 4600 and other gram-positive cocci uniformly susceptible to the first-generation cephalosporins for another 1100. All the resistant gram-positive cocci were group D enterococci. Except for *Staph. epidermidis*, the activity of the penicillinase-resistant penicillins and the cephalosporins was quite comparable for these organisms. During the same period, 11,700 (63 percent) of 18,800 gram-negative bacillary isolates were *E. coli*, *K. pneumoniae*, and *P. mirabilis*; cumulative percentages of susceptibilities of these organisms (plate dilution method) at concentrations of 2, 8, and 16 μg/ml for ampicillin were 23 percent, 58 percent, and 64 percent, and for the first-generation cephalosporins they were 21 percent, 81 percent, and 90 percent. It is often said, and may even be true, that agents other than cephalosporins with a narrower spectrum and equal efficacy should be used for treatment of an infection with a specific organism. Nonetheless, it is difficult to select a single agent, especially one which can be given orally, that is so free from adverse effects and broadly effective as a cephalosporin against the bacterial flora isolated from most outpatient and surgical infections.

Prudence dictates the use of antibiotic combinations before a specific bacteriologic diagnosis to broaden the spectrum of antimicrobial therapy in patients with serious sepsis and probable bacteremia, particularly in the immunocompromised host in whom mortality due to sepsis is both high and rapid. Neither a penicillin, a cephalosporin (including the second-generation broadened-spectrum cephalosporins), nor an aminoglycoside can be optimally employed as single-agent therapy before bacteriological results become available. The lack of evidence (except in the case of *Pseudomonas*) that combinations of antibiotics are more efficacious than single agents to which an organism is susceptible for the management of specific bacteremias is not helpful in designing the empirical treatment of sepsis before precise knowledge of the causative agent is available. Even after the organism causing bacteremia is known, the decision to discontinue an aminoglycoside in favor of a cephalosporin or a penicillin alone would by no means be unanimous unless aminoglycoside toxicity were an important consideration. The higher survival of patients with *P. aeruginosa* sepsis treated with synergistic combinations of antibiotics also prompts a desire to exploit similar activity for infections with other bacteria. Unfortunately, except for enhanced serum bactericidal activity the benefit of in vitro synergism in infections due to bacteria other than *Pseudomonas* has either not been demonstrated or has been only suggestive in terms of survival (18).

The common antibiotic combinations, which usually include an aminoglycoside, employed for the initial empirical treatment of serious sepsis, do not usually pose any problem except for an occasional patient at high risk for nephrotoxicity or ototoxicity. Although preliminary data for human beings are available showing the high effectiveness of such antibiotics as piperacillin and third-generation antipseudomonal cephalosporins used singly, considerably more experience is necessary to evaluate their efficacy compared with that when they are combined with an aminoglycoside. The role of problems related to the emergence of resistant organisms will be an important aspect of any future evaluation.

The empirical choice of drugs is often influenced somewhat by the probable source of infection. In a septic patient with community-acquired disease and a portal of entry likely to be the skin, soft tissues, or respiratory tract the causative organisms are often *Staph. aureus*, beta-hemolytic streptococci, or *Strep. pneumoniae*. These considerations would prompt a choice of penicillin G, a penicillinase-resistant penicillin, or a cephalosporin. Similarly, *Staph. aureus* or *K. pneumoniae* may be suspected as causal agents in acute pulmonary infections in patients with chronic lung disease, chronic alcoholism, diabetes mellitus, or postinfluenzal infections. A cephalosporin with or without an aminoglycoside would be logical choices for such individuals. In none of these instances, however, would a second-generation cephalosporin be a better choice than cefazolin, which actually has greater activity against *Staph. aureus* than the second-generation agents. For the patient with community-acquired aspiration pneumonia who is allergic to penicillin, cefoxitin could be regarded as an alternative choice to clindamycin in preference to the first-generation cephalosporins. For the patient with hospital-acquired pneumonia (where *Staph. aureus*, gram-negative bacilli, and anaerobes are usually regarded as the likely pathogens) cefoxitin, with or without an aminoglycoside, would be one of the antimicrobial options.

One approach to putting the cephalosporins in perspective might be to address questions which would relate the first-generation agents to those in the second generation. The following questions seem appropriate:

1 Are the new cephalosporins acceptable for the treatment of meningitis or other infections of the central nervous system?

2 Does the broadened spectrum of the second-generation agents make them useful for treating infections caused by *Enterobacter*, indole-positive *Proteus*, *Serratia*, or

Pseudomonas, for which the penicillins have traditionally been the cell-wall-active antimicrobials of choice?

3   Should the second-generation agents (usually combined with an aminoglycoside) replace the first-generation compounds for the empirical treatment of septicemia?

4   Can cefoxitin or cefamandole be regarded as an alternative choice for the management of abdominal or pelvic infections in which anaerobes, specifically *B. fragilis*, are likely to be involved?

5   Do cefamandole and cefaclor represent advances for the management of non-meningeal infections in which *H. influenzae* may be involved? To what extent should cefaclor replace ampicillin or amoxicillin with or without sulfonamides for the therapy of infections of the upper respiratory tract in infants and children?

6   Should the newer cephalosporins replace cefazolin for prophylactic uses?

Do the second-generation cephalosporins have a role in the treatment of meningitis?

The cephalosporins penetrate poorly into the cerebrospinal fluid, and cefamandole and cefoxitin are no exception. Conspicuous failures of cefamandole have been reported in *H. influenzae* meningitis (19). Meningitis due to bacteria susceptible to cephalosporins has developed during treatment of infections due to *Strep. pneumoniae, Listeria,* and *Neisseria meningitidis* (20). Such observations require that patients with bacteremic infections likely to involve the central nervous system, including *Staph. aureus* sepsis, should be closely observed for early evidence of such involvement which would dictate a change in antimicrobial therapy.

The role of second-generation cephalosporins in the treatment of infections due to *Enterobacter,* indole-positive *Proteus, Serratia,* and *Pseudomonas*

The reported experience with the second-generation cephalosporins, singly or combined with an aminoglycoside, in the treatment of serious infections due to *Enterobacter,* indole-positive *Proteus,* and *Serratia marcescens* (species against which they possess greater in vitro activity) is quite limited. The practical usefulness of the broadened spectrum of the second-generation cephalosporins is restricted primarily to:

1   The activity of cefoxitin against *B. fragilis* and about one-third of the strains of *S. marcescens*

2   The activity of cefoxitin and cefamandole against cephalothin-resistant strains of the common Enterobacteriaceae

3   The activity of cefaclor against *H. influenzae,* including many of the ampicillin-resistant strains

The last of these will be considered below. Ordinarily, the activity of a compound against a particular species of bacteria would not be regarded as particularly useful if it was confined to only one-third of the strains. Carbenicillin and ticarcillin, however, are the only beta lactam agents active against *Serratia marcescens*, and 40 percent of the strains are resistant to them. Therefore, providing a specific strain is susceptible, cefoxitin offers an important option for combination therapy with an aminoglycoside. Such combinations have been shown to be synergistic in vitro and have been used to treat *Serratia marcescens* endocarditis successfully (21). Both cefoxitin and cefamandole, particularly the former, are usually active against cephalothin-resistant strains of *E. coli*, *K. pneumoniae*, and *P. mirabilis*. Thus, in the unique hospital setting where the bacterial population tends to be resistant to the first-generation cephalosporins, these agents might be quite useful. For example, Meyer and associates (Table 3) tested the isolates from Wadsworth Veterans Hospital, where aminoglycoside and cephalosporin resistance has been unusually substantial for several years (22). Although cefoxitin appears superior for this group of isolates, the difference between cefamandole and cefoxitin may not always be so striking. More clinical experience is necessary to establish the efficacy of these agents in infections due to organisms resistant to the first-generation cephalosporins.

First- versus second-generation cephalosporins in the empirical treatment of septicemia

Unlike some of the third-generation antipseudomonal cephalosporins, the second-generation agents and the older cephalosporins have such serious gaps in their gram-negative coverage that they should not be used alone for empirical treatment of patients with suspected gram-negative septicemia. In fact, so little clinical experience is available in treating serious infections caused by *En-*

Table 3 Cephalothin-resistant (MIC ≥ 32 µg/ml) organisms selected from 1974 to 1978*

	% strains	Percent susceptible (MIC ≤ 32 µg/ml)	
		Cefamandole	Cefoxitin
E. coli	9	67	99
Klebsiella	38	11	89
P. aeruginosa	47	0	0
Serratia	50	0	34
Providencia	23	88	100
Proteus	11	27	63
Total no.†	178		

* 172 resistant to gentamicin (MIC ≥ 16 µg/ml).   † Total no. of strains; not a percent.
SOURCE: From Reference 22.

terobacter, indole-positive *Proteus*, and *Serratia* (organisms against which the second-generation agents possess greater in vitro activity) that it is difficult to justify the use of cefamandole or cefoxitin, alone or combined with an aminoglycoside, until the responsible organism has been identified and shown to be susceptible to the latter agents and resistant to the first-generation cephalosporins. A penicillin, notably carbenicillin or ticarcillin, combined with an aminoglycoside remains the best regimen for empiric treatment of serious sepsis possibly due to gram-negative bacteria. This is particularly true for the neutropenic patient. In the rather infrequent situation where a patient presents a history of penicillin allergy strong enough to preclude cautious trial of a penicillin, a choice would be necessary between chloramphenicol and a second-generation cephalosporin to combine with an aminoglycoside.

What is the role of second-generation cephalosporins in the management of abdominal and pelvic infections?

It is essential to recognize the mixed character of the bacterial flora associated with infections of the pulmonary, gastrointestinal, and female genitourinary systems, infections which usually arise in association with some damage to their epithelial surfaces. Anaerobes can be cultured from 75 to 95 percent of these infections, and *B. fragilis* is present in the vast majority. Facultative aerobic gram-negative bacilli are also present in the majority of such infections. The relative importance of these different classes of bacteria in the pathogenesis of the infections from which they can be isolated has not been defined. In fact, evidence from studies of experimental infections suggests that synergy between aerobes and anaerobes may be important, that early bacteremia and early mortality may be associated mainly with aerobic gram-negative bacilli, and that abscess formation and late bacteremia may be due mainly to anaerobes, especially *B. fragilis* (23). This complexity of bacterial flora and the variety of antimicrobials which are active against it has led to the use of quite an array of antibiotic regimens. One conclusion which appears well documented is that drug regimens with activity against both aerobic and anaerobic components of the bacterial flora are attended with statistically better results than those active against only one or the other (24). Obviously the optimal treatment should be based on the results of controlled trials in human subjects; comparisons based on retrospective case analyses (historical comparisons) are notoriously unreliable. Unfortunately, not only are comparative data difficult to obtain in numbers sufficient to establish statistical significance but their interpretation is also complicated because of the differences in host defenses and underlying disease, and especially because of the critical role which surgical therapy plays in the management of these infections. The assessment of drug efficacy may therefore be extremely difficult in such a setting. For example, how is one to interpret the favorable clinical and bacteriologic response of 92 percent of patients treated with cefamandole for anaerobic infections in which *B. fragilis* was involved when most strains of this organism are resistant in vitro? This may be rendered somewhat easier by the observations in an animal model of intraabdominal sepsis in which abscess formation is clearly related to *B. fragilis*. Abscesses formed in 35 percent, 7 percent, and 5 percent, respectively, of animals treated with cefamandole, cefoxitin, and clindamycin ($p \leq 0.05$ cefamandole versus cefoxitin). Abscess formation occurred in 100 percent of the untreated controls and in 38 percent and 50 percent of animals treated with cephalothin and cefazolin (p not specified) indicating that even cefamandole and the first-generation cephalosporins had some (about the same) therapeutic effect (23). Thus, the most relevant questions with respect to these and similar new agents still under study may not be whether they are simply effective, because all of them are more or less likely to be. The important question is whether a new compound which might be more cost-effective or present less toxicity is as effective as the optimal or most rational of the current regimens with which we have had extensive experience.

Only three studies known to me have developed data from this point of view. Stone et al. randomized patients with mixed anaerobic and aerobic peritoneal (124 patients) and soft tissue (39 patients) sepsis between regimens consisting of clindamycin and gentamicin, metronidazole and gentamicin, and cefamandole and erythromycin. In conjunction with surgical therapy the regimens were equally and highly effective in controlling the primary sepsis although recurrence of infection was significantly less frequent with the metronidazole-gentamicin regimen (greater effectiveness against anaerobes?) and the patients receiving gentamicin were the only ones who manifested nephrotoxicity (25). Tally et al. randomized patients with infections due to anaerobes (from the majority of which *B. fragilis* was isolated) between cefoxitin (20 patients, 6 of whom also received amikacin) and clindamycin-amikacin (18 patients). Both regimens were highly and equally efficacious (26). Drusano et al. compared cefoxitin (26 patients) with clindamycin-gentamicin (20 patients) for anaerobic abdominal and pelvic infections with equally good results. Four of six failures were due to poorly drained abscesses, and there was one instance of nephrotoxicity (in a clindamycin-gentamicin patient) requiring dialysis (27). Several points should be borne in mind when assessing the reports of various investigators concerning anaerobic infections of the abdomen and pelvis:

1 Patients with bacteremia originating in the gastrointestinal tract have a higher mortality rate than those whose bacteremia originates in the genital tract.

2 Mortality is considerably higher in patients over 40 years old.

3 In patients who have undergone appropriate surgical drainage, the outcome has been the same regardless of whether the antibiotic treatment was appropriate (based on the organisms isolated from associated bacteremias) or inappropriate.

It is not possible to take an unassailable position on the place of the second-generation cephalosporins in the treatment of abdominal and pelvic infections. The open studies, which are very difficult to interpret, support the effectiveness of both agents, but they are not very useful in a comparative evaluation with older chemotherapeutic regimens. The preliminary and evolving controlled prospective studies with cefoxitin are very encouraging with regard to its relative efficacy and lack of toxicity when compared with the clindamycin-gentamicin combination. This is especially true in the early management of these infections, before antibiotic therapy and exposure to the hospital environment may promote superinfection with *Pseudomonas*. Cefamandole cannot be similarly recommended in the absence of such comparative studies and its relative inactivity against *B. fragilis*. The significance of the latter finding tends to be confirmed by the complications due to this organism which have been observed when cefamandole has been used prophylactically (28). The major cause of antibiotic failure will continue to be inadequate drainage of abscesses.

Do cefamandole and cefaclor represent advances in the management of nonmeningeal infections in which *H. influenzae* may be involved?

Cefamandole, cefuroxime, and cefaclor are the first cephalosporins with useful activity against *H. influenzae*, including beta-lactamase–producing strains. The virulence of *H. influenzae* is associated with its capsule, most commonly type b, which interferes with phagocytosis. This type of *H. influenzae* is responsible for disease in infants and young children. The strains of *H. influenzae* causing disease in adults, which can also be isolated from the upper respiratory tract of 75 percent of healthy individuals, are unencapsulated, non-type-specific bacteria. A safe antibiotic effective against *Streptococcus pyogenes*, *Staph. aureus*, and *H. influenzae* is important for the treatment of infections of the skin and associated structures and the respiratory tract in infants and children. Otherwise, combination therapy with ampicillin and chloramphenicol for variable periods of time would ordinarily be required. Cefamandole has been effective in the treatment of *H. influenzae* bacteremia. The experience with cefaclor in skin and soft tissue infections due to *Haemophilus* is so limited that recommendations are difficult. Unfortunately, the evaluation of antibiotics in these infections is extremely difficult. For example, there are reports from two experienced investigators of cures with cefoxitin, an agent to which *H. influenzae* is resistant, of 14 patients with cellulitis (3 of whom had bacteremia) from whom *H. influenzae* was cultured. No failures were observed (29, 30). The use of either of these agents for cellulitis involving the face should be undertaken with due consideration of supervening meningitis. Even though cefamandole has been shown to be effective for *H. influenzae* bacteremia, many physicians would not wish to use a cephalosporin, especially in view of the unfavorable results with cefamandole in the treatment of meningitis due to *H. influenzae* (19).

Any consideration of oral antimicrobials for minor respiratory infections should emphasize that most pharyngotonsillitis is nonbacterial. When bacterial infection is involved, group A beta hemolytic streptococci are the most common pathogens. *H. influenzae* is an important consideration in infants and children but seldom in adults. Contrariwise, otitis media is generally associated with bacterial infection. *Strep. pneumoniae* is involved in about 75 percent of the cases and *H. influenzae* (usually nontypable) in about 20 percent of cases in both children and adults. Group A streptococci, *Neisseria meningitidis*, *Staph. aureus*, and *Neisseria catarrhalis* occur less commonly. In patients with bilateral otitis media the cultures from the two ears may be different in as many as 25 percent of patients. Bacteriologic diagnosis is an easy and inexpensive routine procedure for pharyngotonsillitis but is impractical for the management of otitis media. Culture of exudate from the ear canal is also unrewarding unless performed at the time of rupture of the tympanic membrane since colonizers quickly prevail in this exudate. Cultures of the pharynx or nasopharynx are also not helpful since they frequently reveal *Strep. pneumoniae* and non-type-specific *H. influenzae*.

The frequency of ampicillin-resistant *H. influenzae* is variable in different geographic locations. Clinical laboratories should routinely test for penicillinase-producing strains. The importance of using an antimicrobial agent initially to cover the possibility of an ampicillin-resistant strain will depend on the severity of the disease and the local epidemiologic considerations. The use of cefaclor for otitis media or sinusitis in which *H. influenzae* may be involved may not be indicated in areas where ampicillin resistance is uncommon.

The course of otitis media has undoubtedly been influenced favorably by antibiotics, and the need for mastoidectomy and the incidence of chronic tympanic perforations have both decreased during the antibiotic era. Although it would be attractive to assume that antibiotic therapy of otitis media might prevent some cases of meningitis, there is no direct evidence to confirm this supposition. From bacteriological considerations, otitis media should be treated with a regimen effective against both *Strep. pneumoniae* and *H. influenzae*. Penicillin, ampicillin, and erythromycin are effective in eradicating *Strep. pneumoniae* from otitis media; ampicillin and amoxacillin are effective in eradicating *H. influenzae*. The usual regimens employed for treatment of otitis media consist of ampicillin or amoxacillin orally or benzathine penicillin by injection. A sulfonamide such as sulfasoxazole is often given concurrently. Erythromycin combined with a sulfonamide is used for patients with a history of penicillin allergy. Trimethoprim-sulfamethoxazole has also been employed, but comparative studies have failed to demonstrate any significant advantage over a sulfonamide alone. Although cephalexin and cephradine have been permitted claims for efficacy in otitis media, their relative lack of activity against *H. influenzae* (and the questionable reliability of some of the data supporting the assertions) fail to support an enthusiastic endorsement of this claim.

It is helpful in evaluating the current clinical studies with new agents which may be recommended for otitis media to consider the natural course of the disease before specific chemotherapeutic agents became available. Spontaneous recovery often occurs without treatment and usually without antimicrobial agents. In 1940 Heller (31) evaluated 588 cases of otitis media and found that 50 percent subsided spontaneously. The drum ruptured spontaneously in 16 percent of cases, and myringotomy was performed in 34 percent. Mastoidectomy was performed in 3 percent of his cases. Otitis media therefore is a disease in which almost any form of therapy might be attended with a success rate well over 90 percent in terms of eventual patient outcome. In order to assess the comparative efficacy of different modalities of treatment critically, enormous numbers of patients would be necessary (as well as other methods of evaluation such as the appearance of the tympanic membrane, the rapidity of disappearance of organisms from repeated aspirates of middle ear fluid, and the frequency of relapse) to make the comparison precise. Clinical criteria such as duration of symptoms after institution of treatment, while supportive, will probably contribute little to the evaluation of relative efficacy. Middle ear effusion, i.e., sterile fluid collections after effective treatment of acute otitis media, is estimated to occur in 50 percent of patients. Although it may be more frequent after otitis media due to *H. influenzae*, it is equally frequent after ampicillin, amoxacillin, erythromycin-sulfa, or cotrimoxazole treatment of the acute otitis (32). These observations might also suggest that minimizing the cost of treatment is especially productive if many patients may need to be treated to prevent complications or sequelae in a few.

The comparative microbiological and clinical effectiveness of cefaclor in controlling otitis media in which ampicillin-resistant *H. influenzae* is a participant (the only compelling reason to use this agent) remains to be assessed. Although cefaclor has been shown to be effective for otitis media in open studies, the data from comparative studies with the older therapeutic regimens are not yet available. At a symposium held in September 1978 to introduce cefaclor three groups of investigators reported on 80 cases of acute otitis media, from 29 of which *H. influenzae* was cultured. Two ampicillin-resistant strains were observed; one was cured with cefaclor (but one ampicillin-susceptible strain in another patient persisted after cefaclor treatment), and the code for the other patient had not yet been broken (33–35). This illustrates the difficulties in generating the clinical data to support claims for efficacy in an illness such as this, but anything less is unacceptable. At best, the only justifiable current recommendation for cefaclor in view of its relatively high cost is that it is the agent of choice if a cephalosporin is required (which should not be frequently) for the treatment of acute otitis media.

The place for cefamandole and cefaclor in the treatment of pulmonary infections in adults, in which gram-positive cocci and *H. influenzae* may be involved, is even less clear. Open noncomparative studies leave little doubt about their effectiveness, but there is little need for another agent without obvious advantages for the management of acute bacterial pneumonia which responds extremely well to the penicillins and first-generation cephalosporins and which is rarely caused by *H. influenzae*. The major question relevant to disease in adults, because it will be an area of considerable promotional effort by industry, concerns the usefulness of cefaclor in the treatment of acute exacerbations of infection in patients with chronic obstructive pulmonary disease (COPD) from whose sputum *H. influenzae* can be cultured. The first question is whether in a particular patient these organisms which can be cultured from a specimen of sputum really come from the tracheobronchial tree since they can be isolated from the nasopharynx of most healthy people. The next question is whether these non-type-specific organisms are primarily fellow travelers or play an important role in acute exacerbations of disease. They can certainly be isolated repeatedly, even by transtracheal aspiration, over many months from the respiratory tract of such patients during periods of stable chronic disease as well as during acute exacerbations of infection.

In addition to adequate serum and sputum levels of an antibiotic and good activity of the agent against the potential bacterial pathogens, other factors contribute to clinical improvement of these patients. Furthermore, acute exacerbations of infection in these patients respond well to ampicillin, tetracycline, and trimethoprim-sulfamethoxazole, which are outstandingly safe and inexpensive agents. The comparative merit of a new agent is very difficult to evaluate under such circumstances. Until the results from satisfactory comparative studies become available, it is difficult to see how cefaclor can be recommended except for patients who are allergic to penicillin or who have failed to respond to other older agents.

H. influenzae is an infrequent cause of serious infections in adults with the exception of immunocompromised hosts. It may be involved in sinusitis; cause suppurative arthritis, pneumonias, or cellulitis; or be associated with bacteremia. Were such an infection to be due to an ampicillin-resistant strain, cefamandole would be an attractive alternative to chloramphenicol. It should be obvious, however, that cefamandole or cefaclor seldom would be necessary for the treatment of infections in adults based upon a consideration of *H. influenzae*; and even then it would be necessary only if the patient were likely to have an ampicillin-resistant strain proved susceptible to these cephalosporins.

The relative merits of second- and first-generation cephalosporins for prophylactic uses

Any indication which accounts for such a large portion of antibiotic use as prophylaxis is bound to draw the attention of both physicians and those who purvey antibiotics to the medical community. It is therefore particularly important that physicians critically evaluate the goals of prophylaxis, the type of bacteria most likely to cause the infection one seeks to prevent, data supporting the usefulness of one regimen over another, cost comparisons, and potential adverse effects (both to the individual patient and to the hospital environment). The last of these includes the role of prophylactic use in the development of infections due to unusual organisms as well as delay in the detection of intraabdominal or pelvic infections. Considerable sentiment exists for the claim that antibiotics which are valuable for the treatment of clinical infections should not be used for prophylaxis, in order to minimize the emergence and spread in the hospital environment of resistant organisms. This is particularly applicable to the second-generation cephalosporins and the likelihood that resistance may appear among gram-negative bacteria against which they are active. Nothing less than controlled comparative studies should be acceptable for evaluation of antimicrobials for prophylaxis, and even then careful attention should be paid to the conditions of the study. For example, there should be similarity in the competence of the participating surgeons, the technical features of the procedure with regard to drains, the degree of contamination or hematoma formation, the structures subjected to surgery, etc. It does not seem appropriate to combine cases in which normal or inflamed appendixes are removed with cases in which the appendix is gangrenous or ruptured; operations on the biliary tract or stomach should not be analyzed with those performed on the colon; and the favorable results of prophylaxis in vaginal hysterectomy cannot be transposed to abdominal hysterectomy (36).

Fortunately, the prophylactic uses of the cephalosporins have been reserved almost exclusively for surgical patients. Utilization reviews have greatly improved the major abuses of surgical prophylaxis; namely, use in clean procedures, starting antibiotics after a surgical procedure rather than immediately preoperatively, and unnecessarily prolonged administration.

The goals of prophylaxis, or at least what is likely to be achieved, may be quite variable. General agreement exists that even the small number of infections complicating clean procedures such as the insertion of prosthetic orthopedic devices, vascular grafts, or prosthetic heart valves are so catastrophic that antibiotic prophylaxis is indicated. If this prophylaxis is associated with negligible adverse effects, such a proposition seems acceptable but there may be a point at which the perfection of techniques and experience of surgeons renders antibiotic prophylaxis essentially ineffective. Contrariwise, infectious complications of colon surgery must be a fact of life. Reducing these complications to a 5 to 8 percent level may represent the maximal or at least optimal accomplishment. Further investigation might be directed mainly to improving cost effectiveness and minimizing adverse effects.

If one recognizes the difficulty of establishing the efficacy of prophylactic antibiotics in procedures, such as hip arthroplasty, where the incidence of early infection is extremely low, it should not be surprising that comparative studies to determine the best chemoprophylaxis regimen to accomplish this do not exist. The major determinant of the choice of antibiotics for such a procedure has been the in vitro susceptibility of the bacteria most likely to be involved in the infection and the demonstration of adequate concentrations of a particular agent in the blood and tissues involved for the duration of a surgical procedure. *Staph. aureus* and *Staph. epidermidis* are the major bacteria involved in postoperative infections complicating orthopedic and cardiovascular procedures. Since about 15 percent of strains of *Staph. epidermidis* are resistant to the penicillinase-resistant penicillins, the cephalosporins are recommended for prophylaxis. Thanks to its longer effective serum concentration, its more dependable tissue concentrations during the surgical procedure, and its cost effectiveness, cefazolin has become the agent of choice. The presence of minority populations in some cultures of *Staph. epidermidis* which are resistant to the cephalosporins as well as the penicillinase-resistant penicillins has prompted speculation whether other active agents (e.g., gentamicin, vancomycin, or rifampin) should be added to the usual cephalosporin prophylaxis. Reliable answers to this problem, if it is a problem, are unlikely to be forthcoming soon, but the new cephalosporins do not offer any advantages in this regard over the first-generation agents and cefazolin in particular.

The other major areas of chemoprophylaxis where the cephalosporins have been extensively tested are in abdominal and pelvic surgery. The administration of antibiotics to the patient who is undergoing surgery and who has a gangrenous or ruptured appendix or who has suffered trauma with a perforated viscus should not be regarded as chemoprophylaxis but as therapy of early infection.

The bacterial contamination associated with these and similar events is certain to be gross and mixed and will always include anaerobes; clostridia must be considered, and facultative aerobic gram-negative bacilli such as *Pseudomonas* susceptible mainly to the aminoglycosides are possibilities. Significant gaps in the antimicrobial activity of all of the penicillins, cephalosporins, clindamycin, and chloramphenicol weigh against their use alone for the initial treatment of such serious situations. Carbenicillin or ticarcillin, clindamycin, cefoxitin, or chloramphenicol combined with an aminoglycoside would be recommended for these patients unless the risk factors for an aminoglycoside were exceptional. The first-generation cephalosporins and cefamandole are not good choices because of their inactivity against anaerobes. Clostridial myonecrosis has been observed during treatment with cephalothin, admittedly usually at inadequate dosage levels, and bacteremia due to *B. fragilis* has been reported in patients receiving cefamandole (37, 38).

That properly given antimicrobial agents can decrease the infectious complications of colorectal surgery and, in selected cases, those complicating biliary tract and gastric surgery is not in question. The question is which agents and how they should be given. This discussion is limited to the role of the cephalosporins. Not unexpectedly in colorectal surgery a regimen which includes antibiotics active against both aerobic gram-negative bacilli and anaerobic bacteria has proved most effective, and it is clear that the reduction of anaerobic bacteria in the bowel heavily influences the incidence of postoperative infection. Two successful and widely used oral regimens are neomycin-erythromycin and kanamycin-metronidazole. It is not clear whether parenterally administered agents are more effective and have fewer adverse effects than an oral regimen. A recent study comparing kanamycin-metronidazole orally and parenterally was highly favorable to the latter route, but additional studies are needed (38).

Since 1969, when cephaloridine was reported to decrease the rate of wound and/or intraabdominal infections complicating colorectal surgery, many surgeons have shown an almost supernatural devotion to certain cephalosporins for chemoprophylaxis. Although a comparison of cefazolin-neomycin-erythromycin with neomycin-erythromycin showed a lower infection rate in the former the difference was not statistically significant (25). A recent controlled prospective Veterans Administration Cooperative study found no difference in the infectious complications in patients given oral neomycin-erythromycin with or without cephalothin (39). Nonetheless, the survey of surgical practices related to colorectal surgery performed as a part of this study revealed that 49 percent of the surgeons responding employed parenteral antibiotics, predominantly cephalosporins, in addition to oral antibiotics. It is unlikely that this will change. Considerations related both to the antimicrobial spectrum and to cost weigh heavily against cefamandole for this purpose (28). One would hesitate to recommend cefoxitin in addition to, or as a substitute for, the older regimens for chemoprophylaxis considering the slight further reduction which might be possible in infectious complications, the risks to the individual patient, and the hospital environment and cost/benefit factors. I am aware that cefoxitin is being used for this purpose and can understand the arguments in its favor, but since resistance to the cephalosporins has occurred readily in the past, until controlled studies attest to a significant benefit for cefoxitin compared with cefazolin, a benefit itself unsettled, prophylactic use should be restricted. On the other hand, in a situation where the risk of septic complications is markedly increased (e.g., a perforated appendix or a ruptured diverticulum) and recognizing that antibiotics should be started preoperatively if they are to be effective, cefoxitin with an aminoglycoside would be an appropriate regimen (therapeutic rather than prophylactic).

Since bacteria are commonly recovered from bile and peritoneal fluid during biliary tract surgery or appendectomies, cephalosporins have been widely used prophylactically. No evidence exists to support the superiority of one cephalosporin over another or over ampicillin (except for the cost effectiveness of cefazolin and ampicillin).

Several well-controlled studies of prophylaxis in gynecologic surgery have demonstrated a significant reduction in wound infections complicating vaginal hysterectomy. The antibiotic-treated groups in the various studies have shown wound or cuff infections in 0 to 9 percent of patients (40). Various first-generation cephalosporins, ampicillin, penicillin G, tetracycline, and metronidazole have been employed. Other reports concern the favorable effect of prophylaxis on wound infections and endometritis after cesarean section, although it is not so clear that the less frequent serious infectious complications of cesarean section are similarly influenced. Although the results of clinical trials of antibiotic prophylaxis in women undergoing elective abdominal hysterectomy are not entirely in agreement, the studies with adequate sample sizes have shown a significant reduction in pelvic and wound infections in the group receiving antibiotics. No studies with the second-generation cephalosporins are available, but the comments interdicting cefoxitin as a prophylactic agent in gastrointestinal surgery are even more compelling for gynecologic surgery. The role of anaerobes, particularly *B. fragilis* or other anaerobes resistant to the first-generation cephalosporins or ampicillin, may be less important in postoperative pelvic infection than in postoperative infections after gastrointestinal surgery. The first-generation cephalosporins—cefazolin in particular because of its cost effectiveness—should remain the agents of choice for prophylaxis in gynecologic surgery until new studies emerge proving another regimen to be superior. The antibiotic should be started shortly before surgery and should be discontinued 24 h thereafter (41).

ADVERSE EFFECTS

This discussion of adverse effects will be limited to local reactions, enhancement of aminoglycoside nephrotoxicity, and reactions of patients with a history of penicillin allergy. All cephalosporins can be administered intramuscularly for a few doses, but only cefazolin is realistically an intramuscular agent. The others are primarily intravenous compounds because of the daily dose required for effective treatment and/or the pain incident to intramuscular injection. Comparative studies of phlebitis have reported conflicting results.

Clinically significant nephrotoxicity due to the cephalosporins (except for cephaloridine) is extremely infrequent, but several controlled studies in human subjects have demonstrated a significantly greater incidence of nephrotoxicity in patients concurrently treated with cephalothin and an aminoglycoside (gentamicin, tobramycin) than in similar patients treated with a combination of a penicillin and an aminoglycoside or cephalothin and a penicillin (42). In the largest study, that of the European Organization for Research in the Treatment of Cancer, in which the cooperative investigator group was concerned primarily with the treatment of sepsis in neutropenic patients, the higher incidence of nephrotoxicity in the patients receiving cephalothin and an aminoglycoside was especially striking in those over 50 years old, suggesting a possible association with preexisting renal disease (43). A similar association was not found in one of the other studies (44). The EORTC group subsequently introduced into their controlled study a regimen consisting of cefazolin-carbenicillin-aminoglycoside, which has shown no greater incidence of nephrotoxicity than regimens which do not contain a cephalosporin. One might alternately conclude that cefazolin either does not potentiate aminoglycoside nephrotoxicity or that carbenicillin in some way, for example, by promoting osmotic diuresis, exerts an ameliorating effect on the potentiating phenomenon. Whatever the explanation, it would seem prudent to avoid the cephalothin-aminoglycoside combination and use cefazolin when the cephalosporin-aminoglycoside regimen is indicated. No data are available with respect to the second- and third-generation cephalosporins. Since patients receiving any cephalosporin combined with an aminoglycoside generally have serious sepsis, which itself may be complicated by renal impairment, and are often receiving other potentially nephrotoxic drugs including potent diuretics, their renal function should be monitored with special care.

The relative freedom of the cephalosporins from adverse effects believed to be related to hypersensitivity constitutes one of their major indications. About 5 percent of courses of penicillin are associated with "allergic" manifestations and about 0.02 percent with immediate life-threatening reactions. Although the incidence of similar reactions associated with administration of the cephalosporins seems lower, according to anecdotal experience, the data base is considerably less precise than for the penicillins. The investigation and use of cephalosporins such as cefoxitin and cefuroxime in large numbers of patients for the treatment of sexually transmitted diseases, especially gonococcal infection, may provide better data on this point. No resolution is available of the question of "cross reactivity" between penicillins and cephalosporins, since cross-reacting antibodies are frequently present in patients who experience no adverse effects. The risk of allergic reactions to a cephalosporin in patients with a history of penicillin allergy is probably higher than in patients without such a history, but whether this is related to cross reactivity or to the increased likelihood in this population group of drug reactions to unrelated compounds is unknown. Recent preliminary results indicate that patients with positive skin tests to both major and minor penicillin determinant antigens, who would be at high risk for immediate and serious reactions to penicillin, can be given a cephalosporin without adverse effects (45). This is not to say that patients with a history of penicillin allergy should be given a cephalosporin cavalierly. Since anaphylactic reactions may occur in such patients, prudence dictates that another equally effective agent be sought, especially if the other compound is equally safe and the illness is not too serious. If the illness is serious and the alternate agents have inherent toxicity, a cephalosporin may be tried under conditions where adequate supportive treatment can be given should an immediate reaction occur. Neutropenia and elevated serum levels of transaminases are much less common in association with cephalosporin therapy than with the penicillinase-resistant penicillins. Interstitial nephritis, such as occurs following methicillin therapy, is not well documented. Pseudomembranous enterocolitis, usually related to an enterotoxin produced by C. difficile and appearing during and after a variety of antibiotics, has been observed in association with several of the cephalosporins, including the second-generation compounds.

REFERENCES

1 **Winston DJ, Young LS:** Cephalosporins, in Kagan BM (ed): Antimicrobial Therapy, ed. 3. Philadelphia, Saunders, 1980.

2 **Tomasz A:** Mechanism of the irreversible antimicrobial effects of penicillins. Annu Rev Microbiol 33:113, 1979.

3 **Matthew M:** Plasma-mediated beta lactamases of gram-negative bacteria: Properties and distribution. J Antimicrob Chemotherapy 5:349, 1979.

4 **Kaye D et al:** Treatment of experimental Staphylococcus aureus abscesses: Comparison of cefazolin, cephalothin, cefoxitin, and cefamandole. Antimicrob Agents Chemotherapy 15:200, 1979.

5 **Duye A et al:** Comparative activity of two newer cephalosporins, cefoxitin and cephalothin, against selected Enterobacteriaceae and correlation with enzymatic resistance mechanisms. J Antimicrob Chemotherapy 5:293, 1979.

6 **Richmond MH:** Factors influencing the antibacterial action of beta lactam antibiotics. J Antimicrob Chemotherapy 4 (B):1, 1978.

7 **Ericsson HM, Sherris JC:** Antibiotic sensitivity testing: Report of an international collaborative study. Acta Pathol Microbiol Scand (B) Suppl 217:1, 1971.

8 **Gray BM, Dillon HC:** In vitro evaluation of cefaclor for Hemophilus influenzae infection. 19th Intersci Conf Antimicrob Agents Chemotherapy, abstract 744, 1979.

9 **Adams HG et al:** In vitro evaluation of cefoxitin and cefamandole. Antimicrob Agents Chemotherapy 9:1019, 1976.

10 **Findell CM, Sherris JC:** Susceptibility of Enterobacter to cefamandole: Evidence for a high mutation rate to resistance. Antimicrob Agents Chemotherapy 9:970, 1976.

11 **Benner EJ et al:** Natural and acquired resistance of Klebsiella aerobacter to cephalothin and cephaloridine. Proc Soc Exp Biol Med 119:536, 1965.

12 **Washington JA:** The effects and significance of subminimal inhibitory concentrations of antibiotics. Rev Infect Dis 1:781, 1979.

13 **Borgå O:** Läkemedelsinteraktion vid proteinbindning och distribution. Soci komm läkemedelsinform 1:24, 1974.

14 **Gerding DN et al:** Cephalosporins and aminoglycoside concentrations in peritoneal capsular fluid in rabbits. Antimicrob Agents Chemotherapy 10:902, 1976.

15 **Carbon C et al:** Penetration of cefazolin, cephaloridine, and cefamandole into interstitial fluid in rabbits. Antimicrob Agents Chemotherapy 11:594, 1977.

16 The choice of antimicrobial drugs. Med Lett Drugs Ther 22:5, 1980.

17 Antimicrobial prophylaxis for surgery. Med Lett Drugs Ther 21:73, 1979.

18 **Winston DJ et al:** Antimicrobial therapy of septicemia due to Klebsiella pneumoniae in neutropenic rats. J Infect Dis 139:377, 1979.

19 **Steinberg EA et al:** Failure of cefamandole in treatment of meningitis due to Haemophilus influenzae type b. J Infect Dis Suppl 137:S180, 1978.

20 **Mangi RJ et al:** Development of meningitis during cephalothin therapy. Ann Intern Med 78:347, 1973.

21 **Cooper R, Mills J:** Serratia endocarditis. A follow-up report. Arch Intern Med 140:199, 1980.

22 **Louie MH et al:** In vitro susceptibility of cephalothin-resistant Enterobacteriaceae and Pseudomonas aeruginosa to a 1-oxa cephalosporin (LY127935 or moxalactam), amikacin and selected cephalosporins. Curr Microbiol 3, 1980 (in press).

23 **Onderdonk AB et al:** Microbial synergy in experimental intra-abdominal abscess. Infect Immun 13:22, 1976.

24 **Chow AW et al:** A double-blind comparison of clindamycin with penicillin plus chloramphenicol in the treatment of septic abortion. J Infect Dis Suppl 135:S35, 1977.

25 **Stone HH et al:** Clinical comparison of antibiotic combinations in mixed aerobic-anaerobic surgical sepsis. 19th Intersci Conf

Antimicrob Agents Chemotherapy, abstract 657, 1979.

26 **Tally FP et al:** Randomized comparison of cefoxitin and clindamycin in suspected anaerobic sepsis. *19th Intersci Conf Antimicrobial Agents Chemotherapy*, abstract 822, 1979.

27 **Drusano G et al:** Cefoxitin vs. clindamycin/gentamicin for penicillin-resistant anaerobic infection. *19th Intersci Conf Antimicrobial Agents Chemotherapy*, abstract 823, 1979.

28 **Slama TG et al:** Comparative efficacy of prophylactic cephalothin and cefamandole for elective colon surgery. Results of a prospective, randomized, double-blind study. *Am J Surg* 137:593, 1979.

29 **Santos JI et al:** Cefoxitin (cx) vs. multiple antibiotic therapy (MRx) for cellulitis in children. *19th Intersci Conf Antimicrobial Agents Chemotherapy*, abstract 522, 1979.

30 **Rodriguez WJ et al:** Evaluation of cefoxitin in susceptible pediatric infections. *Intersci Conf Antimicrobial Agents Chemotherapy*, abstract 523, 1979.

31 **Heller G:** Statistical study of otitis media in children. *J Pediatr* 17:322, 1940.

32 **Schwartz RH, Rodriguez WJ:** The incidence of middle ear effusion (MEE) following antimicrobial therapy for acute otitis media (AOM). *19th Intersci Conf Antimicrobial Agents Chemotherapy*, abstract 527, 1979.

33 **Rodriguez WJ et al:** Cefaclor in the treatment of susceptible infections in infants and children. *Postgrad Med J* 55 (suppl 4):35, 1979.

34 **Jacobson JA et al:** Evaluation of cefaclor and amoxycillin in the treatment of acute otitis media. *Postgrad Med J* 55 (suppl 4):39, 1979.

35 **Bluestone CD et al:** Cefaclor compared with amoxycillin in acute otitis media with effusion: A preliminary report. *Postgrad Med J* 55(suppl 4):42, 1979.

36 **Hirschmann JV, Inui TS:** Antimicrobial prophylaxis: A critique of recent trials. *Rev Infect Dis* 2:1, 1980.

37 **Mohr JA et al:** Clostridial myonecrosis during cephalosporin prophylaxis. *JAMA* 239:847, 1978.

38 **Keighley MRB et al:** Comparison between systemic and oral antimicrobial prophylaxis in colorectal surgery. *Lancet* 1:894, 1979.

39 **Condon RE et al:** Preoperative prophylactic cephalothin fails to control septic complications of colorectal operations: Results of controlled clinical trial. A Veterans Administration cooperative study. *Am J Surg* 137:68, 1979.

40 **Chodak GW, Plaut ME:** Wound infections and systemic antibiotic prophylaxis in gynecologic surgery. *Obstet Gynecol* 51:123, 1978.

41 **Polk BF et al:** Randomized clinical trial of perioperative cefazolin in preventing infection after hysterectomy. *Lancet* 1:437, 1980.

42 **Marsh FP:** Do cephalosporins potentiate or antagonize aminoglycoside nephrotoxicity? *J Antimicrob Chemotherapy* 4:103, 1978.

43 **European Organization for Research and Treatment of Cancer:** Three antibiotic regimens in the treatment of infection in febrile granulocytopenic patients with cancer. *J Infect Dis* 137:14, 1978.

44 **Wade JC et al:** Cephalothin plus an aminoglycoside is more nephrotoxic than methicillin plus an aminoglycoside. *Lancet* 2:604, 1978.

45 **Solley GO et al:** Evaluation of skin tests in patients with penicillin allergy. *J Allergy Clin Immunol* 63:184, 1979.

The diagnosis and treatment of gangrenous and crepitant cellulitis

DAVID S. FEINGOLD

INTRODUCTION

Infections considered in this chapter are those involving soft tissues (the skin, subcutaneous tissue, fascia, and skeletal muscle) and characterized by extensive necrosis of tissue and/or production of discernible quantities of tissue gas. Infections, so defined, constitute a small subset of pyodermas and cellulitides but an often alarming and confusing subset. They are dramatic in the speed with which they may progress, the extent of necrosis, and the frequent requirement for aggressive surgery. They are confusing in both delineation and classification, as will be amplified below.

The purpose of this article is to present an updated scheme of classification of gangrenous and crepitant cellulitis with a discussion of some of the clinical findings, especially those helpful for differential diagnosis. Emphasis will be placed on bedside observations and rapid diagnostic measures which can guide the internist, dermatologist, or surgeon to prompt, proper therapy.

CLASSIFICATION

Gangrenous and crepitant cellulitis are difficult to classify since they are clinical entities rather than specific bacterial infections. One clinical syndrome (e.g., necrotizing fasciitis) may be caused by more than one bacterium. The same microorganism(s) can cause infections in different loci or tissue compartments with strikingly different characteristics (e.g., *Clostridium perfringens* infections of subcutaneous tissues or muscle) and a single organism (e.g., phycomycetes) can infect several tissue compartments. To render classification even more difficult the clinical findings in different entities may overlap.

Some of the vagaries of older classification schemes were probably caused by deficiencies in clinical microbiology, especially in the isolation of anaerobic

Supported by the Veterans Administration.

bacteria. Modern techniques for the culture and identification of anaerobes became generally available during the 1960s and 1970s and resulted in a better understanding of the pathogenic role of these organisms, especially in mixed infections with facultative bacteria. In 1938 Altemeier argued convincingly that the putrid odor of pus in peritonitis was due to anaerobes (1). Yet today, one still hears physicians refer to putrid *"Escherichia coli* pus," a concept generated by failure to identify anaerobes in mixed infections. In fact, a putrid aroma from tissue infection should be an important clue implicating anaerobic microorganisms, although the metabolites generating the odor have not been identified.

The clinical entities covered in this article, including a partial listing of synonyms, are shown in Table 1. Discussion will be selective rather than exhaustive. Pyodermas such as impetigo or erysipelas will not be discussed, nor will the usual cellulitis caused primarily by *Staphylococcus aureus* and/or *Strep-*

Table 1   Gangrenous and crepitant cellulitis—clinical entities

Clinical entity	Synonyms
Clostridial cellulitis*	Clostridial crepitant cellulitis, anaerobic cellulitis
Nonclostridial crepitant cellulitis*	Nonclostridial anaerobic cellulitis, anaerobic cellulitis, aerobic aerogenic infections, gas abscess
Necrotizing fasciitis*	Hemolytic streptococcal gangrene, streptococcal necrotizing fasciitis, gangrenous or necrotizing erysipelas, perineal phlegmon, Fournier's gangrene (or syndrome)
Progressive bacterial synergistic gangrene	Bacterial synergistic gangrene, Meleney's gangrene, postoperative progressive gangrene
Clostridial myonecrosis*†	Gas gangrene
Nonclostridial myositis*†	(Anaerobic) streptococcal myositis, nonclostridial gas gangrene
Synergistic necrotizing cellulitis*†	Nonclostridial gas gangrene, synergistic nonclostridial anaerobic myonecrosis, perineal phlegmon, Fournier's gangrene (or syndrome), necrotizing cutaneous myositis, gram-negative anaerobic cutaneous gangrene
Phycomycotic gangrenous cellulitis†	Necrotizing cutaneous phycomycosis
Infected vascular gangrene*†	
Pyoderma gangrenosum	
Miscellaneous types of gangrenous cellulitis in the compromised host*	

* Tissue gas accumulation may be detected in these entities.
† Muscle involvement is prominent in these entities.

tococcus pyogenes. Small areas of skin necrosis may be seen with these infections, but necrosis is rarely prominent.

SOME UNIFYING PRINCIPLES

Predisposing conditions

Since the infections under discussion constitute a heterogeneous group, it is best to identify predisposing conditions in each case; a few general comments are in order, however.

With some exceptions gangrenous and crepitant cellulitis are not caused by opportunistic organisms, which usually cause infection only in hosts with impaired humoral or cellular defense mechanisms. Instead primarily local tissue conditions related to the type and dose of bacterial contamination determine infection. Any of dozens of conditions which create a local decrease in oxidation-reduction potential (E_h) predispose to anaerobic infections. Since potentially pathogenic anaerobes are the predominant microflora on mucous membranes, there is usually no paucity of pathogens and the vast majority of infections with anaerobes is endogenous. Conditions of hypoxia also foster infection with facultative bacteria since polymorphonuclear leukocytes function poorly under decreased oxygen tension. In turn, the growth of facultative organisms may further lower E_h, allowing growth of more fastidious anaerobes. Thus, one sees most gangrenous and crepitant cellulitis in areas of trauma, surgery, ischemia, burns, malignancy, foreign body introduction, or other forms of tissue damage.

Diabetes is present in an impressively large number of the patients with the types of infection under discussion. Infected vascular gangrene (2), synergistic necrotizing cellulitis (3), nonclostridial crepitant cellulitis (4), necrotizing fasciitis (5), and phycomycotic gangrenous cellulitis (6) have all been reported to be more common in patients with diabetes mellitus. One reason for this association is the premature atherosclerosis and resultant ischemic vascular disease which occurs in this condition. However, the frequency with which diabetes is reported [e.g., 75 percent of the 63 patients with synergistic necrotizing cellulitis reported by Stone and Martin (3)] suggests that other factors may also be involved, such as small blood vessel disease, poor leukocyte function related to acidosis or hyperglycemia, or other chemical abnormalities in tissues of the diabetic patient. It has also been suggested that generation of tissue gas is more prominent when such infections occur in the setting of diabetes mellitus. A facultative gram-negative bacillus may be capable of producing tissue gas in a patient with diabetes because rapid bacterial growth is favored both by the presence of abundant substrate for fermentation and by the inhibition of leukocyte function due to relative local hypoxia.

The gas

Gas in infected tissues is an important clinical sign since it almost always reflects tissue hypoxia, which must be remedied to control the infection. The end products of aerobic metabolism in which energy sources are completely oxidized, usually via iron-containing cytochrome systems and environmental oxygen, are carbon dioxide and water. Carbon dioxide will rarely accumulate in tissue because of its ready solubility in aqueous media. Less complete oxidation is carried out by anaerobic and facultative bacteria. Incomplete oxidation can result in accumulation of a diverse array of intermediates including gaseous components. Hydrogen, which is the major gas produced by intestinal bacteria (7), is about 40 times less water-soluble than is carbon dioxide (8). Almost certainly hydrogen is the major tissue gas in crepitant cellulitis (9), although this has not been established. Hydrogen is not a noxious agent in tissues except indirectly by increasing tissue pressure and hence anoxia. However, its presence usually means that rapid bacterial multiplication is taking place at a low E_h.

Rarely, extensive soft tissue gas may occur after trauma, and its presence may falsely suggest crepitant infection (10). Gas resulting from trauma occurs within a few hours of the trauma and in the absence of signs and symptoms of bacterial infection. Subcutaneous emphysema can also result from a ruptured alveolus or hollow viscus.

The gangrene

Extensive tissue necrosis (gangrene), the other unifying sign of the infections being discussed, can take several forms: (1) necrosis primarily of skin, as in progressive bacterial synergistic gangrene; (2) necrosis of subcutaneous tissue, as in clostridial or nonclostridial crepitant cellulitis; (3) necrosis of fascia, as in necrotizing fasciitis; or (4) necrosis of muscle, as in the myonecrosis of gas gangrene.

The necrosis associated with infection can occur by several mechanisms. Pressure necrosis is seen secondary to extensive inflammatory swelling possibly augmented by tissue gas. This is most prominent when the affected area is relatively contained by fascia or skin. Digital necrosis and necrosis of male genitals secondary to rapidly progressing cellulitis probably reflect simple pressure necrosis from intense inflammation in closed spaces.

Necrosis may result from thrombosis of vessels; anaerobic organisms may be especially capable of causing vascular thrombosis, possibly by production of heparinase (11) or by direct acceleration of coagulation (12). Phycomycetes directly invade vessels causing vascular occlusion. Extracellular enzymes or toxins produced by bacteria, such as the lecithinase produced by *C. perfringens*, may be a prominent cause of tissue necrosis. There is substantial evidence that certain organisms in combination can cause extensive gangrene whereas the individual organisms do not (13). The presence of extensive tissue necrosis, whatever the cause, is of central importance for therapy. Necrotic tissue usually must be removed since neither host defenses nor antibiotics are effective in necrotic areas. Myonecrosis may be a unique problem since it has been suggested that products of muscle degradation cause important cardiovascular toxicities, but this is poorly documented.

Necrosis of tissue may also occur from several noninfectious causes, the most important of which are ischemia and thermal burns. Other causes include necrosis from tissue infiltration of sympathomimetic amines (14) or pitressin

(15), beta blockade employed in the treatment of patients with hypertension (16), or as a rare complication of the use of coumarin derivatives (17). Disseminated intravascular coagulation may cause extensive dermal necrosis, as may vascular occlusion with cryoprecipitates.

Therapy

It should be clear from the foregoing that surgery is almost always essential for treatment of these infections. Necrotic tissue must be removed, and the hypoxia, responsible for gas production, must be remedied. Also, adequate exposure of the infected site is required for diagnosis. Some surgeons have classified cellulitis according to the requisite surgical therapy (18). For example, extensive surgical incision and drainage is required in clostridial cellulitis and necrotizing fasciitis while excision of tissue is required in gas gangrene and synergistic necrotizing cellulitis.

CLOSTRIDIAL CELLULITIS

Following local trauma or surgery resulting in devitalized tissue, wound contamination (especially from bowel flora) can result in a necrotizing infection of subcutaneous tissue caused by clostridia, usually *C. perfringens*. Certain of the clinical features of this entity are outlined in Table 2. Often the wound is unimpressive except for serous to purulent drainage. Pain is mild and toxicity is minimal. The presence of tissue gas, which may be extensive, leads the physician to consider the differential diagnosis of crepitant soft tissue infections (starred items in Table 1).

Surgical exploration of the wound is mandatory at this point to establish the diagnosis. The involved soft tissue must be laid open so that the underlying muscle can be examined. With clostridial cellulitis the surgeon is reassured by normal appearing muscle; necrotic tissue should be removed, pus drained, and

Table 2 Clinical features of crepitant cellulitis

	Clostridial cellulitis	*Nonclostridial crepitant cellulitis*
Pain	Little	Little
Tissue gas	Extensive	Extensive
Skin changes	Little	Little
Odor of exudate	Foul at times	Foul regularly
Systemic toxicity	Little	Moderate
Progression	May be rapid	May be rapid
Predisposing factors	Local trauma	Diabetes frequently present

the wound opened widely. Examination of a Gram-stained smear of the exudate is required for presumptive bacteriologic diagnosis and initiation of appropriate antibiotic therapy. The finding of thick gram-positive rods consistent with clostridia confirms the diagnosis of clostridial cellulitis. High doses of penicillin (10 to 20 million units daily in the adult) intravenously are indicated.

NONCLOSTRIDIAL CREPITANT CELLULITIS

A crepitant, usually minimally toxic infection similar to clostridial cellulitis can be caused by a variety of anaerobic and facultative bacteria including peptostreptococci, *Bacteroides* spp., or Enterobacteriaceae. Cultures frequently reveal more than one bacterial agent. Involvement of anaerobes is responsible for the foul smell not usually found with pure clostridial cellulitis. Patients with diabetes appear to be more susceptible to this syndrome of nonclostridial crepitant cellulitis. Among diabetic patients with crepitant cellulitis, bacteria other than clostridia are much more frequent than *Clostridia* spp. as etiologic agents (2, 19). Even *Staph. aureus* alone has been reported to cause the syndrome in the setting of diabetes (20).

Operative findings are similar to those found in clostridial cellulitis. After debridement of necrotic tissue, antibiotic therapy should initially be based on the results of examination of Gram-stained smears of exudate while awaiting the determination of antimicrobial susceptibilities of the organisms isolated. Antibiotic combinations are usually indicated. If the area is contaminated by bowel flora, clindamycin or chloramphenicol is often a good choice for one of the therapeutic agents in the combination. If Enterobacteriaceae are implicated, an aminoglycoside or a cephalosporin (cefoxitin or cefamandole) is probably best.

NECROTIZING FASCIITIS

This entity is an acute necrotizing cellulitis involving primarily the superficial fascia and subcutaneous tissue and resulting in extensive undermining of surrounding structures. The diagnosis is made at operation by visualizing the necrotic fascia and demonstrating the undermining. The latter is evidenced by the lack of resistance to passage of a blunt instrument along the fascial plane. It is a rare, life-threatening infection, originally described by Meleney (21) as hemolytic streptococcal gangrene, presumably caused by the group A streptococcus (*Strep. pyogenes*). Although his clinical description was accurate, it is now clear that many other organisms as well can cause the same complex of signs and symptoms (outlined in Table 3). Some authors use the term *streptococcal gangrene* when this entity is caused by *Strep. pyogenes* and *necrotizing fasciitis* when other organisms are involved. It is important to distinguish clearly between streptococcal gangrene (a type of necrotizing fasciitis) and streptococcal myositis, an entity caused by anaerobic streptococci, discussed below.

Most cases of necrotizing fasciitis follow minor trauma or surgery. Of 44 cases reported in 1970 from Parkland Hospital in Dallas (5), 8 occurred with no history of trauma, 27 followed minor trauma, and 9 occurred after surgery; 8 of

Table 3   Clinical features of necrotizing fasciitis

	Streptococcal (Gp A) infection	*Mixed infection*
Pain	Painful	Painful
Tissue gas	Absent	May be present
Odor to exudate	Little	Foul
Skin changes	Variable amounts of erythema, anesthesia and gangrene; cellulitis with extensive undermining due to necrosis of fascia and subcutaneous tissue	Variable amounts of erythema, anesthesia, and gangrene; cellulitis with extensive undermining due to necrosis of fascia and subcutaneous tissue
Systemic toxicity	Prominent	Prominent
Progression	Rapid	Rapid
Predisposing factors	Spontaneous or secondary to minor trauma	Often secondary to abdominal surgery or perirectal infection

the 44 patients had diabetes mellitus. From 19 of the 44 patients (43 percent) group A streptococci, alone or with other organisms, were cultured. In the Parkland Hospital series a staphylococcus was isolated from 19 patients and gram-negative bacilli from only 5; anaerobic organisms were not reported. The most detailed recording of the bacteriology in necrotizing fasciitis was reported by Giuliano et al. from San Francisco in a prospective study of 16 patients from whose lesions careful aerobic and anaerobic cultures, as well as gram-stained smears, were taken at the time of operative debridement (22). Cultures from 3 of their 16 patients contained group A streptococci either alone or with staphylococci. The remaining 13 revealed facultative bacteria (non-group A streptococci and Enterobacteriaceae) and an anaerobe. They suggested that there are two forms of the disease: one caused by *Strep. pyogenes* and the other due to a synergistic infection of facultative and anaerobic bacteria. Unusual organisms, including group B streptococci (23) and *Haemophilus aphrophilus* (24), have been reported to be etiologic agents in rare cases of necrotizing fasciitis.

The infection spreads rapidly along the superficial fascia. In the early stage of the infection the skin may appear normal. As blood supply to the skin is compromised, erythema and edema occur and may progress to cyanosis, blister formation, and eventually gangrene. Skin anesthesia occurs as the subcutaneous gangrene progresses. Complete involvement of the fascial envelope of the muscle may result in muscle necrosis, but this is uncommon. Crepitus was present in only 2 of 44 cases in the Parkland Hospital series. Foul odor was not commented upon in most reports but certainly may occur when anaerobic bacteria are present. Hypocalcemia may occur and is most likely related to extensive fat necrosis. Bacteremia is common, especially with *Strep. pyogenes*, and metastatic foci of infection may be seen (25). When the lower extremity is involved, differentiation of early necrotizing fasciitis from phlegmasia cerulea dolens may be difficult.

The presence of crepitus will usually initiate prompt surgical exploration. Since crepitus is usually absent in necrotizing fasciitis, the clue for surgical intervention is an acutely ill patient with a cellulitis that is spreading in spite of antibiotic therapy. The cellulitis may be atypical because of cutaneous anesthesia in the absence of cutaneous gangrene or because of extensive cutaneous gangrene. On incision, the diagnosis is made from the findings of extensive undermining of skin by necrotic superficial fascia and subcutaneous tissue. Delay in diagnosis results in increased mortality. In the 30 percent of patients in the Parkland Hospital series who died, the average time from onset to diagnosis and treatment was 7 days. In those surviving the interval was 4 days (5).

At the time of incision, findings on examination of Gram-stained smears of the exudate can guide antibiotic therapy, but surgical treatment is most important. Longitudinal incisions are used to unroof all undermined areas and to remove all necrotic subcutaneous tissue and fascia. Repeated debridements may be necessary. Secondary closure and/or skin grafting is usually required after the infection is cured (26).

Fournier's gangrene (or syndrome) is usually considered as a form of necrotizing fasciitis that initially affects the perineum and genitalia. Infection spreads rapidly between Buck's fascia and the dartos fascia of the genitals or its extensions, Colles' fascia of the perineum, and Scarpa's fascia of the abdominal wall (28). Either group A streptococci or mixed bacterial species may be the etiology. Fournier's original description (27) was of an idiopathic or spontaneous gangrene unassociated with anorectal disease or major trauma. *Strep. pyogenes* is the usual etiologic agent in this spontaneous variant. The mixed infections frequently follow localized infections in the anorectal region, anorectal surgical procedures, or problems associated with extravasation of urine.

Like other forms of necrotizing fasciitis, Fournier's gangrene is an acute process with extensive fascial and subcutaneous necrosis that may become further complicated by extensive gangrene of the scrotum and penis. However, especially in obese diabetic patients, fulminant spread up the abdominal wall can be observed. With multiplication of anaerobic bacteria, tissue gas and foul-smelling exudate may be prominent. The infections may be limited to perineum and scrotum.

The principles of treatment outlined for necrotizing fasciitis apply as well to infections in the anogenital region, with the added consideration that reconstruction of the genitalia may be a major problem if extensive dermal gangrene has ensued.

PROGRESSIVE BACTERIAL SYNERGISTIC GANGRENE (PBSG)

Meleney described and named this unusual but distinctive ulcerating lesion (29). *Postoperative progressive gangrene* might be a better term, since the infection almost always begins at an abdominal or thoracic operative wound site and frequently where wire retention sutures are employed. The appearance and bacteriology are characteristic. A few days to a few weeks after operation a tender, red, swollen, and indurated area develops near the wound. This slowly evolves into a shaggy ulcer with gangrenous purple margins fading into an edematous, erythematous periphery. Without treatment the course is one of relentless spread to enormous size with severe pain but little accompanying toxicity. Multiple fistulous tracts and extensive undermining may occur; this lesion, also described by Meleney, has been called *chronic burrowing ulcer* or *Meleney's ulcer*.

Descriptions of PBSG consistently report the same bacteriology. From the gangrenous margins, a streptococcus (peptostreptococcus) requiring a low E_h is isolated and *Staph. aureus* or Enterobacteriaceae are cultured from the central portion. This bacterial combination in experimental animals causes gangrenous lesions which cannot be reproduced by the individual bacteria (29). Pyoderma gangrenosum is the lesion that most closely resembles PBSG. It usually occurs in a different setting, lacks the characteristic bacterial findings observed in PBSG, and does not respond to antibiotic therapy.

Some authors state that excision of the lesion is required to cure PBSG, but cures have been reported with antibiotics. Thus, penicillin plus oxacillin or an aminoglycoside, depending on the organisms cultured, along with debridement and removal of involved sutures, should be tried before more radical excision.

CLOSTRIDIAL MYONECROSIS

"Where there is any doubt whether a lesion is clostridial gas gangrene, then it almost certainly is not . . . ." (19). This statement emphasizes the dramatic nature of clostridial myonecrosis or gas gangrene. Some of the features are summarized in Table 4; the disease has been very well described in the literature (20, 30, 31).

Clostridia can cause a wide range of soft tissue infections but the acute, toxemic, and fulminating course of clostridial myonecrosis must be appreciated. It occurs in areas of penetrating trauma, at operative sites (especially when associated with bowel surgery), as a complication of thermal burns, and, rarely, without any antecedent trauma (usually associated with intraabdominal disorders such as bowel infarctions, perforation, or neoplasm). Pain at the involved site, rapid progression, and extreme toxicity are characteristic. Crepitus, although not prominent, can at times be detected, and gas, often in a feathery pattern (about fascial planes and muscle bundles), can be seen in the tissues by x-ray. Initially the skin may be tense and blanched. It then takes on a bronze discoloration and develops grey-brown bullae with areas of necrosis. The rapid tissue necrosis which occurs is caused by clostridial toxins. The systemic toxicity is thought to relate to breakdown products of muscle, although they have not been identified. The paucity of leukocytes in the serosanguinous exudate may relate to cell lysis caused by lecithinases. If a mixed infection is present, the odor may be foul. In true gas gangrene, however, the odor is

Table 4 Some clinical features of clostridial myonecrosis and nonclostridial myositis

	Clostridial myonecrosis	*Nonclostridial myositis*
Onset	Acute (at times even less than 12–24 h following injury)	Over several days
Pain	Severe and appears early	May be severe later in illness
Tissue gas	Present but may not be prominent	Present only rarely (slight amount)
Odor of exudate	Not particularly foul or prominent	Variable; may be foul
Cutaneous changes	Bronze discoloration, edema, bullae, and necrosis	Erythema
Systemic toxicity	Extreme and evident early; may be decreased promptly by use of hyperbaric oxygen	Present only late; not benefited by hyperbaric oxygen
Progression	Extremely rapid	Variable; may be slow
Findings on Gram-stained smear of exudate	Thick, gram-positive rods and few neutrophiles	Gram-positive cocci in chains and numerous neutrophiles
Predisposing factors	Local trauma, surgery, or bowel pathology	Local trauma

described as sweet or "mousy." *C. perfringens* is the most common species of clostridia causing gas gangrene but *C. septicum*, *C. novyi*, *C. hemolyticum*, and other clostridial species can cause the syndrome.

As the infection rapidly progresses with attendant systemic toxicity, hypotension may become prominent. Renal failure may then rapidly develop. Bacteremia is uncommon, occurring in only 10 to 15 percent of cases (32, 33). Hemolytic anemia (due to intravascular hemolysis) may occur, particularly in patients with associated bacteremia, but it is uncommon. This complication is more likely to develop in patients with uterine infection (septic abortion) where a complicating bacteremia is more frequent and more likely to be intense.

Clostridial bacteremia without any soft tissue infection or other apparent sequelae is quite common. This bacterial species was found in 2.6 percent of 2168 positive blood cultures obtained over a 14-month period at Cook County Hospital in Chicago, and in more than half the instances the bacteremia seemed only incidental to the primary clinical illness (34). Clostridial bacteremia with metastatic foci of infection, including myonecrosis, also occurs spontaneously; it often is associated with perforations of the colon and carcinomas of the colon (35). Even silent, nonperforating carcinomas can cause bacteremia and metastatic myonecrosis and cellulitis; in this setting, C. *septicum* is often the clostridial species involved (36, 37).

The diagnosis of clostridial myonecrosis can be suspected from the clinical picture. Incision in the involved area is required for confirmation. Early, incised muscle appears pale, friable, and edematous and then becomes brick red. It does not bleed from the cut surface, contractility is lost, and gas is often found between the muscle bundles. On Gram-stained smears of exudate large gram-positive rods are seen. In gas gangrene due to C. *perfringens*, spores are not seen, but occasionally they may be observed when this syndrome is due to other toxigenic species of clostridia.

The management of clostridial gas gangrene includes three essential elements: (1) surgical debridement (usually extensive, aimed at removal of all involved muscle, and frequently requiring multiple incisions and fasciotomies or amputation), (2) intravenous penicillin G (12 to 20 million units daily in divided doses every 4 h), and (3) supportive measures (monitoring of central venous pressure, serum electrolytes, and renal function; volume expansion; treatment of renal failure and marked anemia). Hyperbaric oxygen, if immediately available, may have a role in treatment, particularly when gas gangrene involves the trunk and where extensive excision of involved muscle would be mutilating (38). In this situation, decompression by fasciotomy and antibiotic therapy with intravenous penicillin should be instituted promptly. Shortly thereafter exposure to 100% oxygen at 3 atm pressure may cause a substantial decrease in clinical manifestations ascribed to toxicity. Oxygen itself does not neutralize clostridial toxins but does inhibit further toxin production. The use of hyperbaric oxygen permits a staged approach to surgery in that it may limit the necessity to remove certain masses of muscle tissue initially by allowing a delay in removal of muscle of uncertain viability. In no other anaerobic infection is the apparent response to hyperbaric oxygen nearly as salutory; the response to hyperbaric oxygen may also help in differential diagnosis (39). The value of polyvalent clostridial antitoxin in the treatment of clinical gas gangrene has never been established even though it was used almost routinely in treatment for decades. It is now no longer commercially available for clinical use.

NONCLOSTRIDIAL MYOSITIS

Myositis or myonecrosis can be caused by a variety of bacteria other than clostridia. The anaerobic streptococcus (peptostreptococcus) is the most common cause. Clinically, anaerobic streptococcal myositis usually acts like subacute gas gangrene. Following local trauma there is a latent period of several days before edema and erythema are observed. Systemic toxicity is minimal. Local pain is not prominent but may become marked late in the infection when the process accelerates rapidly. Gas may be present but is not a prominent feature.

It is essential to distinguish anaerobic streptococcal myositis from gas gangrene. Whereas involved muscle must be removed in gas gangrene, such is not the case in streptococcal myositis. Although discolored and edematous, the muscle reacts to stimuli with contraction and may recover (40). In addition to the slower pace of the process, the finding of a purulent exudate containing gram-positive cocci helps in diagnosis. The foul smell of the exudate in anaerobic streptococcal myositis contrasts with the usual finding in gas gangrene. Darke et al. (39) state that the differential diagnosis may be difficult but that hyperbaric oxygen therapy, when available, is extremely helpful in making this differentiation; only clostridial infections responded favorably.

Treatment should consist of surgical decompression, drainage of purulent material, and limited removal of grossly necrotic tissue but not of muscle with lesser degrees of involvement. Intravenous penicillin is the antibiotic of choice in the treatment of peptostreptococcal infections.

Often other organisms are found along with the anaerobic streptococci. The presence of mixed infection may modify the course and makes these syndromes especially difficult to classify. For example, group A streptococci may also be present and, according to Finegold (20), may make the disease more acute with cutaneous erythema, bright red muscles, and frequently a terminal septicemia. In the presence of enteric gram-negative bacilli, in addition to the anaerobes, synergistic necrotizing cellulitis may be the most appropriate label.

SYNERGISTIC NECROTIZING CELLULITIS

Table 5 lists the major features of synergistic necrotizing cellulitis, described and named by Stone and Martin in 1972 in a group of 63 patients from Grady Memorial Hospital (3). The patients commonly had diabetes mellitus and cardiorenal disease and were obese. The process usually started in the vicinity of the perineum (perirectal abscess in 40 percent) or in the leg and resulted in an

Table 5 Clinical features of synergistic necrotizing cellulitis

Pain	Severe; marked tenderness
Tissue gas	Crepitus in 25% of cases
Odor of exudate	Foul
Cutaneous changes	Patchy secondary necrosis of skin and subcutaneous tissues
Changes in deeper structures	Extensive muscle and fascial necrosis
Systemic toxicity	Marked
Progression	Rapid progression once infection established
Findings on Gram-stained smear of exudate	"Dishwater" pus with mixture of organisms on Gram-stained smear and culture
Predisposing factors	Diabetes mellitus; perirectal infections
Mortality	76%

acute, painful, toxemic infection. Inspection of the lesions showed variable areas of patchy skin necrosis. In most of the cases there were one or more small ulcers draining "dishwater," foul-smelling pus. Local crepitus was observed in 25 percent of the patients. On incision there was always extensive fascial and muscle necrosis in the absence of major vascular embarrassment. The primary and prominent involvement of muscle in synergistic necrotizing cellulitis differentiates it from necrotizing fasciitis. Subcutaneous tissue and skin are affected secondarily. In necrotizing fasciitis there is primary involvement of superficial fascia and subcutaneous tissue with undermining and secondary skin necrosis.

In all cases reported by Stone and Martin (3) a facultative bacterium (a gram-negative enteric bacillus) *and* an anaerobe (peptostreptococcus and/or *Bacteroides* spp.) were isolated. However, the suggestion that a synergistic necrosis of muscle occurs in this entity is conjectural. Blood cultures were positive in approximately one-half of the patients.

Some of the cases described as Fournier's gangrene (or syndrome) are probably best included with synergistic necrotizing cellulitis. Without myonecrosis, Fournier's gangrene would fit under the heading of necrotizing fasciitis; with myonecrosis, it might best be considered as a form of synergistic necrotizing cellulitis.

The majority (76 percent) of the patients described from Grady Memorial Hospital died (3). The only survivors were those who underwent extensive debridement and drainage of involved tissue. Amputation, where possible, was most effective. This along with aggressive antibiotic therapy and treatment of diabetic acidosis is essential.

PHYCOMYCOTIC GANGRENOUS CELLULITIS

The Phycomycetes are a class of fungi characterized by broad, branching, nonseptate hyphae. *Rhizopus*, *Mucor*, and *Absidia* are pathogenic genera of the family Mucoraceae within the class. Infections with these organisms have been called *mucormycosis* as well as phycomycosis. Spores of these organisms are ubiquitous. Serious pulmonary, rhinocerebral, or disseminated infection by Phycomycetes occurs in severely compromised hosts, especially those with leukemia, lymphoma, or diabetes mellitus (41, 42). In an experimental rabbit model phycomycosis occurred after challenge with the fungus only when diabetes had been induced earlier (43). Phycomycotic gangrenous cellulitis has been reported in patients with extensive burn wounds (44), in patients in whom elasticized adhesive tape has been applied over operative or other wounds (45–48), and in compromised hosts, especially those with diabetes, with some form of cutaneous tissue injury (6).

Bruck reported 22 cases of phycomycotic infection of burn wounds (44). The development of ulceration, tenderness, purplish nodules, black spots, swelling, and fever were characteristic. In over a quarter of the patients dissemination of the fungus occurred resulting in death.

The problem with elasticized adhesive tape (Elastoplast) was first reported in 1978 (45, 46). Twenty-three patients, apparently normal immunologically, developed cutaneous lesions which varied from erythematous papules, pustules,

Table 6   Clinical features of phycomycotic gangrenous cellulitis

Pain	Little pain
Tissue gas	Absent
Odor of exudate	Absent
Cutaneous changes	Central black necrosis or ulcer; may have peripheral raised purple margin; cutaneous anesthesia always present
Systemic toxicity	Variable; little fever
Progression	Rapid
Predisposing factors	Diabetes mellitus; infection initiated at site of local trauma

and plaques to necrosis of skin with ulceration and eschar and abscess formation. Epidemiological investigation revealed that contamination of the bandages with *Rhizopus* spp. occurred during manufacture and was not eliminated by ethylene oxide sterilization of the rolled bandages. The manufacturer and the Center for Disease Control recommended that these bandages "should not be used over open wounds and should not come in contact with sterile fields if the maintenance of sterility is vital" (46). This recommendation is especially important in infection-prone patients. In normal individuals the infections promptly cleared after removal of the bandages. At most, minor debridement was required. In some cases the phycomycotic infections were confused with allergic contact dermatitis.

In the absence of burns, rapidly progressive phycomycotic gangrenous cellulitis is rare but extremely important to keep in mind since diagnosis is difficult, and prompt, aggressive therapy is essential. In 1976 Wilson et al. reported two new cases and culled nine similar ones from the literature (6). Seven of the patients had diabetes mellitus; in three of them the diabetes was reported to have been under good control. At the site of infection, all had prior tissue injury including compound fractures, open or closed soft tissue trauma, or ileostomy stomas. The characteristic lesion is a central, black, anesthetic ulcer or area of necrosis surrounded by a purple, edematous margin (Table 6). Spread may be extremely rapid. Toxicity may be severe. Four of the eleven patients died. The hallmark of this infection is vascular invasion by hyphae, thrombosis, and necrosis extending to involve all tissue compartments.

The diagnosis of phycomycotic gangrenous cellulitis is difficult on several counts. Since the disease is rare, it has been seen by few physicians. There may be overlap in the clinical picture between this entity, necrotizing fasciitis, and synergistic necrotizing cellulitis. If crepitus is present, one can eliminate phycomycosis from the differential diagnosis. Phycomycosis may be seen complicating previous bacterial infection, or bacterial growth may occur in the necrotic tissue so only bacteria may be seen on Gram-stained smears of exudate;

the fungi stain poorly. The fungi are frequently not isolated from phycomycotic lesions. Furthermore, the organisms may be grown from normal skin or occur as laboratory contaminants; thus, one cannot count on the usual microbiologic diagnostic measures.

Diagnosis is best made from histologic examination of a biopsy specimen, usually of the margin of the lesion, showing the nonseptate hyphae invading tissue. The hematoxylin-eosin stain does not reliably identify fungi in tissue sections. Periodic-acid-Schiff (PAS) and methenamine-silver stains are most helpful. Rapid diagnosis by microscopic examination of a frozen section is possible (44). The hyphae can at times be identified microscopically in crushed tissue specimens treated with 20% potassium hydroxide.

Bruck et al. (44) found that phycomycotic infection of burns was best treated by an aggressive surgical approach, reserving amphotericin B for multifocal involvement or disseminated infection. Progressive phycomycotic cellulitis must be treated by removal of the involved tissue and parenteral therapy with amphotericin B.

INFECTED VASCULAR GANGRENE

Infection frequently complicates the distal gangrene seen with peripheral vascular insufficiency. Often it is marked by the development of a putrid odor and accumulation of gas in the gangrenous tissue. Pain and/or systemic toxicity, which are usually minimal, can become prominent, especially if cellulitis spreads to viable tissue. Bessman and Wagner reviewed the hospital admission of 278 diabetic patients with vascular gangrene or neuropathic ulcerative problems (2). Tissue gas was present in 49 (17 percent). Although infection was usually limited to the gangrenous tissue, neglect at times resulted in spreading gangrenous cellulitis. Evolution of this type of process into true gas gangrene has been reported (30, 49).

Louie et al. at Tufts–New England Medical Center have reported detailed bacteriologic studies on diabetic foot ulcers, emphasizing the important role of anaerobes (50). Over five species per culture were isolated with the following frequency of organisms in decreasing order: *Bacteroides* spp., peptococci, *Proteus* spp., enterococci, *Staph. aureus*, *Clostridium* spp., and *E. coli*. Similar careful bacteriologic studies have not been reported in a series of patients with infected vascular gangrene, but clearly anerobes are of major significance, as evidenced by the frequent crepitus and foul smell. Again it should be emphasized that gas in the tissues does not mean gas gangrene or even clostridial infection, especially in patients with diabetes. Only 1 of the 49 patients reported by Bessman and Wagner had a clostridial gas-producing infection.

It is important to draw the distinction between gangrene and infection in a cold or warm foot. In the former, gangrene is primary and amputation is usually required; efforts to improve the circulation with grafts bypassing occlusions of major vessels may be in order. In the latter, infection may be primary, and although debridement and appropriate antibiotics are required, amputation may be avoided.

PYODERMA GANGRENOSUM

Pyoderma gangrenosum usually presents as an elevated plaque, sometimes with bullae, that develops progressive central necrosis and may evolve into a deep ulcer with a bluish-red necrotic border. There is no evidence that infection is the cause of this entity although secondary bacterial growth is regularly seen. More than 50 percent of the cases are associated with inflammatory bowel disease or connective tissue disorders. The rate of progression of this necrotizing process is usually slow, and systemic toxicity is minimal. The mechanism by which this skin lesion is produced is unknown. Of the various necrotizing processes being considered in this review, confusion with PBSG is most likely.

MISCELLANEOUS GANGRENOUS CELLULITIS IN THE IMMUNOLOGICALLY COMPROMISED HOST

Certain opportunistic infections of this group of patients may present as gangrenous and/or crepitant cellulitis. They will be discussed briefly.

Pseudomonas sepsis may be complicated by metastatic gangrenous cellulitis, especially in patients with extensive burns and those with impaired cellular or humoral defense mechanisms. Skin and subcutaneous necrosis and various combinations of edema, erythema, and bullae may be seen; ecthyma gangrenosum represents a specific morphologic form of metastatic pseudomonas infection. Rarely, other gram-negative facultative bacilli may cause similar lesions. The diagnosis is best established by Gram stain of an aspirate from the skin lesion or with a biopsy showing extensive invasion of blood vessel walls by the bacteria.

Necrotic dermal plaques and ulcers, multiple or solitary, have been described during aspergillus sepsis (51) and in primary aspergillus infection (52) in immunosuppressed patients. Morphologically these usually cannot be differentiated from skin lesions due to *Pseudomonas*. If an aspirate does not show abundant gram-negative rods, a biopsy is indicated. Branching, septate hyphae much narrower than phycomycetes will often be seen on PAS stain; culture is confirmatory. Phycomycosis (53), cryptococcosis (54), and *Aeromonas hydrophilia* sepsis (55) can also cause dermal necrotic plaques in these patients. The septic skin lesions in candidiasis tend to be nodular and erythematous rather than necrotic (56, 57).

Crepitant cellulitis has been reported with A. *hydrophila* (58) and *Bacillus cereus* (59) in compromised hosts. A rapidly lethal crepitant myonecrosis was described with *Klebsiella pneumoniae* in a diabetic patient with alcoholic liver disease (60). It is clear that a wide range of organisms can cause gangrenous and/or crepitant cellulitis in the immunosuppressed patient. In many cases of sepsis, skin lesions may afford the best chance for early diagnosis. Hence, in these patients one should be very aggressive in trying to identify the causative organism.

SUMMARY OF PRACTICAL DIAGNOSTIC MEASURES

In the entities discussed in this article, prompt diagnosis is urgent to expedite mandatory therapy (often extensive debridement) and to avoid unnecessary mutilating surgery. Appropriate diagnostic measures were mentioned in the discussion of specific entities. The flow sheet in Table 7 may be helpful as a guide in the approach to patients with gangrenous and/or crepitant cellulitis.

If tissue gas is detected, it is always wise to incise the lesion. If no gas is present, if necrosis of skin is minimal, and if the rate of spread of the cellulitis is slow and the host is normal, one may treat with antibiotics and observe. If the response to antibiotics is poor or spread is rapid, surgical incision is required. Gas may not be detected early in clostridial myonecrosis, and relatively normal appearing skin may mask extensive underlying necrosis in necrotizing faciitis. If after inspection and Gram stain phycomycotic gangrenous cellulitis or other fungal infection remains in the differential diagnosis, one must specifically look for fungi. This is most reliably done by punch biopsy and PAS or methenamine-silver stain. At times examination of an aspirate using KOH and India ink preparations will yield the diagnosis.

Table 7   Some diagnostic procedures in gangrenous and/or crepitant cellulitis

1   History

2   Physical examination

3   Blood cultures

4   Soft tissue radiographs

5   If crepitus or gas in tissue by x-ray
    Surgical incision of infected area
    (1)   Inspect subcutaneous tissue
    (2)   Inspect fascia; attempt to pass blunt instrument along superficial fascial planes
    (3)   Inspect muscle
    Obtain exudate for examination
    (1)   Odor
    (2)   Gram stain
    (3)   Culture: aerobic and anaerobic

6   If progressive necrosis or rapidly spreading cellulitis without tissue gas
    Proceed as outlined in 5, above; if diagnosis not made, search for fungus
    (1)   Examination of aspirate or crushed tissue by KOH preparation, Wright stain, India ink
    (2)   Punch biopsy of margin of lesion; PAS and methenamine-silver-stains most helpful; frozen sections may yield diagnosis

REFERENCES

1 **Altemeier WA:** The cause of the putrid odor of perforated appendicitis with peritonitis. *Ann Surg* 107:634, 1938.

2 **Bessman AN, Wagner W:** Nonclostridial gas gangrene: Report of 48 cases and review of the literature. *JAMA* 233:958, 1975.

3 **Stone HH, Martin JD Jr:** Synergistic necrotizing cellulitis. *Ann Surg* 175:702, 1972.

4 **Swartz MN:** Subcutaneous tissue infections and abscesses, in Mandell GL et al (eds): *Principles and Practice of Infectious Diseases.* New York, Wiley 1979, p 813.

5 **Rea WJ, Wyrick WJ Jr:** Necrotizing fasciitis. *Ann Surg* 172:957, 1970.

6 **Wilson CB et al:** Phycomycotic gangrenous cellulitis. A report of two cases and a review of the literature. *Arch Surg* 111:532, 1976.

7 **Bond JH, Levitt MD:** A rational approach to intestinal gas problems. *Viewpoints Digest Dis* 9:1, 1977.

8 **VanBeek A et al:** Nonclostridial gas-forming infections. A collective review and report of seven cases. *Arch Surg* 108:552, 1974.

9 **Davis BD et al (eds):** *Microbiology.* New York, Harper & Row, 1967, p 62.

10 **Filler RM et al:** Post-traumatic crepitation falsely suggesting gas gangrene. *N Engl J Med* 278:758, 1968.

11 **Gesner BM, Jenkin CR:** Production of heparinase by bacteroides. *J Bacteriol* 81:595, 1961.

12 **Bjornson HS, Hill EO:** Bacteroidaceae in thromboembolic disease: Effects of cell wall components on blood coagulation in vivo and in vitro. *Infect Immun* 8:911, 1973.

13 **Gorbach SL, Bartlett JG:** Anaerobic infections. *N Engl J Med* 290:1177, 1974.

14 **Greene SI, Smith JW:** Dopamine gangrene. *N Engl J Med* 294:114, 1976.

15 **Greenwald RA et al:** Local gangrene: A complication of peripheral pitressin therapy for bleeding esophageal varices. *Gastroenterology* 74:744, 1978.

16 **Gokal R et al:** Peripheral skin necrosis complicating beta-blockage. *Br Med J* 1:721, 1979.

17 **Bahadir I et al:** Soft tissue necrosis and gangrene complicating treatment with the coumarin derivatives. *Surg Gynecol Obstet* 145:497, 1977.

18 **Finegold SM et al:** Management of anaerobic infections. *Ann Intern Med* 83:375, 1975.

19 **Bird D et al:** Non-clostridial gas gangrene in the diabetic lower limb. *Diabetologia* 13:373, 1977.

20 **Finegold SM:** Infections of skin, soft tissue and muscle, in *Anaerobic Bacteria in Human Disease.* New York, Academic, 1977.

21 **Meleney FL:** Hemolytic streptococcal gangrene. *Arch Surg* 9:317, 1924.

22 **Giuliano A et al:** Bacteriology of necrotizing fasciitis. *Am J Surg* 134:52, 1977.

23 **Ramamurthy RS et al:** Necrotizing fasciitis and necrotizing cellulitis due to group B streptococcus. *Am J Dis Child* 131:1169, 1977.

24 **Crawford SA et al:** Necrotizing fasciitis associated with *Haemophilus aphrophilus. Arch Intern Med* 138:1714, 1978.

25 **Wilson D, Haltalin KC:** Acute necrotizing fasciitis in childhood. Report of 11 cases. *Am J Dis Child* 125:591, 1973.

26 **Grossman M, Silen W:** Serious post-traumatic infections with special reference to gas gangrene, tetanus and necrotizing fasciitis. *Postgrad Med* 32:110, 1962.

27 **Fournier JA:** Gangrene foudroyante de la verge. *Medicole pratique (Paris)* 4:589, 1883.

28 **Flanigan RC et al:** Synergistic gangrene of the scrotum and penis secondary to colorectal disease. *J Urol* 119:369, 1978.

29 **Meleney FL:** Bacterial synergism in disease processes with a confirmation of the synergistic bacterial etiology of a certain type of progressive gangrene of the abdominal wall. *Ann Surg* 94:961, 1931.

30 **MacLennan JD:** The histotoxic clostridial infections of man. *Bacteriol Rev* 26:177, 1962.

31 **Weinstein L, Barza M:** Gas gangrene. *N Engl J Med* 289:1129, 1973.

32 **Caplan ES et al:** Gas gangrene—Review of 34 cases. *Arch Intern Med* 136:788, 1976.

33 **Duff, HJ et al:** Treatment of severe anaerobic infections. *Arch Surg* 101:314, 1970.

34 **Gorbach SL, Thadepalli H:** Isolation of clostridium in human infections: Evaluation of 114 cases. *J Infect Dis* 131:S81, 1975.

35 **Jendrzejewski JW et al:** Nontraumatic clostridial myonecrosis. *Am J Med* 65:542, 1978.

36 **Alpern RJ, Dowell VR, Jr:** *Clostridium septicum* infections and malignancy. *JAMA* 209:385, 1969.

37 **Gorbach SL:** Case records of the Massachusetts General Hospital. *N Engl J Med* 301:1276, 1979.

38 **Slack WK et al:** Hyperbaric oxygen in the treatment of gas gangrene and clostridial infections. *Br J Surg* 56:505, 1969.

39 **Darke SG et al:** Gas gangrene and related infection: Classification, clinical features and aetiology, management and mortality. A report of 88 cases. *Br J Surg* 64:104, 1977.

40 **Anderson CB et al:** Anaerobic streptococcal infections simulating gas gangrene. *Arch Surg* 104:186, 1972.

41 **Meyer RD et al:** Phycomycosis complicating leukemia and lymphoma. *Ann Intern Med* 77:871, 1972.

42 **Krick JA, Remington JS:** Opportunistic invasive fungal infections in patients with leukaemia and lymphoma. *Clin Haematol* 5:249, 1976.

43 **Bauer H et al:** Experimental cerebral mucormycosis in rabbits with alloxan diabetes. *Yale J Biol Med* 28:29, 1955.

44 **Bruck HM et al:** Opportunistic fungal infection of the burn wound with phycomycetes and *Aspergillus. Arch Surg* 102:476, 1971.

45 Nosocomial outbreak of *Rhizopus* infections associated with Elastoplast wound dressings—Minnesota. *MMWR* 27:33, 1978.

46 Follow-up on *Rhizopus* infections associated with Elastoplast bandages—United States. *MMWR* 27:243, 1978.

47 **Mead JH et al:** Cutaneous *Rhizopus* infection. Occurrence as a post-operative complication associated with an elasticized adhesive dressing. *JAMA* 242:272, 1979.

48 **Sheldon DL et al:** Cutaneous mucormycosis. Two documented cases of suspected nosocomial cause. *JAMA* 241:1032, 1979.

49 **Bornstein DL et al:** Anaerobic infections—Review of current experience. *Medicine* 431:207, 1964.

50 **Louie TJ et al:** Aerobic and anaerobic bacteria in diabetic foot ulcers. *Ann Intern Med* 85:461, 1976.

51 **Findlay GH et al:** Skin manifestations in disseminated aspergillosis. *Br J Dermatol* 85 (suppl 7):94, 1971.

52 **Prystowsky SD et al:** Invasive aspergillosis. *N Engl J Med* 295:655, 1976.

53 **Meyer RD et al:** Cutaneous lesions in disseminated mucormycosis. *JAMA* 225:737, 1973.

54 **Schupbach MD et al:** Cutaneous manifestations of disseminated cryptococcosis. *Arch Dermatol* 112:1734, 1977.

55 **Ketuver BP et al:** Septicemia due to *Aeromonas hydrophilia:* Clinical and immunologic aspects. *J Infect Dis* 127:284, 1973.

56 **Balandran L et al:** A cutaneous manifestation of systemic candidiasis. *Ann Intern Med* 78:400, 1973.

57 **Bodey GP, Luna M:** Skin lesions associated with disseminated candidiasis. *JAMA* 229:1466, 1974.

58 **Levin ML:** Gas-forming *Aeromonas hydrophila* infection in a diabetic. *Postgrad Med* 54:127, 1973.

59 **Groschel D et al:** Gas gangrene-like infection with *Bacillus cereus* in a lymphoma patient. *Cancer* 37:988, 1976.

60 **DiGiola RA et al:** Crepitant cellulitis and myonecrosis caused by klebsiella. *JAMA* 237:2097, 1977.

Management of acute and chronic otitis media

JEROME O. KLEIN

INTRODUCTION

Surveys of office practices of physicians who provide care to children show that otitis media is the most frequent diagnosis recorded for illness and the most frequent reason (after well baby and child care) for office visits (1). By 3 years of age more than two-thirds of children have had one or more episodes of acute otitis media and one-third of children have had three or more episodes (2). Fluid persists in the middle ear long after the onset of acute otitis even though symptoms usually resolve within a few days after initiation of antimicrobial therapy. About 70 percent of children with otitis media have demonstrable fluid in the middle ear at the conclusion of a 2-week antimicrobial regimen; 40 percent of children have such fluid 1 month after onset of disease; and 10 percent still have fluid 3 months after the first signs of middle ear infection (3). Hearing is impaired to some degree whenever fluid is present in the middle ear, and many pediatricians and otolaryngologists are concerned about the effects of persistent middle ear fluid associated with otitis media during the first years of life, when perception of language is critical to the development of speech and to the learning processes.

Otitis media is less common in the school-age child, adolescent, and adult. Nevertheless, infection of the middle ear may be the cause of fever, significant pain, and impaired hearing in these age groups. In addition, adults suffer from the sequelae of otitis media of childhood; these include hearing loss, cholesteatoma, adhesive otitis media, and perforation of the tympanic membrane (TM).

This review focuses on issues of management of otitis media. For the purposes of discussion, the review is divided into issues of management of acute episodes of otitis media, management of the patient with recurrent episodes of

This work was supported in part by the National Institute of Allergy and Infectious Diseases, Contract no. N01-AI-5235, and a grant from the Mancini Charitable Foundation.

acute infection, and medical and surgical treatment of the patient with persisting fluid in the middle ear that results from otitis media.

PATHOGENESIS

Otitis media is a disease involving several contiguous structures: the nares, nasopharynx, eustachian tube, middle ear, and the mastoid. Whatever affects one element affects others as well. These structures are lined with a respiratory epithelium which contains ciliated cells, mucus-secreting goblet cells, and cells capable of secreting local immunoglobulins.

The middle ear resembles a flattened box which is approximately 15 mm from top to bottom, 10 mm wide, and only 2 to 6 mm deep. The superior wall lies over the jugular bulb; the lateral wall includes the tympanic membrane; the medial wall includes the oval and round windows; the mastoid air cells lie behind, and the orifice of the eustachian tube is in the superior portion of the front wall.

The eustachian tube connects the middle ear with the posterior nasopharynx. The lateral one-third of the tube lies in bone and is open. The medial two-thirds is in cartilage, and the walls are in apposition except during swallowing or yawning. In the young child the eustachian tube is shorter and proportionately wider than in the older child, and the cartilaginous and osseous portions of the tube form a relatively straight line. In the older child the angle of the tube is more acute, and the tube is longer and narrower. These anatomic differences may be one reason why most infections of the middle ear occur in early childhood.

Anatomic or physiologic dysfunction of the eustachian tube appears to play a critical role in the development of infection of the middle ear. The eustachian tube has at least three physiologic functions with respect to the middle ear: (1) protection of the ear from nasopharyngeal secretions, (2) drainage into the nasopharynx of secretions produced within the middle ear, and (3) ventilation of the middle ear to equilibrate air pressure inside the ear cavity with pressure in the environment (as represented by pressure in the external ear canal). When one or more of these functions is compromised, the result may be development of fluid and infection in the middle ear. Congestion of the mucosa by infection or allergy may result in obstruction of the isthmus, the narrowest portion of the eustachian tube between the bony and cartilaginous sections. Secretions that are constantly formed by the mucosa of the middle ear accumulate behind the obstruction, and if a bacterial pathogen is present, a suppurative infection may result.

CLINICAL MANIFESTATIONS

Acute otitis media is defined by the presence of middle ear fluid accompanied by a sign or symptom of acute illness such as ear pain, ear drainage, or fever. Infants may have only general signs of disease such as lethargy, irritability, feeding problems (anorexia or vomiting), and diarrhea. Vertigo, nystagmus, and tinnitus may occur. Hyperemia of the tympanic membrane is an early sign of otitis media, but redness of the tympanic membrane may be caused by inflammation of the mucosa elsewhere in the upper respiratory tract. Thus "red ear" alone does not establish the diagnosis of otitis media; the diagnosis requires the presence of fluid in the middle ear.

The presence of fluid in the middle ear is best determined by use of pneumatic otoscopy, a technique that permits assessment of mobility of the tympanic membrane. The motion of the tympanic membrane is proportional to the pressure applied by gently squeezing and then releasing the rubber bulb attached to the head of the otoscope. Normal mobility is apparent when positive pressure is applied and the membrane moves rapidly inward; with release of the bulb and the resulting negative pressure, the membrane moves outward. The presence of fluid in the middle ear (or high negative pressure) dampens mobility of the tympanic membrane.

Tympanometry uses an electroacoustic impedance bridge to record compliance of the tympanic membrane and middle ear pressure. This technique provides objective evidence of the status of the middle ear and the presence or absence of fluid. A small probe is inserted into the external canal by means of a snug-fitting cuff; a tone of fixed characteristics is delivered by an oscillator-amplifier via the probe. The compliance of the tympanic membrane is measured by a microphone while the external canal pressure is varied by a pump-manometer. The tone is delivered at a given intensity as the air pressure in the canal is varied over a negative and positive range. The recording that results, the tympanogram, reflects the dynamics of the middle ear system. The technique is reliable, simple, and readily carried out by nonprofessional personnel. The data obtained by use of tympanometry correlate well with documentation of fluid present in the middle ear at the time of surgery or aspiration of middle ear fluid (4).

MICROBIOLOGY OF ACUTE OTITIS MEDIA

The microbiology of otitis media has been defined by culture of middle ear fluids obtained by needle aspiration. Many studies of the bacteriology of acute otitis media have been performed, and the results are remarkably consistent in demonstrating the importance of *Streptococcus pneumoniae* and *Haemophilus influenzae* as pathogens. Although epidemiologic evidence associates virus infection with otitis media, viruses are isolated infrequently from middle ear fluids. Similarly, *Mycoplasma* are seldom associated with otitis media. *Chlamydia* may be important in the etiology of otitis media in young infants.

Bacteria

Studies of the bacteriology of otitis media conducted in Sweden, Finland, and the United States all gave similar results (5) (Figure 1). *Strep. pneumoniae* is the most common agent in all age groups and *H. influenzae* is second in importance. Group A *Streptococcus* was the pathogen in a significant number of cases studied in Scandinavia but not in the United States. *Staphylococcus aureus* and

BACTERIOLOGY OF
OTITIS MEDIA WITH EFFUSION

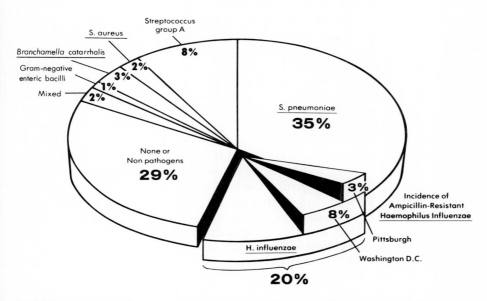

FIGURE 1 Bacteriology of acute otitis media with effusion based on reports from centers in the United States, Finland, and Sweden, 1953–1975, including 3583 children.

gram-negative enteric bacilli are infrequent causes of acute otitis media in children and adults but are responsible for about 25 percent of cases in newborn infants. These bacteria may be the agent of infection in patients with chronic perforation of the tympanic membrane.

Because *Strep. pneumoniae* is the most important cause of otitis media, investigators have carefully studied the types responsible for infections of the middle ear. The results of studies of approximately 2000 children indicate that relatively few types are responsible for most disease (6 –8). The most common types in order of decreasing frequency are 19, 23, 6, 14, 18, 4, 1, and 7. All are included in the currently available dodecavalent pneumococcal vaccines (Pneumovax, Merck, Sharp and Dohme; and Pnu-Imune, Lederle Laboratories).

Most cases of otitis media due to *H. influenzae* are attributable to nontypable strains. Type b strains are present in about 10 percent of cases of otitis media due to *H. influenzae*. Children with infection due to type b *H. influenzae* appear toxic, and about one-quarter of these children have concomitant bacteremia or meningitis (9). Until recently *H. influenzae* appeared to be limited in importance to preschool children, but new information indicates that this organism is a significant cause of otitis media in older children, adolescents, and adults (5).

Recent studies of Brook et al. suggest that anaerobic bacteria may cause otitis media (10). *Peptococcus*, an organism that colonizes the upper respiratory tract and may cause lower respiratory tract disease, and *Proprionibacterium acnes*, a component of the normal skin flora, were the most frequently isolated anaerobic organisms. In some studies, the external canal was not cleaned before aspiration of the middle ear fluid; it therefore is possible that the organisms isolated represent contaminants from the external canal rather than pathogens causing otitis media. In a study of children with persistent middle ear effusion, Teele et al. used appropriate methods of cleaning the canal and failed to isolate anaerobic bacteria from the middle ear (11).

Disparate results of bacterial cultures of middle ear fluid obtained by needle aspiration from children with bilateral otitis media have been reported by several investigators. In most cases culture of the effusion from one ear is sterile, but a bacterial pathogen is isolated from the other ear. In some cases, a different bacterial pathogen is isolated from each of the two ears. Pelton et al. (12) cultured middle ear fluid from both ears of 122 children with bilateral acute otitis media; disparate results were found in 27 (22 percent) of the children. These data indicate that investigative studies of the microbiology of bilateral otitis media must include aspiration of both ears to determine the efficacy of methods of treatment (i.e., trials of antimicrobial agents) or prevention (i.e., evaluation of vaccines or drugs).

Viruses

Epidemiologic data suggest that virus infection is sometimes associated with acute otitis media. In a longitudinal study of respiratory illnesses and complications in children 6 weeks to 11 years of age, Henderson et al. (13) demonstrated a correlation between isolation of viruses from the upper respiratory tract and the clinical diagnosis of otitis media. Outbreaks of viral infection coincided with epidemics of otitis media. In contrast to this epidemiologic association are the results of studies of fluid obtained for viral culture from middle ear effusions of children and adults with acute and chronic otitis media. Viruses were infrequently isolated from the middle ear effusions: a virus was isolated from only 29 (4.4 percent) of 663 fluids (14). Respiratory syncytial virus and influenza virus were the most common isolates, and they were most likely to be present in middle ear fluid during periods of epidemic infection in the community. The low frequency of isolation of viruses from middle ear fluids does not support the belief that these agents play a direct role in the etiology of acute otitis media. However, there are three possibilities:

1 Viruses present early in the course of the disease were no longer present when the patients sought medical attention.

2 The viruses were present in low concentrations and were not readily isolated from the ear fluids.

3 Inhibitory material, such as antibody, interferon, or lysozyme, prevented successful isolation of the virus.

Mycoplasma

A report of a study with adult volunteers suggested a role for *Mycoplasma pneumoniae* in otitis media. Myringitis, associated with hemorrhage and bleb formation, was observed in nonimmune volunteers inoculated with this organism (15). However, when specimens of the middle ear fluid of a large number (771) of patients were cultured for isolation of *M. pneumoniae*, this organism was isolated from the fluid of only one patient (14). Thus, results of this study suggest that mycoplasmas do not play a significant role in the vast majority of cases of acute otitis media. Some cases of respiratory infection due to *M. pneumoniae* are accompanied by inflammation of the tympanic membrane, either alone or in association with middle ear effusion.

Chlamydia

Chlamydia trachomatis causes a mild but prolonged pneumonitis in young infants. This organism has been isolated from middle ear fluids of some infants with pneumonitis (16). Dawson and colleagues isolated *C. trachomatis* from the middle ear fluid of a patient with inclusion cell conjunctivitis (17) and produced otitis in adults experimentally infected with the organism by the ocular route (18). These studies suggest a significant role for *C. trachomatis* as a cause of otitis media.

MICROBIOLOGY OF CHRONIC OTITIS MEDIA

The results of recent studies of the bacteriology of chronic otitis media with effusion suggest that the middle ear fluids of asymptomatic children with persistent effusion harbor bacterial pathogens. At the time of myringotomy or the placement of tympanostomy tubes, cultures of middle ear fluid revealed bacteria in about half of the children; *Strep. pneumoniae, H. influenzae,* and group A *Streptococcus* were isolated from 10 to 20 percent of these asymptomatic children. There were only minimal differences in the rates of isolation of bacteria from serous, mucoid, or purulent fluids (19–21). The significance of this finding is, at present, uncertain. The bacteria may colonize the persistent fluid without producing pathologic changes, or the organisms may be responsible for a low-grade or subclinical infection that may be a factor in the development and persistence of the middle ear fluid.

MICROBIOLOGIC DIAGNOSIS

The correlation between bacterial cultures of the nasopharynx and the oropharynx and cultures of middle ear fluids is poor. Thus, cultures of the upper respiratory tract are of limited value in specific bacteriologic diagnosis of otitis media. In contrast, the consistent results of the microbiologic studies of middle ear fluid of children with acute otitis media provide an accurate guide to the most likely pathogens. If the patient is toxic or has a localized infection elsewhere, culture of the blood and of the focus of infection should be performed.

Needle aspiration of middle ear effusion of patients with acute otitis media provides immediate and specific information about bacterial pathogens and should be considered in the following circumstances: if the patient is critically ill when first seen, if the patient fails to respond appropriately to initial therapy for acute otitis media, or if the patient has altered host defenses. The latter group includes the newborn infant and the patient with malignancy or immunologic disease since these patients may be infected with unusual agents.

MANAGEMENT OF ACUTE OTITIS MEDIA

In vitro activity of antimicrobial agents of value in otitis media (Table 1)

The antimicrobial agent prescribed for the patient with otitis media must be active against *Strep. pneumoniae* and *H. influenzae*. The penicillins, cephalosporins, erythromycin, clindamycin, and trimethoprim-sulfamethoxazole (TMP-SMZ) are effective against *Strep. pneumoniae*. Only the aminoglycosides are relatively ineffective against this organism. Ampicillin, amoxicillin, carbenicillin, ticarcillin, TMP-SMZ, chloramphenicol, and the aminoglycosides are active against *H. influenzae*, but relatively high concentrations of penicillin V, the penicillinase-resistant penicillins, cephalothin, erythromycin, and clindamycin are required for inhibition of this organism. Penicillin G is intermediate in activity between ampicillin and penicillin V and may be sufficiently active against *H. influenzae* to be efficacious for therapy of otitis media due to some strains of this species. Cefaclor, cefamandole, and cefoxitin are more active against *H. influenzae* than previously available cephalosporins.

Recent reports of multiresistant strains of *Strep. pneumoniae* in South Africa (22) and of the isolation of a penicillin G –resistant strain of type 14 in Minnesota (23) suggest the possibility of a major change in the pattern of antimicrobial susceptibility of *Strep. pneumoniae*. The South African strains are remarkable in being not only significantly resistant to penicillin G but also resistant to most of the other antimicrobial agents considered as alternatives, including erythromycin, tetracycline, clindamycin, and TMP-SMZ. These strains have a minimal inhibitory concentration (MIC) ≥ 4 μg/ml, which is far greater than the usual MIC of 0.005 to 0.05 μg/ml. Of equal importance has been the identification of strains intermediate in susceptibility to penicillin G with MICs of 0.1 to 1.0 μg/ml.

We studied 173 strains of *Strep. pneumoniae* obtained from middle ear fluids and nasopharyngeal secretions of children with acute otitis media during the period 1975–1980. Three had MICs of 0.1 to 0.4 μg/ml, but all the others were more susceptible to penicillin G. Thus, at present, the highly resistant strains noted in South Africa have not been identified in Boston, Massachusetts, and the strains of intermediate susceptibility are of low incidence in that location.

Strains of *H. influenzae* resistant to ampicillin were first isolated in 1973. At

Table 1   Sensitivity of *Strep. pneumoniae* and *H. influenzae* isolated from middle ear fluids of children with acute otitis media, 1976– 1979

| | Minimal inhibitory concentration (median), μg/ml[a] | | | |
| | Strep. pneumoniae | | H. influenzae | |
Antimicrobial agent	Sensitive[b]	Resistant[c]	Sensitive[d]	Resistant[e]
Penicillin G	0.01	0.4	1.6	>100
Penicillin V	0.01	0.4	12.5	>100
Ampicillin	0.03	0.1	0.8	>100
Methicillin	0.1	6.4	3.1	50
Nafcillin	0.01	0.8	25	50
Carbenicillin	0.2	6.4	0.4	>100
Cephalothin	0.1	1.6	25	12.5
Cephalexin	3.2	3.2	100	50
Cefoxitin	1.6	6.4	6.3	6.3
Cefamandole	0.1	1.6	0.4	3.1
Cefaclor	0.4	1.6	12.5	25
Erythromycin	0.05	0.03	3.1	3.1
Clindamycin	0.05	0.05	3.1	6.3
Chloramphenicol	3.2	3.2	0.4	0.8
Tetracycline	0.2	25	0.4	0.4
Amikacin	>100	100	3.1	6.3
Trimethoprim	1.6	3.2	0.8	1.6
Sulfamethoxazole	100	>100	>100	>100
Trimethoprim/ sulfamethoxazole[f]	0.3:6	0.3:6	0.2:3	0.2:3

[a] Inocula replictor method: 10^0 dilution for *Strep. pneumoniae*; 10^{-2} *Strep. pneumoniae*; *H. influenzae*.
[b] Twenty-two strains with MIC for penicillin G < 0.1 μg/ml.
[c] One strain with MIC for penicillin G ≥ 0:1 μg/ml.
[d] β-lactamase-negative strains including 3 type b and 20 nontypable.
[e] β-lactamase-positive strains including 3 type b and 4 nontypable.
[f] 1 part trimethoprim/19 parts sulfamethoxazole.
SOURCE: Teele DW, Norton C, Klein JO: unpublished data.

present, approximately 15 percent of nontypable strains of *H. influenzae* isolated from the middle ear fluid of children with otitis media in our clinic are resistant to ampicillin.[1] Resistance to ampicillin is attributable to production of a penicillinase that hydrolyzes ampicillin, amoxicillin, penicillin G and V, and, to a lesser extent, carbenicillin. Sulfonamides, TMP-SMZ, and the new cephalosporins, cefamandole and cefoxitin (both administered parenterally) and cefaclor (administered orally), are effective in vitro against these strains of ampicillin-resistant, nontypable *H. influenzae*.

[1] Teele DW, Norton C, Klein JO: unpublished data.

Diffusion of antimicrobial agents into middle ear fluids

Although studies of concentrations of various drugs in serum and middle ear fluid (Table 2) used different dosage schedules, times of collection, and methods of assay, the results all indicate that most antimicrobial agents of value for treatment of acute otitis media achieve significant concentrations in middle ear fluid (24–27). Penicillin G and V produce concentrations in middle ear fluid that are 13 to 22 percent of levels in serum. Approximately half of the concentration in serum is present in middle ear fluid after oral administration of ampicillin, amoxicillin, erythromycin, and sulfonamides. Concentrations of ampicillin in middle ear fluid of patients with serous otitis media are lower than concentrations in fluid of patients with acute disease, but concentrations of amoxicillin are similar in acute suppurative and serous effusions. Thus, usual dosage schedules of penicillins and erythromycin produce concentrations of antimicrobial activity in middle ear fluid that are sufficient to inhibit *Strep. pneumoniae*, but concentrations in middle ear fluid produced by intramuscular administration of benzathine penicillin G, penicillin V, and erythromycin are not adequate to inhibit most strains of *H. influenzae*.

The in vivo sensitivity test

Drs. Virgil Howie and John Ploussard, pediatricians in practice in Huntsville, Alabama, have contributed significant information about the epidemiology, diagnosis, and management of otitis media. The *in vivo sensitivity test* is one of their most valuable studies (28). The middle ear fluid of children with acute otitis media was aspirated and cultured before starting therapy with antimicrobial agents. All drugs were prescribed in their usual dosage schedules, and patients were advised to return in 2 to 5 days. If fluid was still present at the second visit, a second culture of the fluid was obtained. The results of these studies are consistent with results expected on the basis of data from in vitro

Table 2   Concentration of orally administered antimicrobial agents in serum (S) and middle ear fluids (MEF) of children with acute otitis media

Agent	Dosage, mg/kg	Concentration, μg/ml*			Ref.
		S	**MEF**	**MEF/S**	
Penicillin V	13	8.1	1.8	0.22	24
Ampicillin	10	4.3	1.2	0.28	25
Amoxicillin	10	4.8	2.2	0.46	26
Erythromycin estolate	7.5	3.9	1.3	0.33	26
Sulfonamide (trisulfapyrimidine)	30	13.4	8.3	0.62	26

* Measured 0.5 to 2 h after administration.

studies (Table 1) and achievable concentrations of drug in middle ear fluid (Table 2). Penicillins G and V, benzathine penicillin G (administered intramuscularly as a single dose), and erythromycin were all successful in eradicating *Strep. pneumoniae* from middle ear fluid. Sulfonamides and tetracyclines did not sterilize middle ear fluid infected with *Strep. pneumoniae*. *H. influenzae* was eradicated by ampicillin but not by penicillin V, intramuscular benzathine penicillin G, or erythromycin. The high MIC of penicillin V for *H. influenzae* and the relatively low concentrations of benzathine penicillin G achieved in serum (and by extrapolation in middle ear fluid) probably explain the failure of these two penicillins to eradicate *H. influenzae* from middle ear fluid. An oral form of penicillin G was not studied.

New antimicrobial agents

Although few data are available regarding the efficacy of the new antimicrobial agents trimethoprim-sulfamethoxazole (TMP-SMZ) and cefaclor, both appear to be effective in treatment of acute otitis media. Both agents have a spectrum of activity that includes the major pathogens responsible for otitis media, i.e., *Strep. pneumoniae* and *H. influenzae* (including both β-lactamase-negative and -positive strains).

There is a paucity of published information on the clinical efficacy of TMP-SMZ for middle ear infection. In a randomized trial in which TMP-SMZ was compared with ampicillin, Shurin et al. (29) treated 132 children with acute otitis media. The antibacterial efficacy of the drugs was assessed from results of cultures of middle ear aspirates obtained during or after therapy. The number of microbiologic failures (including persistent, recurrent, and new infections of the middle ear) was similar for both groups. The drug regimens were well accepted by the patients and were not associated with significant side effects. Schwartz et al. evaluated TMP-SMZ for otitis media and found that the combination was effective against strains due to ampicillin-resistant *H. influenzae*; resolution of the infection occurred promptly after therapy with TMP-SMZ (30). These data indicate that TMP-SMZ is an effective alternative to ampicillin for initial treatment of acute otitis media and may be recommended when the presence of ampicillin-resistant strains of *H. influenzae* is known or suspected. TMP-SMZ is also useful for patients who are allergic to penicillins. The combination can be given twice daily, compared with 3 times per day for amoxicillin and 4 times per day for ampicillin. However, TMP-SMZ would not be expected to be effective for otitis media due to group A *Streptococcus* since, like other sulfonamides, the combination drug is inadequate for treatment of streptococcal tonsillopharyngitis.

Cefaclor, an orally administered cephalosporin with stability to β-lactamases, was introduced in 1979. Until that time oral cephalosporins, including cephalexin and cephradine, had poor activity against most strains of *H. influenzae* and only limited effectiveness in therapy of acute otitis media. Nelson et al. found that cefaclor was similar in efficacy for treatment of acute otitis media to amoxicillin or a combination of a sulfonamide plus erythromycin or penicillin V (31).

Recommendations for initial choice of antimicrobial therapy for patients with acute otitis media

Amoxicillin or ampicillin are the currently preferred drugs for initial treatment of otitis media since they are active both in vitro and in vivo against *Strep. pneumoniae* and *H. influenzae*. Other regimens that are satisfactory include combinations of a sulfonamide with benzathine penicillin G (administered by the intramuscular route as a single injection), oral penicillin G or V, or erythromycin, and TMP-SMZ and cefaclor. For the child who is allergic to penicillins, cefaclor or erythromycin combined with a sulfonamide or TMP-SMZ provides equivalent antimicrobial coverage.

With appropriate antimicrobial therapy, most children with acute bacterial otitis media are significantly improved within 48 to 72 h. The physician should be in contact with the patient (or the patient's parents) to ascertain that improvement has occurred. If the patient remains toxic or the condition worsens, he or she must be reevaluated and a change in antimicrobial therapy, myringotomy for drainage, or needle aspiration for diagnosis should be considered.

The current incidence of strains of ampicillin-resistant *H. influenzae* is low (only 3 to 8 percent of all cases of acute otitis media) and does not require a change in recommendations for initial therapy (Figure 1). However, if the patient does not respond to initial therapy with ampicillin or amoxicillin, infection with a resistant strain of *H. influenzae* should be considered. If the patient is not toxic, a change in therapy to include a sulfonamide, TMP-SMZ, or cefaclor is appropriate. If the patient is toxic, tympanocentesis should be performed to determine the microbiology of the infection.

The bacteriology of middle ear infections in children who have recurrent episodes of acute otitis media is similar to that found in first episodes; the predominant pathogens are *Strep. pneumoniae* (though of different serotypes) and nontypable strains of *H. influenzae*. Thus, the child with a recurrent episode of otitis media should be treated initially with the same antimicrobial regimens as the child with a first episode of middle ear infection.

MANAGEMENT OF CHRONIC OTITIS MEDIA

The term *chronic otitis media* includes recurrent episodes of acute infection and prolonged effusion of the middle ear resulting from acute infection. For prevention of recurrent episodes of acute otitis media, management should include consideration of chemoprophylaxis (use of antimicrobial agents for prolonged periods) or immunoprophylaxis (use of pneumococcal vaccine). For management of persistent middle ear effusions, four methods are considered: myringotomy, adenoidectomy, placement of tympanostomy tubes, and use of steroids. Although there is evidence for the support of each method for management of chronic otitis media, the data are incomplete. Management of chronic otitis media is a subject of current interest in many centers in the United States, Canada, western Europe, and Japan, and new information is expected to clarify some of the unresolved issues.

Management of recurrent episodes
of acute otitis media

Chemoprophylaxis   Recent studies of children in Alaskan Eskimo villages (32) and in Rochester, New York (33), suggest that chemoprophylaxis may be of value in prevention of acute illness in children who have suffered from recurrences of middle ear infections. Eskimo children were enrolled in a 1-year double-blind prospective trial in which ampicillin and a placebo were used. Children treated with a course of ampicillin (four times daily for 10 days) had a smaller number of episodes of otorrhea compared with controls. The children in the Rochester study were enrolled in a randomized, double-blind control trial in which sulfisoxazole and a placebo were used. After 3 months, children who received the antimicrobial agent had significantly fewer episodes of otitis media than children who received the placebo. The groups were switched for the following 3 months, and the results again indicated efficacy of sulfisoxazole in prevention of new clinical episodes. Although these data are persuasive, there are significant limitations in the design of each study, including failure to evaluate persistence of middle ear effusion.

Pneumococcal vaccine   Prevention of disease by use of bacterial vaccines has been considered because of the limited number of pathogens responsible for otitis media. Since most strains of *H. influenzae* are nontypable and current vaccines are prepared from capsular polysaccharide, there is no immediate prospect for a vaccine against this organism. A polyvalent (14 types) pneumococcal vaccine has been shown to be effective in preventing new episodes of pneumonia and bacteremia. The types present in the vaccine are responsible for about 90 percent of cases of otitis media caused by *Strep. pneumoniae*.

Studies of the immune response to the pneumococcal vaccine have indicated that, as with the polysaccharide vaccines prepared from capsular materials of *H. influenzae* type b and *Neisseria meningitidis* group A and C, children under 2 years of age exhibit low and irregular serologic responses to a single dose of vaccine. Borgano et al. immunized infants with a pneumococcal (12-type) vaccine; 50 percent of the children had a significant antibody response to 10 of the 12 types (34). Children over 2 years of age respond satisfactorily to this vaccine, but the titers of antibody to most types were lower after immunization than the titers in adults.

Investigations currently underway are designed to test the efficacy of the pneumococcal vaccine in children with otitis media; physicians in Boston, Massachusetts, Huntsville, Alabama, and Helsinki, Finland, are conducting the trials. Preliminary results are available only from the Finnish study (35); they show that children 2 years of age and older who received the vaccine had significantly fewer subsequent episodes of otitis media due to pneumococcal types present in the vaccine than children who had received the placebo (*H. influenzae* type b polysaccharide vaccine); children under 2 years of age at the time of immunization had some protection against new episodes of type-specific otitis media compared with controls, but the differences were not statistically significant. Thus, the limited microbiologic efficacy of the pneumococcal vaccine in young children is consistent with the data about their immunologic response.

Management of persistent middle ear effusion

Myringotomy Myringotomy, or incision of the tympanic membrane, is a method of draining middle ear fluid. A curvilinear blade is used to make a semilunar incision in the inferior posterior quadrant of the membrane. This procedure produces immediate relief of pain in the patient with acute otitis media as pus under pressure exudes from the middle ear. The incision usually remains open for 1 to 2 days, allowing continued drainage; however, the membrane is elastic and vascular and the hole heals rapidly.

Before the introduction of antimicrobial agents, myringotomy was the main mode of management of acute otitis media. Today, it is used only under selected circumstances. Current usage of myringotomy includes relief of intractable ear pain, hastening resolution of mastoid infection, drainage of persistant middle ear effusion that is unresponsive to medical therapy, and management of acute otitis media that is accompanied by signs of cranial nerve (VI or VII) involvement.

Adenoidectomy Enlarged adenoids may obstruct the orifice of the eustachian tube in the posterior nasopharynx and interfere with adequate ventilation and drainage of the middle ear. While the results of studies of adenoidectomy are inconsistent, they suggest that the procedure is of value for some children.

An extensive study in progress at Children's Hospital in Pittsburgh, Pennsylvania, may provide significant information about the use of adenoidectomy in children with chronic middle ear disease (36). The preliminary results indicate that adenoidectomy does not prevent recurrent otitis media, but it remains uncertain whether the procedure reduces the rate, severity, or duration of recurrent episodes. The issue is complex because of the large number of variables that must be taken into account, and it has become apparent that large numbers of subjects will be required in order to reach firm conclusions.

Tympanostomy tubes Tympanostomy tubes that resemble small collar buttons are placed through an incision in the tympanic membrane to provide drainage of fluid and ventilation of the middle ear. The criteria for placement of the tubes include persistent middle ear effusions that are unresponsive to adequate medical treatment over a period of 3 months, persistent tympanic membrane retraction pockets with impending cholesteatoma, persistent negative pressure, and any of the above in lesser degrees when accompanied by impairment of hearing.

Hearing improves dramatically after placement of the ventilating tubes. The tubes have also been of value in patients who have difficulty maintaining ambient pressure in the middle ear. Thus, barotrauma occurring in airline personnel frequently resolves when tubes are placed in the tympanic membrane. Placement of the tympanostomy tubes is treatment of an effect and not a cause of chronic ear disease. Controlled trials are needed to provide specific criteria for use and maintenance of tympanostomy tubes in patients with chronic otitis media.

Use of steroids Schwartz et al. reported preliminary results of a short course of prednisone for treatment of persistent middle ear effusion following otitis media (37). Children with effusion for 1 month or more after appropriate antimicrobial therapy were enrolled in a double-blind study and were randomly assigned to receive either prednisone or lactose placebo concomitant with a sulfisoxazole suspension for 7 days. Of the 24 children who received prednisone and sulfisoxazole as the initial treatment, 15 (62.5 percent) experienced resolution of the effusion, which was observed for only 1 of the 17 children who received lactose and sulfisoxazole. Of the 16 children who failed to be cured initially by treatment with lactose and sulfisoxazole, 13 (81 percent) showed resolution following therapy with prednisone, whereas only 1 of 9 children who failed initially on therapy with prednisone cleared when subsequently given the lactose placebo. These preliminary results suggest that prednisone may be an important adjunct to chemotherapy in resolution of fluid that persists after acute otitis media.

COMPLICATIONS

Suppurative complications

Suppurative complications of acute infection of the middle ear are now uncommon, but contiguous spread of infection may be responsible for mastoiditis, petrositis, labyrinthitis, brain abscess, and meningitis. Infection can spread to the intracranial structures by one of the following routes: vascular channels; direct extension; or preformed pathways such as the round window, skull fracture, or congenital or surgically acquired dehiscences. Any patient who develops persistent headache, severe otalgia, or localized or general signs of a central nervous system lesion should be suspected of having a suppurative intracranial complication of otitis media.

Inflammation of the mastoid air cells often accompanies otitis media. A clouding of the mastoid area appears on radiologic examination. Appropriate medical treatment of the middle ear effusion usually reverses the process in the mastoid. Local signs of mastoid infection sometimes accompany otitis media. The pinna is displaced downward and forward, there may be some swelling of the posteriosuperior external canal wall, and the mastoid area is tender, red, and swollen. Treatment consists of immediate tympanocentesis or myringotomy and initiation of chemotherapy that is based on results of examination of Gram-stained smears of the purulent material. Mastoid surgery is necessary if a subperiosteal abscess has developed or if the infection breaks through the mastoid tip into the neck or forms a fistula into the external ear canal.

Suppurative labyrinthitis may arise by direct bacterial invasion through the round or oval windows during an episode of otitis media. Signs consistent with labyrinthitis include vertigo, nystagmus, tinnitus, hearing loss, nausea, and vomiting. Medical treatment may be sufficient, but surgical labyrinthectomy is usually indicated.

Aural cavity complications

Cholesteatoma appears as a white, shiny, greasy debris (keratin or desquamating epithelium) lining a saclike structure behind a marginal posteriosuperior or an attic perforation of the eardrum. Tympanomastoid surgery should not be delayed, because the disease can spread with destructive effects to other structures of the temporal bone and to the intracranial cavity.

Although the eardrum usually seals after a spontaneous or surgically induced perforation, in some patients the perforation persists and tympanoplasty may be required for closure.

Fibrous tissue may proliferate as a result of inflammation of the middle ear. The mucous membrane becomes thickened and may obstruct movement of the ossicles, with the possible result of conductive hearing loss. The condition may be irreversible, and early consultation with an otolaryngologist is important for appropriate management.

Hearing impairment

Patients with acute otitis media and those with persistent middle ear effusion may suffer temporary loss of hearing. Olmsted et al. (38) studied children $2\frac{1}{2}$ to 12 years of age with acute otitis media; of 82 children included in the study, 33 (40 percent) had impaired hearing (15 dB) for from 1 to 6 months and an additional 10 (12 percent) had hearing loss throughout the 6-month period of observation. The significance of hearing loss associated with acute infection or persistent middle ear effusions in the young child is uncertain. Retrospective studies (39–42) suggest that chronic middle ear disease with effusion during the first few years of life has adverse effects on development of speech and language, intelligence, and performance in school. Most of the studies on this topic had significant deficiencies in design. Thus, at present, there is concern for the results of impairment of hearing that accompanied otitis media during the first years of life, but the precise effect on intellectual development is uncertain.

REFERENCES

1 **Koch H, Dennison NJ:** *Office Visits to Pediatricians.* National Ambulatory Medical Care Service, National Center for Health Statistics, 1974.

2 **Teele DW, Klein JO, Greater Boston Collaborative Otitis Media Program:** Epidemiology of otitis media during first two years of life. *Pediatr Res* 12:428, 1978.

3 **Teele DW et al:** Epidemiology of acute and chronic otitis media. *Ann Otol Rhinol Laryngol* 89(suppl 68):5, 1980.

4 **Shurin PA et al:** Persistence of middle-ear effusion after acute otitis media in children. *N Engl J Med* 300:1121, 1979.

5 **Klein JO:** Microbiology of acute and chronic otitis media. *Ann Otol Rhinol Laryngol* 89(suppl 68):98, 1980.

6 **Austrian R et al:** The bacteriology of pneumococcal otitis media. *Johns Hopkins Med J* 141:104, 1977.

7 **Gray BM et al:** Serotypes of *Streptococcus pneumoniae* causing disease. *J Infect Dis* 140:979, 1979.

8 **Kamme C:** Distribution of *Diplococcus pneumoniae* types in acute otitis media in children and influence of the types on the clinical course in penicillin V therapy. *Scand J Infect Dis* 2:183, 1970.

9 **Harding AL et al:** *Hemophilus influenzae* isolated from children with otitis media, in Sell SHW, Karzon DT (eds): *Hemophilus Influenzae*. Nashville, Vanderbilt University Press, 1973, p 21.

10 **Brook I et al:** Aerobic and anaerobic bacteriology of acute otitis media in children. *J Pediatr* 92:13, 1978.

11 **Teele DW et al:** Persistent middle ear effusions in young children: cultures for anaerobic bacteria. *Ann Otol Rhinol Laryngol* 89(suppl 68):102, 1980.

12 **Pelton SI et al:** Disparate cultures of middle ear fluids in bilateral otitis media. *Am J Dis Child*, in press.

13 **Henderson FW et al:** The epidemiology of acute otitis media in childhood. *Abstr Intersci Conf Antimicrob Agents Chemother*, 1977.

14 **Klein JO, Teele DW:** Isolation of viruses and mycoplasmas from middle ear effusions. A review. *Ann Otol Rhinol Laryngol* 85:140, 1976.

15 **Rifkind DR et al:** Ear involvement (myringitis) and primary atypical pneumonia following inoculation of volunteers with Eaton agent. *Am Rev Respir Dis* 85:479, 1962.

16 **Tipple MA et al:** Clinical characteristics of afebrile pneumonia associated with *Chlamydia trachomatis* infections in infants less than 6 months of age. *Pediatrics* 63:192, 1979.

17 **Dawson C, Schachter J:** TRIC agent infections of the eye and genital tract. *Am J Ophthalmol* 63:1288, 1967.

18 **Dawson C et al:** Experimental inclusion conjunctivitis in man: III. Keratitis and other complications. *Arch Ophthalmol* 78:341, 1967.

19 **Liu YS et al:** Chronic middle ear effusions. Immunochemical and bacteriological investigations. *Arch Otolaryngol* 101:278, 1975.

20 **Healy GB, Teele DW:** The microbiology of chronic middle ear effusions in children. *Laryngoscope* 57:1472, 1977.

21 **Riding KH et al:** Microbiology of recurrent and chronic otitis media with effusion. *J Pediatr*, in press.

22 **Ward J:** Epidemiology of antibiotic-resistant strains of *Streptococcus pneumoniae*. *Rev Infect Dis*, in press.

23 **Cates KL et al:** A penicillin-resistant pneumococcus. *J Pediatr* 93:624, 1978.

24 **Kamme C et al:** The concentration of penicillin V in serum and middle ear exudate in acute otitis media in children. *Scand J Infect Dis* 1:77, 1969.

25 **Lahikainen EA et al:** Azidocillin and ampicillin concentrations in middle ear effusion. *Acta Otolaryngol* 84:227, 1977.

26 **Howard JE et al:** Otitis media of infancy and early childhood. *Am J Dis Child* 130:965, 1976.

27 **Lundgren K et al:** The concentration of penicillin-V in middle ear exudate. *Int J Pediatr Otorhinolaryngol* 1:93, 1979.

28 **Howie VM, Ploussard JH:** The "in vivo sensitivity test"—Bacteriology of middle ear exudate during antimicrobial therapy in otitis media. *Pediatrics* 44:940, 1969.

29 **Shurin PA et al:** Trimethoprimsulfamethoxazole compared with ampicillin in the treatment of acute otitis media *J Pediatr*, 96:1081, 1980.

30 **Schwartz R et al:** Treatment of otitis media with trimethoprim-sulfamethoxazole. Letter to editor. *J Pediatr* 95:666, 1979.

31 **Nelson JD et al:** Treatment of acute otitis media of infancy with cefaclor. *Am J Dis Child* 132:992, 1978.

32 **Maynard JE et al:** Otitis media in Alaskan Eskimo children. Prospective evaluation of chemoprophylaxis. *JAMA* 219:597, 1972.

33 **Perrin JM et al:** Sulfisoxazole as chemoprophylaxis for recurrent otitis media. A double-blind crossover study in pediatric practice. *N Engl J Med* 291:664, 1974.

34 **Borgano JM et al:** Vaccination and revaccination with polyvalent pneumococcal polysaccharide vaccines in adults and infants. *Proc Soc Exp Biol Med* 157:148, 1978.

35 **Karma P et al:** The efficacy of pneumococcal vaccination against recurrent otitis media: Preliminary results of a field study in Finland. *Ann Otol Rhinol Laryngol* 89(suppl 68):357, 1980.

36 **Paradise JL:** T and A—Nature of the controversy and steps toward its resolution. *Int J Pediatr Otorhinolaryngol* 1:201, 1979.

37 **Schwartz RM et al:** Use of a short course of prednisone for treating middle ear effusion: A double-blind crossover study. *Ann Otol Rhinol Laryngol* 89(suppl 68):296, 1980.

38 **Olmsted RW et al:** The pattern of hearing following acute otitis media. *J Pediatr* 65:252, 1964.

39 **Holm VA, Kunze LH:** Effect of chronic otitis media on language and speech and development. *Pediatrics* 43:833, 1969.

40 **Kaplan GJ et al:** Long-term effects of otitis media. A ten-year cohort study of Alaskan Eskimo children. *Pediatrics* 52:577, 1973.

41 **Lewis N:** Otitis media and linguistic incompetence. *Arch Otolaryngol* 102:387, 1976.

42 **Zinkus PW et al:** Developmental and psychoeducational sequelae of chronic otitis media. *Am J Dis Child* 132:1100, 1978.

ADDITIONAL READING

Bluestone CD, Shurin PA: Middle ear disease in children. Pathogenesis, diagnosis, and management. *Pediatr Clin North Am* 21:379, 1974.

Hanson DG, Ulvestad RF (eds): Otitis media and child development. Speech, language and education. *Ann Otol Rhinol Laryngol*, v 88 (suppl 60), 1979.

Klein JO: Middle ear disease in children. *Hosp Pract* 11:45, 1976.

Lim DJ et al (eds): Recent advances in middle ear effusion. *Proc 2d Int Symp Recent Adv Middle Ear Effusion, Columbus, Ohio, May 9–11, 1979. Ann Otol Rhinol Laryngol* 89:1, 1980.